Emergency Clinical Diagnosis

Ashis Banerjee

Emergency Clinical Diagnosis

Springer

Ashis Banerjee
Royal Free NHS Foundation Trust
London, United Kingdom

ISBN 978-3-319-50717-0 ISBN 978-3-319-50718-7 (eBook)
DOI 10.1007/978-3-319-50718-7

Library of Congress Control Number: 2017932743

Printed on acid-free paper

This Springer imprint is published by Springer Nature
The registered company is Springer International Publishing AG
The registered company address is: Gewerbestrasse 11, 6330 Cham, Switzerland

Introduction

The demands on emergency departments are rising worldwide. Simultaneously, the scope of practice of emergency medicine continues to expand. This is fuelled by an ageing population, complex medical presentations, rising patient expectations, difficulties with access to primary care facilities, and the desire for second opinions in the case of diagnostic delay or failure in primary care settings.

Diagnostic failure is the leading source of clinical complaints and of medico-legal litigation involving emergency departments. The emergency practitioner not only needs to be proficient in the evaluation of common high-stakes conditions, but also has to be aware of malignant disease and rarer conditions that can present to the emergency department and facilitate their diagnosis and subsequent management. This ensures more effective communication with specialists receiving referrals. In particular, the new diagnosis of cancer is increasingly being made in the emergency setting.

Once the correct diagnosis is made, it is recognised that treatment protocols and referral pathways can vary widely and that local guidance is more appropriate. Diagnostic accuracy, however, remains a universal common concern.

This book aims to provide the emergency practitioner with diagnostic aide-memoires and checklists as part of the front-line diagnostic armamentarium.

Contents

1 Cardiovascular Emergencies

Chest pain

A good focused history is essential to the adequate assessment of chest pain. It is important to rapidly exclude potentially life-threatening causes of chest pain to avoid adverse clinical outcomes.This should be preceded by an ABCD (airway, breathing, circulation, disability) assessment. Once cardiac chest pain is determined to be likely, early risk stratification should be achieved in order to guide choice of further management.

The **PQRST history** for chest pain provides a basic framework for history taking:

- Provokes: deep breathing, coughing, movement, physical exertion, cold weather, emotional stress, heavy meal, sexual intercourse
- Palliates: rest; position; food; antacids; over the counter or prescription drugs
- Quality: burning, stabbing, crushing, dull, aching, sharp, heaviness, tightness
- Region: central, lateral; localization by the patient's finger(s) is useful to determine the site of pain
- Radiation: back, neck, upper limb
- Severity: graded from 1 to 10
- Timing: duration of symptoms; time of onset

Associated symptoms of relevance include:

Systemic: fever, chills, fatigue, sweating
Cardio-pulmonary: dyspnoea, palpitations, syncope or near syncope
Gastrointestinal: nausea and vomiting, heartburn

Red flags in chest pain assessment include:

- Severe dyspnoea
- Severe or ongoing pain
- Exertional chest pain
- Haemoptysis
- Syncope
- Multiple cardiovascular risk factors (three or more usually)
- Abnormal vital signs associated with haemodynamic instability
- Signs of hypoperfusion

Focused assessment for patients presenting with possible cardiac chest pain includes

- History of pain characteristics and associated symptoms
- Presence of cardiovascular risk factors
- History of cardiovascular disease, including ischaemic heart diseasse, and any previous treatment for coronary artery disease (coronary revascularization, including thrombolysis, percutaneous coronary intervention, and coronary artery bypass grafting)
- Any other previous investigation/treatment for chest pain

A. Banerjee, *Emergency Clinical Diagnosis*, DOI 10.1007/978-3-319-50718-7_1

- Response to glyceryl trinitrate should not be used to confirm the diagnosis of cardiac chest pain in isolation

Known risk factors for coronary artery disease
Non-modifiable

- Genetics: family history of premature coronary heart disease in first degree relative-before 55 years of age in men (fathers, sons, or brothers) and 60 in women (mothers, daughters, or sisters)
- Age: over 45 years' age in men and over 55 years' age in women
- Male sex

Potentially modifiable

- Hypertension
- Other cardiovascular disease
- Diabetes mellitus
- Cigarette smoking: tobacco use
- Physical inactivity: lack of exercise
- Obesity
- Heavy alcohol consumption
- Metabolic syndrome (central or abdominal obesity, hypertension, elevated fasting plasma glucose, high serum triglycerides, low HDL- cholesterol levels, microalbuminuria)
- Dyslipidaemia: elevated total cholesterol (>4.9 mmol/L); elevated LDL-cholesterol (>3.0 mmol/L); HDL-cholesterol (<1.0 mmol/L in males and <1.2 mmol/L in females); elevated triglycerides (>1.7 mmol/L)
- Hyperhomocystineaemia

Risk factors for premature onset coronary artery disease include:

Recreational drug use: cocaine
Dyslipidaemia (familial hypercholesterolaemia; familial combined hyperlipidaemia)
Positive family history of coronary artery disease in first degree relatives
Metabolic syndrome
Cigarette smoking
Kawasaki's disease
Structural lesions of coronary arteries: anomalous origin of left coronary artery from pulmonary artery; coronary artery ostial stenosis after neonatal arterial switch repair of D-transposition of great arteries
Prothrombotic defects

Physical examination in the presence of suspected cardiac chest pain includes:

- Evaluation of haemodynamic status
- Signs of sympathetic activation (pallor, sweating, tachycardia) or vagal activation (vomiting, bradycardia)
- Signs of complications:pulmonary oedema, cardiogenic shock
- Signs of non-coronary causes of acute chest pain: aortic dissection (asymmetrical pulses, differential blood pressure between left and right upper limbs, acute aortic regurgitation), pericarditis (pericardial friction rub)
- Weight, height and calculation of body mass index, and waist circumference may help identify patients at risk of cardiac chest pain
- Levine's sign of the use of the clenched fist to indicate the site of discomfort may indicate cardiac chest pain

Causes of acute chest pain
Cardiovascular

a. **Cardiac**
   - Acute coronary syndromes: (ST elevation myocardial infarction (STEMI); non-ST elevation acute coronary syndrome (NSTE-ACS)): Angina is often described as crushing, heaviness, squeezing, aching, constricting or vice-like and can radiate to the back (mid-scapula), neck, jaw, and down one or both arms. The pain has a crescendo pattern and reaches a maximal intensity after a few minutes. Angina can be provoked by physical exertion, emo-

tional stress and sexual intercourse, and aggravated by cold weather after heavy meals. Typically, angina is relieved following rest and/or administration of glyceryl trinitrate within around 5min.

- Pericarditis: central or precordial pleuritic chest pain, worse when supine and relieved by sitting forward, and radiating to the trapezius ridge, neck, left shoulder and arm; pericardial rub on auscultation
- Myocarditis (background of recent viral illness): pain may be related to myocardial ischaemia or concurrent pericarditis
- Coronary vasospasm (cocaine; triptans)
- Valvular heart disease (aortic stenosis; mitral valve prolapse)
- Hypertrophic cardiomyopathy
- Angina secondary to cardiac arrhythmia

b. **Aortic**

- Acute aortic syndromes: aortic dissection: abrupt onset of intense tearing or ripping retrosternal pain radiating to the back (inter-scapular region) and extending to the abdomen, hips and legs with distal extension, maximal at the onset; intramural haematoma; penetrating atherosclerotic ulcer; contained traumatic aortic rupture
- Thoracic aortic aneurysm (ascending aortic aneurysms tend to cause anterior chest pain, arch aneurysms cause pain radiating to the neck, and descending thoracic aneurysms cause inter-scapular back pain)
- Aortitis

Pulmonary

- Pneumonia
- Pneumothorax
- Pleurisy
- Pulmonary embolism
- Pneumomediastinum
- Acute chest syndrome (sickle cell crisis)

Oesophageal

- Gastro-oesophageal reflux; reflux oesophagitis
- Oesophageal spasm
- Infective oesophagitis
- Oesophageal rupture with mediastinitis (Boerhaave syndrome): Mackler's triad of **chest pain** following severe **vomiting** or retching related to dietary overindulgence and alcohol consumption, and **subcutaneous emphysema**; crunching precodial sound on auscultation (Hamman's sign); acute dyspnoea; dysphagia; upper gastrointestinal bleeding; abdominal pain; crepitus in the chest wall and neck; pneumothorax and pneumomediastinum, pleural efussion on xrays

Musculoskeletal Localised chest wall pain (often pointed to with one or two fingers), reproduced by pressure over the site of spontaneous pain; positional

Ribs and articulations

- Costochondritis (Tietze's syndrome): painful and tender swelling of one or more upper costal cartilages (usually 2nd and 3rd) at the sterno-chondral junctions, with no overlying skin changes
- Rib fractures: traumatic; metastases
- Slipping rib syndrome (hypermobile inferior-8th,9th and 10th- costal cartilages): subcostal pain, associated with a clicking or popping sound on lifting objects, flexing the trunk or walking, associated with a localized tender area on the costal margin
- Costo-vertebral arthritis

Sternum and articulations

- Costochondritis (Tietze's syndrome): painful and tender swelling of the sternoclavicular joint
- Sternoclavicular arthritis
- Manubriosternal arthritis
- Painful xiphoid syndrome

Myofascial structures

- Pain arising from intercostals or shoulder girdle muscles (traumatic muscle pain)

- Precordial catch syndrome (a syndrome of intermittent and short lived (<5 min) left sided chest pain, recurring frequently for a few hours
- Epidemic myalgia (Bornholm disease or pleurodynia-Coxsackie B virus infection): paroxysms of sharp pain in the chest or abdomen

Referred pain from the thoracic spine
Neuropathic pain secondary to thoracic spine disease may mimic musculoskeletal chest pain, and may be caused by myelopathy (cord compression); radiculopathy (nerve root compression); neuropathy (nerve involvement, such as intercostal nerves)

- Herniated thoracic disc disease
- Costo-vertebral arthritis
- Vertebral crush fractures secondary to osteoporosis
- Metabolic bone disease
- Spinal metastases
- Herpes zoster (intercostal neuropathy, characterized by 1 or 2 weeks of sensory symptoms involving one or two contiguous dermatomes, almost always unilateral, followed by a maculopapular rash which progresses to vesicles with erythematous bases
- Compressive radiculopathy

Referred pain from the upper abdomen

- Biliary tract disease: acute cholecystitis; biliary colic; cholangitis
- Acute pancreatitis
- Perforated peptic ulcer
- Gastritis

Psychogenic

- Panic and anxiety disorder
- Depression

Localisation of chest pain may indicate the underlying cause of pain
Central:

- Cardiac
- Aortic
- Pulmonary/mediastinal
- Oesophageal
- Traumatic

Lateral:

- Pulmonary
- Chest wall
- Psychogenic

Acute coronary syndromes
Categorisation of Acute Coronary Syndromes

- Acute chest pain and persistent (>20 min) ST-segment elevation or new onset left bundle branch block: **STEMI**
- Acute chest pain without persistent ST-segment elevation: persistent or transient ST-segment depression or T wave inversion, flat T waves, pseudo-normalisation of T waves, or no ECG changes at presentation

1. **NSTE-ACS**: defined by elevation of troponins
2. Unstable angina

Potential clinical presentations of NSTE-ACS

- Prolonged (>20 min) angina at rest
- New onset angina
- Recent destabilization of previously stable angina
- Post-myocardial infarction angina

Features of chest pain which are notcharacteristic of myocardial ischaemia
(AHA/ACC guidelines for NSTE Acute Coronary Syndromes, 2014)

- Pleuritic pain (sharp or knife-like pain provoked by respiration or cough)
- Pain localised by the tip of one finger, especially at the left ventricular apex or costochondral junction
- Pain reproducible with movement or palpation of chest wall or arms
- Brief episodes of pain lasting a few minutes or less
- Constant pain persisting for many hours

- Pain radiating into lower limbs
- Pain of maximum intensity at onset (the pain of acute coronary syndrome reaches maximum intensity only after several minutes)

Atypical presentations of acute coronary syndrome

- Pain in the neck, back, jaw, shoulders or arms
- Acute dyspnoea; acute exacerbation of heart failure
- Dizziness, presyncope and syncope
- Sweating
- Weakness and fatigue
- Nausea and vomiting; abdominal discomfort
- Acute confusion
- Stroke

Atypical presentations are commoner in the following circumstances:

- Old age
- Female gender
- Diabetes mellitus
- People of South Asian or African-Caribbean origin

Causes of acute coronary syndrome

Atherosclerosis: plaque rupture; thrombosis
Coronary arterial spasm: primary; cocaine/amphetamine induced
Arteritis: Kawasaki disease (coronary artery aneurysms with thrombotic occlusion or rupture); Takayasu's arteritis; rheumatoid arthritis; lupus
Structural coronary artery abnormalities: radiation fibrosis; aneurysm; ectasia; anomalous origin of coronary artery; trauma; dissection
Coronary embolism

12 Lead ECG in acute coronary syndromes
Criteria for diagnosis of ST elevation myocardial infarction

- ST segment elevation, measured at the J point (junction of termination of QRS complex and beginning of ST segment), 2 mm or greater in two or more contiguous chest leads
- ST segment elevation, measured at the J point, 1 mm or greater in two or more contiguous limb leads
- New or presumed onset left bundle branch block
- ST segment depression in V1-V3 (reciprocal ST elevation in posterior leads V8-V10) (isolated posterior myocardial infarction)
- ST segment elevation in aVR

Universal definition of myocardial infarction
Detection of the rise and/or fall of cardiac biomarkers (preferably troponin) with at least one value above the 99th percentile of the upper reference limit, together with at least one of the following:

- Symptoms of myocardial ischaemia
- ECG changes indicative of new ischaemia (new significant ST-T changes or new left bundle branch block)
- Development of pathological Q waves in the ECG
- Imaging evidence of new loss of viable myocardium or new regional wall motion abnormality
- Identification of an intracoronary thrombus by angiography or autopsy

(Thygesen K, Alpert JS, Jaffe AS, et al.Third universal definition of myocardial infarction. 2012;126:2020–35)

Baseline ECG abnormalities that may obscure interpretation of ST elevation and which require prompt management in patients with signs and symptoms of ongoing myocardial ischaemia include:

- Left bundle branch block
- Ventricular paced rhythm
- Left ventricular hypertrophy
- Brugada syndrome

Changes on ECG which are not diagnostic for infarction, but which may be due to ischaemia

- ST segment depression 1 mm or more with T inversion in lateral leads (can be caused by acute elevation of left ventricular end diastolic pressure, related to subendocardial ischaemia).
- Transient ST segment elevation
- Axis shift-left or right
- Transient T wave inversion
- Deep T waves in V1 to V4
- Increase in R wave voltage.
- Reduction of R wave progression over precordial leads reflects loss of left ventricular musculature.
- Left bundle branch block or right bundle branch block
- 1st degree, 2nd degree, or 3rd degree AV block
- Tachyarrhythmias
- Transient peaked tall T waves due to epicardial artery obstruction or narrowing

Chest pain evaluation may include

- Serial 12 lead ECG; review of previous ECGs, and consideration of recording from additional ECG leads
- Chest xray
- Serial cardiac biomarkers (including high sensitivity troponin)
- Arterial blood gases
- D-dimer (suspected pulmonary embolism-low Wells score of 4 or less)

Risk stratification for acute coronary syndrome
GRACE (Global Registry of Acute Cardiac Events) Score at initial presentation is based on

- Age in years
- Resting heart rate (beats per minute)
- Systolic blood pressure (mm Hg)
- ST segment deviation
- Congestive Heart Failure (Killip Class)
- Serum creatinine

This scoring system is recommended by NICE, the European Society of Cardiology, the American Heart Association and American College of Cardiology. The risk score has been developed into an app, facilitating widespread use. The scoring system was based on a study of 102,000 patients in 30 countries.The GRACE 2.0 risk calculator incorporates a revised algorithm for use when serum creatinine and Killip class are not available,

Fox KAA, Dabbous OH, Goldberg RJ, et al. Prediction of risk of death and myocardial infarction in the six months after presentation with acute coronary syndrome: prospective multinational observational study (GRACE). BMJ. 2006;333:1091–4

Causes of cardiogenic shock following acute myocardial infarction

- **Acute left ventricular failure** (severe contractile dysfunction of the left ventricle with reduced ejection fraction)
- Severe contractile dysfunction of the right ventricle due to right ventricularmyocardial infarction (acute inferior wall STEMI, unexplained hypoxia, high-grade atrioventricular block, cardiogenic shock with the triad of hypotension, elevated jugular venous pressure and clear lung fields, marked sensitivity to preload-reducing agents such as nitrates,morphine and diuretics as cardiac output is preload-dependent; a tricuspid regurgitant murmur, Kussmaul's sign and pulsus paradoxus indicate significant haemodynamic effects due to right ventricular ischaemia)
- **Mechanical complications**: acute aortic regurgitation; ventricular septal rupture; contained left ventricular free wall rupture with pericardial tamponade; papillary muscle rupture and acute mitral regurgitation (recognized by bedside echocardiography)

Predisposing factors for cardiogenic shock (persistent hypotension, systolic blood pressure <80 mm Hg, in the presence of adequate or elevated filling pressure-absence of hypovolaemia) in acute coronary syndrome

- Older age
- Systolic blood pressure: hypertension
- Killip class II (I: no clinical signs of heart failure; II: lung crackles, S3 and elevated jugular venous pressure; III: acute pulmonary oedema; IV: cardiogenic shock)
- Diabetes mellitus
- Anterior infarction
- Previous infarction; multi-vessel coronary artery disease
- Peripheral vascular disease
- Prior diagnosis of heart failure
- Left bundle branch block

Other causes of cardiogenic shock

- Myocarditis
- End-stage cardiomyopathy
- Left ventricular outflow tract obstruction
- Acute aortic regurgitation
- Pulmonary embolism
- Myocardial contusion

Features suggesting oesophageal origin of chest pain (the default position is always cardiac unless proven otherwise):

- History of heartburn
- Dysphagia; odynophagia
- Acid regurgitation
- Water brash: sudden appearance of a slightly sour or salty fluid in the mouth
- Pain relief with antacids
- Post-prandial pain, especially after a large meal
- Worse when lying flat
- Sleep interrupted by pain
- Symptoms lasting longer than 20 min in the absence of exertion
- Retrosternal pain without lateral radiation

Risk factors for aortic dissection

- Hypertension
- Aortic disease: congenital bicuspid aortic valve, thoracic aortic aneurysm, coarctation of the aorta, annulo-aortic ectasia, cystic medial degeneration; previous operative repair of aneurysm/dissection
- Atherosclerosis
- Pregnancy (especially third trimester)
- Genetic connective tissue disease: Marfan syndrome –two or more criteria: reduced upper segment to lower segment ratio: arm span to height ratio >1.05; pectus carinatum or excavatum; high arched palate; arachnodactyly; family history of Marfan syndrome; vascular Ehlers-Danlos syndrome
- Turner syndrome (short stature; premature ovarian failure; skeletal malformations; abnormalities of eyes and ears; heart anomalies; lymphedema; only affects females)
- Trauma: blunt declerating chest trauma (road traffic collision; fall from a height); iatrogenic: cardiac catheterisation, intra-aortic balloon pump, post cardiac surgery (aortic valve replacement for aortic insufficiency; coronary artery bypass grafting)
- Inflammatory/infectious disease of aorta: giant cell arteritis; Takayasu's arteritis; Behcet disease; tertiary syphilis
- Cocaine abuse
- High intensity weight lifting

Possible clinical presentations and signs of aortic dissection (related to rupture into body cavities, branch occlusion or acute and progressive aortic regurgitation

Cardiovascular: chest pain; hypertension; differential pulses (left radial-right radial; radial-femoral); inter-arm blood pressure difference greater than 20 mm Hg; acute aortic regurgitation; acute congestive heart failure; cardiac tamponade; superior vena caval obstruction; acute ST elevation myocardial infarction; sternoclavicular joint pulsation

Respiratory: haemoptysis; pleural effusion; haemothorax; aorto-pulmonary fistula with haemorrhage

Neurological: syncope; ischaemic stroke; spinal cord syndromes: paraplegia/paraparesis, quadriparesis; anterior spinal cord syndrome

Gastrointestinal: mesenteric ischaemia/infarction with abdominal pain
Renal: acute kidney injury; renal infarction (flank pain with haematuria)
Limbs: acute upper or lower limb ischaemia
Painless aortic dissection (5–10%)
Clinical findings of ischaemia may involve several organ systems

Features associated with increased risk of atypical symptoms in acute aortic syndromes

- Age >70 years
- Female gender
- Diabetes mellitus
- Existing aortic aneurysm
- Prior cardiovascular surgery

Causes of inter-arm blood pressure differences greater than 20 mm Hg

- Normal variant
- Upper limb arterial disease
- Coarctation of the aorta
- Inflammatory vascular disease: Takayasu's arteritis (systemic vasculitis involving large and medium-sized arteries, predominantly affecting females of childbearing age, with an onset age between 10 and 40 years; there is a predilection for the aorta and its branches. It can present with systemic symptoms, limb claudication, hypertension, stroke or transient ischaemic attack, Raynaud's syndrome, or congestive heart failure)
- Aortic dissection
- Supravalvular aortic stenosis

Causes of aortitis

- Large vessel vasculitis: giant cell arteritis; Takayasu arteritis; rheumatoid arthritis; SLE; HLA-B27 associated spondyloarthropathies-ankylosing spondylitis
- Infections: bacterial (Salmonella, Staphylococcus, Streptococcus pneumoniae); syphilis; mycobacterial (tuberculosis)
- Sarcoidosis

Potential presentations of aortitis

- Aneurysmal disease: thoracic aortic aneurysm; abdominal aortic aneurysm
- Cardiac abnormalities: aortic regurgitation; stable angina; acute coronary syndrome
- Aortic thrombosis with distal embolisation
- Aortic dissection or rupture
- Upper and/or lower limb claudication
- Secondary hypertension
- Neurological presentations:transient ischaemic attack, stroke

Conditions other than acute coronary syndrome that are associated with raised cardiac troponins
Cardiac Disease and Interventions

- Tachy- or bradyarrhythmia; atrial fibrillation with fast ventricular rate
- Coronary vasospasm
- Dilated cardiomyopathy
- Severe congestive heart failure, acute and chronic
- Aortic dissection; aortic valve disease
- Hypertrophic cardiomyopathy
- Inflammatory cardiac diseases; eg myocarditis; pericarditis; endocarditis
- Infiltrative cardiac disease: amyloidosis; haemochromatosis
- Myocardial contusion
- Cardiac surgery; post-cardiac transplantation
- Cardioversion and implantable cardioverter-defibrillator shocks
- Percutaneous coronary intervention; radio-frequency ablation; endomyocardial biopsy

Non-cardiac diseases

- Critically ill patients, especially with respiratory failure, or sepsis

- High dose cardiotoxic chemotherapy, eg anthracyclines (doxorubicin; daunorubicin); trastuzumab
- Pulmonary embolism; severe pulmonary hypertension
- Pulmonary oedema
- Rhabdomyolysis
- Renal dysfunction: acute kidney injury; chronic kidney disease
- Subarachnoid haemorrhage
- Scorpion envenomation
- Sepsis and septic shock
- Stroke (haemorrhagic and ischaemic)
- Ultra-endurance exercise(triathlon)
- Burns affecting >30% body surface area
- Acute neurological disease, including stroke, or subarachnoid haemorrhage

Causes of acute pericarditis

- Idiopathic
- Viral infections: adenovirus, enterovirus, Coxsackie A and B, cytomegalovirus, influenza, hepatitis B, herpes simplex virus, Epstein-Barr virus, parvovirus B9, HIV
- Bacterial infections: mycobacterium tuberculosis; staphylococcal; streptococcal; pneumococcal
- Fungal infections: aspergillosis; histoplasmosis
- Metabolic: uraemia
- Chest trauma; post-pericardiotomy (cardiac surgery)
- Neoplastic: breast cancer; lung cancer; Hodgkin's lymphoma; leukaemia
- Autoimmune: rheumatoid arthritis; systemic lupus erythematosus; inflammatory bowel disease
- Drugs: doxorubicin, hydralazine, procainamide, penicillins
- Post-acute myocardial infarction (Dressler's syndrome) (a secondary pericarditis that develops weeks to months after a myocardial infarction and associated with pleuro-pericardial chest pain, low grade fever, elevated ESR and white cell count, and pericardial effusion which may lead to cardiac tamponade)
- Acute myocarditis (myopericarditis)
- Aortic dissection
- Mediastinal radiation therapy (breast or lung)
- Post-pericardiotomy syndrome

Clinical presentations of acute pericarditis

- Anterior chest retrosternal or precordial pleuritic pain, relieved by sitting up and leaning forward and increased by lying down (positional), deep inspiration, coughing or swallowing; may radiate to the back, neck, left shoulder or arm
- Low grade fever
- Pericardial rub (a grating, scratching or rasping to-and-fro systolic and diastolic extra heart sound best heard at the left sternal border)
- Cardiac tamponade

Stages of ECG changes in acute pericarditis

- Stage 1: concave upward ST segment elevation in all leads except aVR; no reciprocal ST depression; PR segment depression (atrial injury)
- Stage 2: QRS-ST junction (J point) returns to baseline and T wave amplitude begins to decrease
- Stage 3:T wave inversion
- Stage 4: ECG returns to normal

Adverse prognostic features in acute pericarditis

- Temperature >38 °C
- Subacute course
- Large effusion or tamponade
- Failure of non-steroidal anti-inflammatory therapy

Causes of Myocarditis
Infection:

- Virus: Coxsackie, influenza, adenovirus, echovirus, rubella, cytomegalovirus, HIV

- Bacteria: Corynebacterium diphtheriae, chlamydia, rickettsia, Coxiella burneti
- Protozoa: Trypanosoma cruzi, Toxoplasma gondii
- Rickettsial: Coxiella burnetii
- Fungal: Aspergillus; Histoplasma

Physical:

- Radiotherapy: breast/lung cancer; thymoma; lymphoma

Chemical (toxic):

- Heavy metals: lead, iron, copper
- Drugs: alcohol, amphetamines, anthracyclines

Immune mediated

- Drugs: emetine; chloroquine; vaccines: tetanus toxoid
- Autoimmune: SLE; Kawasaki disease; Wegener's granulomatosis; sarcoidosis; Churg-Strauss syndrome; inflammatory bowel disease

Miscellaneous

- Bites/stings: scorpion; snake

Clinical features and presentations of myocarditis

- Acute chest pain; pericarditic or pseudo-ischaemic
- Tachycardia out of proportion to fever
- Acute coronary syndrome in younger patients, in the absence of coronary risk factors or structural heart disease
- Congestive heart failure
- Cardiogenic shock
- Fulminant heart failure
- Acute dilated cardiomyopathy
- Embolic events
- Conduction system abnormalities
- Ventricular arrhythmias
- Aborted sudden cardiac death

Clinical presentations of infective endocarditis

- Fever and chills; night sweats; malaise; fatigue; myalgia; arthralgia; anorexia; weight loss
- New or changing regurgitant heart murmur
- Vascular phenomena: splinter haemorrhages; Janeway lesions (haemorrhagic lesions on palms and soles); conjunctival haemorrhages; arterial emboli (cerebral, mesenteric, renal, and splenic infarction-left sided cardiac lesions); pulmonary infarcts, lung abscesses (right sided cardiac lesions); mycotic aneurysms; intracranial haemorhage
- Immunological phenomena: Roth's spots on the retina; Osler's nodes; glomerulonephritis
- New or worsening congestive heart failure
- Neurological presentation secondary to cerebral abscess or embolus (transient ischaemic attack or stroke)
- Pneumonia and pulmonary infarction in right sided endocarditis, or left sided if septal defect
- Fever associated with new conduction disturbance

Risk factors for infective endocarditis

- Valvular heart disease
- Structural heart disease
- Prosthetic heart valve
- Implantable device: pacemakers, vascular catheters, implantable cardioverter-defibrillator, ventricular assist device
- Intravenous drug use (right-sided endocarditis)
- Poor dental hygiene; dental procedures
- Diabetes mellitus
- Immunocompromised state
- Previous history of infective endocarditis

Cardiac lesions predisposing to the development of infective endocarditis
High risk

- Prosthetic heart valves, including bioprosthetic and homograft valves
- Previous bacterial endocarditis
- Complex cyanotic congenital heart disease (eg single ventricle, transposition of the great arteries, Tetralogy of Fallot)
- Surgically constructed systemic-pulmonary shunts or conduits

Moderate risk

- Most other congenital cardiac malformations: patent ducturs arteriosus, ventricular septal defect, coarctation of aorta)
- Hypertrophic cardiomyopathy
- Acquired valvular dysfunction (eg rheumatic heart disease; degenerative or age-related valve disease-degenerative aortic stenosis/mitral annular calcification)
- Mitral valve prolapse with valvular regurgitation and/or thickened leaflets

Negligible risk

- Isolated secundum atrial septal defect
- Surgical repair of atrial septal defect, ventricular septal defect or patent ductus arteriosus (without residua beyond 6 months)
- Mitral valve prolapse without valvular regurgitation
- Physiological murmurs
- Previous Kawasaki disease/rheumatic fever without valvular dysfunction
- Atrial myxoma

Causes of non-bacterial endocarditis
This should be suspected in patients with chronic disease who present with symptoms related to arterial embolism, which can be peripheral or cerebral.

- Valve leaflet trauma (venous catheters with intra-cardiac placement)
- Circulating immune complexes
- Vasculitis
- Hypercoagulability
- Mucin-producing metastatic adenocarcinoma (lung, stomach, pancreas)

ECG presentations
Normal 12 lead ECG

- Paper speed: 25 mm/s
- Each large square (5 mm): 0.20 s (width); 0.5 mV (height)
- Each small square (1 mm): 0.04 s (width); 0.1 mV (height)
- There are five large squares per second, and 300 per minute
- Heart rate: divide 1500 by the number of small squares between two consecutive QRS complexes or divide 300 by the number of large squares between two consecutive QRS complexes. With an irregular heart rate, count the number of R waves in 30 large squares (6 s) and multiply by 10 to obtain the rate per minute
- P wave: duration <0.12 s (3 small squares; 3 mm); <2.5 mm (2.5 small squares) (0.25 mV) in height in limb leads; positive (upright) in leads I, II, aVF, and V2 to V6; inverted in aVR
- PR interval, or PQ interval (beginning of P wave to beginning of QRS or rS complex): 0.12–0.20 s (3–5 small squares)
- QRS complex: 0.06–0.10 s; initial septal Q waves in I and V6; predominantly positive QRS complex in I and V6
- There is a gradual incremental increase in the height of the R wave in the chest leads from V1 through to V6. The transition point (normally at V3/V4), where the R and S waves are equal, indicates the position of the interventricular septum.
- QT interval (beginning of QRS or rS complex to end of T wave; the presence of a U wave is not included in the measurement): QTc (QT interval divided by square root of preceding RR interval) <0.42 s
- T wave: normally upright in I, II, V3-V6; normally inverted in aVR and V1; variable in III, aVF, aVL and V2

Correlates of ECG deflections

- P wave: atrial activation; the first and second halves of the P wave correspond roughly to right and left atrial activation, respectively
- PR interval: time delay between atrial depolarisation and ventricular activation; conduction delay in the atrioventricular node
- QRS complex: ventricular activation; phase 0 of the action potential
- J point: phase 1 of the action potential
- ST segment: phase 2 (plateau phase) of action potential
- T wave: ventricular repolarisation
- QT interval: ventricular systole (ventricular depolarisation and repolarisation)
- TQ: phase 4 of action potential
- U wave: His-Purkinje system repolarisation

Abnormalities of P wave

- Peaked (height >2.5 mm) (P pulmonale) (right atrial enlargement)
- Broad (width >3 mm) (P mitrale) (left atrial enlargement) (can be bifid)
- Biphasic (one half positive and the other half negative)
- Inverted or absent in lead II
- Buried within QRS complex
- Follows QRS complex (retrograde)

Causes of absent P waves

- Replacement by fibrillatory waves or flutter waves
- Buried in QRS complexes owing to retrograde conduction: junctional rhythm
- Superimposition on T waves: supraventricular or ventricular tachycardia

Causes of variable P wave shape

- Wandering pacemaker
- Multiple atrial premature beats
- Paroxysmal atrial tachycardia with atrioventricular block
- Multifocal atrial tachycardia

Causes of prolonged PR interval (>0.20 s)

- 1st degree atrio-ventricular block
- 2nd degree AV block (Mobitz type 1 or Wenkebach)
- Metabolic: hypothyroidism; hyperkalaemia; hypercalcaemia
- Hypothermia
- Drugs slowing atrioventricular nodal conduction: digoxin; beta blockers; calcium channel blockers; quinidine
- Increased vagal tone

Analysis of prolonged PR interval (>0.20 s)

- Are all the PR intervals and P waves the same? If yes, 1st degree atrio-ventricular block is likely; if not, think of premature atrial complexes, wandering pacemaker, multifocal atrial tachycardia, or another type of block
- Do the PR intervals vary consistently?
- Are all the P waves the same?
- Are the PR intervals progressively lengthening?
- Is there grouped beating?
- Are the Ps and QRSs dissociated?

Categorization of AV block

- 1st degree: prolonged PR interval; all P waves conducted to ventricles
- 2nd degree: Type 1 (Wenckebach): patterned dropping of QRS complexes-progressive prolongation of PR interval and progressive shortening of RR interval on consecutive beats until a non-conducted P wave (dropped QRS complex); Type 2: constant PR intervals until a non-conducted P wave, not preceded by PR prolongation nor followed by PR shortening; fixed ratio of P waves to conducted beats
- 3rd degree: different atrial and ventricular rates, with P waves and QRS complexes

occurring at regular but independent intervals, with the P wave rate being greater than the QRS rate; PR interval varies, while PP and RR intervals are constant; cardiac function is maintained by an escape junctional (narrow QRS complex) or ventricular (wide QRS complex) pacemaker

Causes of short PR interval (<0.12 s)

- Junctional rhythms with retrograde atrial activation (inverted P waves in II, III, aVF) and low atrial rhythms
- Retrograde junctional P waves
- Wolff-Parkinson-White syndrome (short PR interval, slurred slow rising initial upstroke of QRS complex (delta wave) (Type A: positive QRS in V1; Type B: negative QRS in V1)
- Lown-Ganong-Levine syndrome (short PR interval and normal QRS duration, associated with paroxysmal supraventricular tachycardia)
- Glycogen storage disease

Causes of variable PR interval

- Complete atrio-ventricular block
- Mobitz type 1 (Wenckebach) 2nd degree atrio-ventricular block
- Wandering atrial pacemaker (variable configuration of P wave)

Causes of acquired atrioventricular block

- Idiopathic(senescent) fibrodegenerative AV block: Lenegre-Lev disease (idiopathic bundle branch fibrosis), characterized by progressive alteration of conduction through the His-Purkinje system with right or left bundle branch block and widening of QRS complexes, leading to complete AV block
- Coronary artery disease: myocardial infarction; ischaemic cardiomyopathy
- Calcific valvular disease
- Postoperative or traumatic: coronary artery bypass; aortic, tricuspid, or mitral valve replacement; VSD repair; septal myomectomy; ablation of septal accessory pathways
- AV node ablation: radiofrequency
- Therapeutic radiation to the chest
- Infections: syphilis; diphtheria; Chagas' disease; tuberculosis; toxoplasmosis; Lyme disease; viral myocarditis (Epstein-Barr, varicella); infective endocarditis
- Collagen vascular disease: rheumatoid arthritis; scleroderma; dermatomyositis; ankylosing spondylitis; polyarteritis nodosa; SLE; Marfan's syndrome
- Infiltrative: sarcoidosis; amyloidosis; haemochromatosis; lymphoma; solid tumour
- Neuromuscular: progressive external ophthalmoplegia; myotonic muscular dystrophy; peroneal muscular atrophy; scapuloperoneal syndrome; limb girdle dystrophy
- Drug effect: digoxin; beta blockers; calcium channel blockers; amiodarone; procainamide; Class IC agents (flecainide, propafenone)

Causes of low voltage QRS complexes <10 mm in any chest lead; <5 mm in any limb lead

- Obesity; thick chest wall
- Old age
- COPD (emphysema)
- Hypothyroidism
- Pericardial effusion; chronic constrictive pericarditis
- Diffuse coronary artery disease
- Congestive heart failure
- Amyloidosis

Causes of abnormally wide QRS duration 0.10–0.11 s

- Incomplete right or left bundle branch block
- Non-specific intra-ventricular conduction delay
- Some cases of left anterior or posterior fascicular block

0.12 s (>3small squares)

- Complete bundle branch block, right (rSR′ –triphasic complex in V1, V2; qRS in V6) or left (QS or rS- broad negative complex-in V1; rSR′ or R in V6)
- Wolff-Parkinson-White syndrome
- Non-specific intra-ventricular conduction delay
- Arrhythmias of ventricular origin
- Implanted ventricular pacemaker (paced rhythm)
- Hyperkalaemia
- Hypothermia
- Sodium channel blocking medication: tricyclic antidepressants
- Intermittent rate-related aberrancy

Causes of wide negative QRS in V1

- Left bundle branch block
- Right sided accessory pathway
- Right ventricular pacing

Causes of physiological Q waves (physiological or positional factors)

- Normal variant "septal" Q waves
- Normal variant Q waves in V1 and V2, III, aVF
- Left pneumothorax or dextrocardia (loss of lateral R wave progression)

Causes of pathological Q waves
(>1 mm or one small square wide (>40 msor 0.04 second in duration); >4 mm or 4 small squares deep; >25% of height of subsequent R wave (Q/R wave ratio >25%); present in right precordial leads V1-V3; must be seen in two contiguous leads)

- Myocardial injury: acute myocardial ischaemia with or without infarction; myocarditis; hyperkalaemia
- Pulmonary embolism
- Right ventricular (reversed or poor R wave progression, particularly with COPD) or left ventricular hypertrophy (slow R wave progression)
- Conduction abnormalities: left bundle branch block; WPW pattern
- Cardiomyopathies: hypertrophic cardiomyopathy; infiltrative myocardial disease (amyloidosis)
- Ventricular septal defect in V5 and V6

Causes of tall R in V1 and V2 (R/S ratio >1)
Narrow R wave

- True posterior myocardial infarction
- Increased R wave amplitude and duration (the pathological R is the mirror image of the pathological Q in the posterior leads V8-V10)
- R/S ratio in V1/V2 >1 (prominent anterior forces)
- Hyper-acute ST-T wave changes (ST depression and large inverted T waves in V1-V3)
- Late normalisation of ST-T with symmetrical upright waves in V1-V3
- Right ventricle intra-ventricular conduction delay: rSr′ complexes
- Right ventricular hypertrophy
- Right heart strain with acute right ventricular dilatation: pulmonary embolism; COPD; cor pulmonale)
- Dextrocardia
- Misplaced precordial leads; normal variants
- Hypothermia
- Hypertrophic cardiomyopathy
- Paediatric ECG (normal variant): tall R and inverted T in V1-V3

Wide R wave

- Right bundle branch block- complete or incomplete
- RBBB mimics: pulmonary embolism; Brugada syndrome; arrhythmogenic right ventricular dysplasia; WPW syndrome
- RBBB with LAFB
- Trifascicular block
- Accessory pathway (Type A Wolff-Parkinson-White syndrome)

Features of right ventricular hypertrophy
QRS complex abnormalities

- Right axis deviation
- R wave taller than S in V1 (R/S ratio >1)
- qR complex in V1
- rS complex from V1 to V6

P wave abnormalities

- P pulmonale

ST segment and T wave abnormalities

- ST depression and T inversion in right precordial leads (V1 to V2)

Describing a QRS complex

- A QRS complex can have one (monophasic), two (diphasic), or three (triphasic) individual waveforms
- A negative deflection initiating the QRS complex is a Q wave
- The first positive (upward) deflection is an R wave, whether or not preceded by a Q wave
- A negative deflection following an R wave is an S wave
- A second positive deflection is termed R′ (R prime)
- A second negative deflection is termed S′ (S prime)
- A monophasic negative QRS complex, with no R wave, is termed a QS wave
- Biphasic complexes are either RS or QR
- Triphasic complexes are RSR′ or QRS
- Large amplitude waves are assigned capital letters Q, R and S, while smaller amplitude waves are assigned lower case letters q, r and s. No specific amplitude is uniformly used to mark the transition between the use of lower case letters and capital letters.
- A typical left precordial lead complex is a qR complex
- A typical right precordial lead complex is an rS complex
- The end of the QRS complex and beginning of the ST segment is termed the J point
- An epsilon wave is a small positive deflection in the terminal QRS complex

Causes of RSR′pattern in V1 and V2

- Normal (5% of young adults)
- Straight back deformity
- Incomplete right bundle branch block
- Right ventricular hypertrophy
- Acute cor pulmonale
- Right ventricular diastolic overload
- Wolff-Parkinson-White syndrome
- Duchenne muscular dystrophy

Causes of a wide QRS complex

- Bundle branch block
- Pacemaker
- Sodium channel blockade
- Non-specific intra-ventricular conduction delay
- Metabolic causes

Causes of left bundle branch block (QRS 120 ms or longer; QS or rS in II, III, aVF, V1 to V3-W pattern; absence of the septal q wave and wide, monophasic notched or slurred R, RS, rsR′ or RSR′ in I, aVL, V5 to V6-M pattern; ST-T changes discordant from terminal QRS; with a similar ECG pattern and QRS duration 110–119 ms, incomplete left bundle branch block is diagnosed)

- Coronary artery disease
- Hypertensive heart disease
- Dilated cardiomyopathy; myocarditis
- Left ventricular outflow tract obstruction: aortic stenosis; coarctation of aorta
- Antero-septal ST elevation myocardial infarction
- Idiopathic degenerative disease of the conduction system (Lenegre)
- Hyperkalaemia
- Severe left ventricular hypertrophy

- Right ventricular pacing lead
- Cardiac surgery

Causes of right bundle branch block (QRS 120 ms or longer; rsr′, rsR′, rSR′, RSR′ or RR′ in V1 to V3-M pattern; wide and/or deep slurred S in I, V5 to V6-W pattern; with a similar ECG pattern and QRS 110–119 milliseconds, incomplete right bundle branch block is diagnosed)

- Normal variant
- Right ventricular hypertrophy
- Pulmonary embolism with right ventricular strain
- Cor pulmonale
- Coronary artery disease
- Idiopathic degenerative disease of conduction system (fibrosis-Lev; sclerosis-Lenegre)
- Rheumatic heart disease
- Atrial septal defect (ostium secundum)
- Brugada syndrome (incomplete RBBB with coved ST elevation)
- Myocarditis; cardiomyopathy

Features of fascicular blocks

- Left anterior fascicular block

qR in I, aVL
rS in II, III, aVF
Left axis deviation
QRS duration <120 ms

- Left posterior fascicular block

rS in I, aVL
qR in II, III, aVF
QRS duration <120 ms
Right axis deviation

- Trifascicular block

Right bundle branch block + left anterior/posterior fascicular block + 1st degree AV block (prolonged PR interval)
Left bundle branch block + 1st degree AV block

Causes of deep T wave inversion (>5 mm)

- Normal variants: persistent juvenile T wave pattern; early repolarisation variants (with ST elevation)
- Myocardial ischaemia or infarction; myocardial contusion
- Wellens' syndrome: angina, associated with deep inverted T waves in V3-V5 and biphasic T wave in V2 during chest pain-free intervals, associated with critical stenosis of the proximal left anterior descending coronary artery which can progressive to acute anterior wall myocardial infarction
- Cardiomyopathies, including arrhythmogenic right ventricular dysplasia
- Cerebrovascular accident (especially intracranial bleeding related to subarachnoid haemorrhage) and related neurogenic patterns (eg radical neck dissection, Stokes-Adams syndrome)
- Left ventricular or right ventricular overload: classic left or right ventricular hypertrophy/enlargement with repolarisation abnormalities ("strain" patterns); apical hypertrophic cardiomyopathy (Yamaguchi syndrome)
- Drug effects: digoxin; phenothiazine
- Post-tachycardia T wave pattern
- Idiopathic global T wave inversion syndrome
- Secondary T wave alternans: bundle branch block; WPW patterns
- Intermittent LBBB; Ventricular premature beats or pacing (cardiac memory T waves)

Causes of tall peaked T wave

- Hyperkalaemia
- Hyperacute myocardial infarction
- Acute posterior myocardial infarction

Causes of long QT syndrome

QT prolongation can be the result of either prolonged ST segment duration with normal T wave duration, as seen with hypocalcaemia or hypomagnesaemia, or widening of the T wave, which is associated with the development of torsades des pointes. The T on P phenomenon is seen in the presence of sinus tachycardia when a prolonged QT interval causes the T wave to adjoin or overlap the succeeding P wave.

QT prolonging drugs:

- Antiarrhythmic drugs-class Ia (disopyramide, procainamide, quinidine), Ic (flecainide, encainide) and III (amiodarone, sotalol)
- Antimicrobials (macrolide antibiotics-erythromycin, clarithromycin; azole antifungals: fluconazole, ketoconazole, itraconazole; pentamidine; fluoroquinolones- ciprofloxacin, levofloxacin, moxifloxacin)
- Antihistamines (astemizole, terfenadine, loratadine)
- Psychotropic drugs (phenothiazines, haloperidol, tricyclic and tetracyclic antidepressants, selective serotonin reuptake inhibitors, antipsychotics: risperidone, lithium, olanzapine)
- Cholinergic agonists (cisapride, organophosphates)
- Antimalarial agents: chloroquine; mefloquine
- Antiemetics: ondansetron; domperidone
- Protease inhibitors

Bradyarrhythmias: severe bradycardia (eg complete AV block)

Electrolyte disorders

- Hypokalaemia
- Hypocalcaemia
- Hypomagnesaemia

Congenital long QT syndromes (inherited ion channel disorders which predispose the ventricular myocardium to catecholamine-induced arrhythmias)

- Romano-Ward syndrome(AD), with normal hearing
- Jervell-Lange-Nielsen syndrome(AR), with deafness

Heart disease: acute myocardial ischaemia; congestive heart failure; cardiomyopathy; myocarditis.

Thyroid disease: hypothyroidism.

Cerebrovascular disease: subarachnoid haemorrhage; ischaemic stroke.

Causes of prominent U waves

- Hypokalaemia
- Class IA and III anti-arrhythmic drugs
- Thyrotoxicosis
- Severe hypertension

Causes of left axis deviation

(Positive QRS in I and aVL; negative QRS in II and aVF)

- Normal variant
- Left anterior hemiblock (anterior fascicular block)
- Left bundle branch block
- Left ventricular hypertrophy
- Elevated diaphragm
- Obesity
- Q waves of inferior myocardial infarction
- Paced rhythm
- Hyperkalemia
- Wolff-Parkinson-White syndrome (right sided accessory pathway)
- Tricuspid atresia
- Ostium primum atrial septal defect
- Mechanical shift of the heart in the chest (lung disease, prior chest surgery)
- Inferior myocardial infarction

Causes of right axis deviation

(Positive QRS in II and aVF; negative QRS in I and aVL)

- Normal variant in children and tall thin adults
- Right bundle branch block
- Left posterior hemiblock (posterior fascicular block)
- Right ventricular hypertrophy
- Chronic lung disease
- Acute cor pulmonale-right heart strain/pressure overload (pulmonary embolism)
- Antero-lateral ST elevation myocardial infarction
- Limb lead reversal

- Dextrocardia
- Wolff-Parkinson-White syndrome (left sided accessory pathway)
- Atrial septal defect
- Lateral wall myocardial infarction

Checklist for history taking with palpitations (subjective and uncomfortable awareness of one's own heartbeat)

Palpitations are common, and most often are benign and due to non-cardiac conditions. It is important to try to recognize cardiac and potentially life-threatening causes of palpitations.

- Mode of onset and offset
- Frequency of episodes
- Rate
- Regularity of rhythm (regular or irregular); sensation of missed beats (atrial or ventricular ectopic beats)
- Associated symptoms, suggesting haemodynamic instability: chest pain, shortness of breath, light headedness, near syncope or syncope
- Precipitating factors: physical exertion; change in position; emotional stress
- Relieving factors: Valsalva manoeuvre
- Medications, including over the counter drugs and recreational drug use as well as prescription medication (beta-agonists, calcium channel blockers, anti-arrhythmic drugs, thyroxine)
- Lifestyle factors: excessive caffeine intake; alcohol abuse
- History of heart disease including heart murmurs
- History of thyroid disease
- Family history of recurrent syncope, premature onset coronary artery disease, pacemaker or ICD use, or sudden cardiac death under the age of 40 years

Clinical and electrocardiographic clues to the electrophysiological mechanisms of arrhythmias

Automaticity is suggested by:

- Gradual acceleration with a steady "warm-up" of the rate
- Significant variation in rate that correlates with sympathetic tone or body temperature
- Slight slowing with vagal manoeuvres
- Gradual deceleration or "cool-down" of an arrhythmia

Re-entry is suggested by:

- Usually paroxysmal, with abrupt onset and offset (or cessation)
- Usually initiated by a premature beat
- Very regular rate
- Abrupt cessation of a tachycardia, especially when terminated by an ectopic impulse
- Abrupt termination with vagal manoeuvres is sometimes successful
- Post-episode diuresis (provoked by atrial natriuretic peptide release)

Causes of narrow complex tachycardia (QRS complex < 120 ms)

a. Regular

Atrial activity seen

P: QRS 1.

P wave similar to sinus P wave

Physiological sinus tachycardia

Inappropriate sinus tachycardia (persistent; no identifiable trigger; hypersensitive response to endogenous catecholamines, with rapid heart rate rise after minimal exercise; seen in young healthy adult females)

Sinus node re-entrant tachycardia (normal P wave morphology; abrupt onset and offset)

P: QRS > 1 (atrial rate > ventricular rate)

Abnormal P wave morphology

Unifocal atrial tachycardia

Flutter waves

Atrial flutter (sawtooth waves; with a fixed 2:1, 3:1, 4:1 or greater AV block; most obvious in II, III and aVF)

No atrial activity (P waves)

AV nodal re-entrant tachycardia (P waves buried within QRS complex or inscribed in terminal portion of QRS as pseudo S′ in III and pseudo R′ in V1; P wave inversion (retrograde P waves) in II, III and aVF; rate-related ST segment depression; phasic variation in QRS amplitude)

Focal junctional ectopic tachycardia

Orthodromic AV re-entrant tachycardia

b. **Irregular**

c. **Fibrillation waves**

Atrial fibrillation

d. **Flutter waves**

Atrial flutter with varying atrio-ventricular block

e. **Abnormal P waves**

Atrial tachycardia with variable AV block

f. **3 or more P wave morphologies**

Multi-focal atrial tachycardia (variable P′-P′, P′-R and R-R intervals)

Tachycardia with atrial premature complexes, ventricular premature complexes and junctional premature complexes

Causes of atrial fibrillation

- Systemic disease: chronic pulmonary disease (COPD), hyperthyroidism, sepsis (pneumonia), pulmonary embolism, drugs, acute alcohol ingestion (holiday heart syndrome)
- Cardiac disease: ischaemic heart disease, valvular heart disease (especially mitral), hypertensive heart disease, cardiomyopathy (dilated, hypertrophic, infiltrative), sick sinus syndrome, congestive heart failure, myocardial contusion, pericarditis, myocarditis, pre-excitation syndrome (Wolff Parkinson-White syndrome), post-cardiac surgery
- Idiopathic

Causes of atrial fibrillation with slow ventricular response (slow resting heart rate <50 bpm, or normal resting heart rate with prolonged ventricular pauses)

- Drug effect: digoxin toxicity, beta blocker toxicity, calcium channel blockers toxicity
- Atrial fibrillation with AV block due to severe AV nodal disease
- Sinus node dysfunction: sick sinus syndrome
- Hypothyroidism
- Hypothermia

Presenting rhythms in sick sinus syndrome

- Atrial bradyarrhythmias: sinus bradycardia; sinus arrest (ventricular pauses 3 s or more), with or without junctional escape rhythm; sino-atrial exit block (Mobitz type I or type II block); ectopic atrial tachycardia; atrial fibrillation with slow ventricular response
- Atrial tachyarrhythmias: atrial fibrillation; atrial flutter; atrial tachycardia
- Alternating bradyarrhythmia and tachyarrhythmia
- Ventricular escape tachyarrhythmias
- Additionally, there is an absence of increase in heart rate in response to physical exercise (chronotropic incompetence)

CHAD2DS2VASc score to estimate stroke risk in atrial fibrillation

Risk factor	Points
C: Congestive heart failure	1
H: Hypertension	1
A: Age > 75 years	2
D: Diabetes mellitus	1
S: Stroke/embolism	2
V: Vascular disease	1
A: Age > 65 years	1
Sc: Female sex	1

Analysis of narrow complex tachycardia based on RP interval

The relationship of P waves to R waves is useful in analyzing the type of narrow complex tachycardia. The RP interval reflects time from ventricular activation to atrial activation

Long RP interval (>70 ms): P closer to succeeding QRS.

AVNRT.

Short RP interval (=<70 ms): P closer to and immediately followingpreceding QRS

a. **Short RP-long PR**

Sinus tachycardia, sinus node re-entrant tachycardia (with relatively prolonged AV conduction)

Atrial tachycardia
Atrial flutter with 2:1 AV block
Junctional ectopic tachycardia with retrograde P wave
Typical atrio-ventricular nodal re-entrant tachycardia
AV re-entrant tachycardia with relatively rapid retrograde conduction

b. **Long RP- short PR**
Atrial tachycardia, sinus tachycardia, sinus node re-entrant tachycardia
Atypical AV re-entrant tachycardia
Orthodromic atrio-ventricular re-entrant tachycardia with slow retrograde conduction
Permanent form of junctional reciprocating tachycardia

c. **RP equal in length to PR**
Typical AV nodal re-entrant tachycardia with 2:1 AV block
Atrial flutter with 2:1 AV block
Atrial tachycardia, sinus tachycardia, sinus node re-entrant tachycardia (with fortuitously timed AV conduction)

Sinus tachycardia

The sinus node rate is faster than age-related normal values. The mechanism is accelerated phase 4 diastolic depolarization in sinus nodal cells, ie enhanced automaticity

Causes of sinus tachycardia

Physiological: Pain; recent physical exertion (catecholamine surge); anxiety; pregnancy

Pharmacological: Sympathomimetics (recreational drugs: cocaine, amphetamines); caffeine; bronchodilators; high doses of beta-agonist medication; inotrope infusion; alcohol; nicotine

Pathological: Fever; hypoxaemia; hypovolaemia; anaemia; shock; sepsis; pulmonary embolism; hyperthyroidism; heart failure; myocardial infarction, myocarditis; serotonin syndrome.

Causes of bradycardia

Atrial
Sinus bradycardia (sinus rhythm; <60 beats per minute)
Sinus arrest (transient absence of P waves)
Sino-atrial block (sinus node exit block) (absence of P waves; the pause is a multiple of the preceding P-P interval)
Sick sinus syndrome

Atrioventricular nodal
Junctional bradycardia

Ventricular
Idioventricular or ventricular escape rhythm

Causes of sinus bradycardia

- Physical conditioning: eg athletes
- Vagal stimulation: eg vomiting
- Carotid sinus pressure/hypersensitivity
- Excess parasympathetic stimulation: acute inferior myocardial infarction
- Raised intracranial pressure (Cushing response)
- Hypothyroidism
- Hypothermia
- Hypoxaemia
- Drugs: beta blockers; calcium channel blockers; digoxin; amiodarone; opiates; cholinergic toxicity
- Sinus node disease: sick sinus syndrome
- Severe Gram negative sepsis

Broad complex tachycardia

(QRS complex 120 msor longer)

Regular

- No AV dissociation

Antidromic AVRT
Assess QRS morphology
Typical LBBB or RBBB: probably SVT
Atypical BBB, criteria for aberrancy not seen: probably VT

- AV dissociation present

P: QRS <1
Ventricular tachycardia
P: QRS >1
Atrial flutter
Atrial tachycardia

Irregular

- Atrial fibrillation in WPW syndrome: a very rapid ventricular response over an accessory pathway with short refractory periods can lead to ventricular fibrillation

- Atrial fibrillation with bundle branch block
- Atrial fibrillation with aberrancy
- Atrial flutter with variable AV block
- Atrial tachycardia with variable AV block with BBB or aberrancy
- Polymorphic VT (torsades de pointes) (twisting of the peaks of the QRS complexes around the isoelectric baseline)

Broad complex tachycardia

The default diagnosis when origin of the rhythm is unclear is always VT

Favours SVT

- Initiation with a premature P wave
- QRS complexes identical to those in resting rhythm
- Long-short sequence preceding initiation
- Changes in P-P interval precede changes in R-R interval
- QRS contours consistent with aberrant conduction (V1, V6)
- Slowing or termination with vagal manoeuvres

Favours VT

- History of ischaemic heart disease, congestive heart failure, cardiomyopathy
- Initiation with premature QRS complex
- Tachycardia beats identical to those of ventricular premature beats during sinus rhythm
- Changes in R-R interval precede changes in P-P interval
- QRS contours inconsistent with aberrant conduction (V1, V6): monophasic or biphasic QRS in V1; RS or QS in V6
- AV dissociation or other non 1 A: V relationships; clinical signs of AV dissociation include cannon a waves in the jugular venous pulse, and varying intensity of the first heart sound and in systolic blood pressure
- Fusion beats (intermediate width and morphology to supraventricular and ventricular complexes)
- Capture beats (QRS complex of normal duration and morphology)
- QRS duration >140 ms (0.14 s)
- Left axis deviation (especially −90 to −180°)
- Concordant R wave progression pattern
- Contralateral bundle branch block pattern from resting rhythm
- Absence of rS complex in any precordial lead

Specific syndromes of monomorphic VT associated with left and right bundle branch block QRS morphologies

Outflow tract ventricular tachycardias are the most common type of idiopathic ventricular tachycardia in patients with structurally normal hearts.

Differential diagnosis of **left bundle branch block pattern regular broad complex tachycardia**

- Ventricular tachycardia

Right ventricular outflow tract tachycardia (LBBB with rightward/inferior axis; sensitive to adenosine and verapamil)

Bundle branch re-entrant tachycardia: associated with dilated cardiomyopathy; bundle branch block or intra-ventricular conduction defect in sinus rhythm

- Pre-excited tachycardia

Mahaim fibre tachycardia: typically, minimal or no pre-excitation in sinus rhythm

- Supraventricular tachycardia: any form with left bundle branch block; may have LBBB in sinus rhythm

Differential diagnosis of **right bundle branch block pattern regular broad complex tachycardia**

Idiopathic left posterior fascicular ventricular tachycardia

Bundle branch re-entrant tachycardia

Fascicular re-entrant tachycardia (RBBB morphology with left axis deviation)

Causes of ventricular tachycardia

Structural heart disease

- Coronary artery disease
- Cardiomyopathies: dilated cardiomyopathy; hypertrophic cardiomyopathy; arrhythmogenic right ventricular dysplasia

- Aortic stenosis
- Complex congenital heart disease
- Cardiac sarcoidosis

Structurally normal heart

- Electrolyte disorders: hypokalaemia; hyperkalaemia
- Drugs: digoxin
- Channelopathies: long QT syndrome, Brugada syndrome
- Idiopathic ventricular tachycardia: RVOT tachycardia, idiopathic left ventricular tachycardia
- Long QT syndromes: torsade de pointes
- Neurological disease

Characteristics of ventricular premature beats that may need suppression

- Two or more in a row
- Multi-form (multi-focal)
- Increased ventricular ectopic activity with exercise
- R on T phenomenon

Causes of accelerated idioventricular rhythm

- Drug toxicity: digoxin; cocaine
- Electrolyte abnormalities
- Myocarditis
- Dilated cardiomyopathy
- Athlete's heart
- Return of spontaneous circulation post-cardiac arrest
- Reperfusion following thrombolysis or percutaneous coronary intervention after acute myocardial infarction

Causes of ST segment elevation

Normal: male pattern: the majority of men have ST elevation of 1 mm or more in the precordial leads. The ST segment is concave. This is most marked in V2.

Benign early repolarisation pattern (ST elevation of normal variant)

Acute trans-mural myocardial infarction (STEMI)

Left ventricular aneurysm (dyskinetic area) or large scar (akinetic area)-persistent elevation

Coronary artery vasospasm: Prinzmetal's or variant angina (recurrent episodes of angina, usually at rest and often occurring in the early morning hours, associated with trasient ST elevation, responsive to short-acting nitrates and calcium channel blockers)

Trans-mural ischaemia: tight coronary stenosis, during exercise testing

Takotsubo cardiomyopathy (transient cardiac syndrome presenting with chest pain that mimics acute coronary syndrome, often with a precipitating emotional or physical stressor; regional systolic dysfunction of the left ventricle, including reversible left ventricular apical ballooning, and normal coronary arteries; named as the narrow neck and wide base of the left ventricle in systole resemble a Japanese octopus pot or takotsubo)

Coronary artery dissection (Marfan's syndrome; Ehlers-Danlos syndrome)

Myocardial injury: trauma to ventricle (myocardial contusion)

Left ventricular hypertrophy, in right precordial leads with large S waves

Hypertrophic cardiomyopathy

Left bundle branch block, in right precordial leads with large S waves

Acute pericarditis

Myocarditis

Aortic dissection

Tumour invading left ventricle

Severe hyperkalemia

Brugada syndrome (RBBB like pattern and ST elevation in right precordial leads, associated with susceptibility to ventricular tachyarrhythmias and sudden cardiac death)

Anomalous origin of left coronary artery from pulmonary artery (Q waves, ST elevation and T inversion in I, aVL, V4-V6)

Pulmonary embolism

Hypothermia

After DC cardioversion

Intracranial haemorrhage

Hyperkalaemia

Type 1c anti-arrhythmic drugs
Ventricular paced rhythm

Types of contour of ST segment elevation

Convex upward (coved)
  Abrupt takeoff following QRS complex
  ST segment rounded in contour
  Associated with injury current seen with ST elevation myocardial infarction
Concave upward
  Takeoff more gradual
  ST segment describes much gentler upward sloping curve on its way to the
  summit of the T wave

Features associated with common causes of ST elevation
Acute Myocardial Infarction (STEMI)

Slow ECG evolution with localisation
Convexity upwards, or straightened
Reciprocal ST-T changes
Development of Q waves with QTc prolongation
ST elevation is maximal 1 h after onset. In the absence of re-vascularisation, there is a gradual return to the baseline over about 10–20 h
In the presence of left bundle branch block, the ST changes in the same direction as the QRS, and the ST elevation is more than would be expected from LBBB alone, eg>5 mm in V1 to V3

Acute Pericarditis

- Generalized, non-anatomical ST-T changes in all leads except aVR and V1
- Concavity upwards
- Often with normal QTc
- PR segment depression, a manifestation of atrial injury
- No reciprocal ST segment depression
- T waves usually low amplitude; ST elevation >25% of total T height
- Heart rate usually increased

Left Ventricular Aneurysm

- Chronic (>2 weeks after acute myocardial infarction) with no evolution
- Localised ST elevation with variable ST-T changes
- Often prolonged QTc

Coronary Arterial Spasm (Prinzmetal's Angina)

- Rapid ECG evolution
- Localised ST elevation
- Normal QTc

Early repolarisation

- ST elevation is most prominent in mid- to left precordial leads V2-V5. ST elevation is less often seen in the limb leads. All leads with an upright T have elevated ST-T segments, and all leads with negative T waves have depressed ST-T segments. This is associated with a relatively tall T wave.
- J point elevation above the isoelectric line, the J point being the junction where the QRS complex ends and the ST segment begins (forming a sharp angle with the terminal QRS). It is the first point of inflexion on the upstroke of the S wave when the ST segment is sloped or the QRS segment is wide. The ST segment elevation begins at the J point. The ST segment may takeoff several mm above the baseline at this point, with preservation of the normal upward concavity of the initial, up-sloping portion of the ST segment/T wave complex. The degree of J point elevation is usually less than 3.5 mm
- Notching or irregular contour of the J point, where the ST joins the QRS. The notch is not part of the QRS and should not be included in its width.
- Normal corrected QT interval
- Absence of reciprocal ST depression
- Early repolarisation is found in 2–5% of the population, mainly in young adult males, and there is a similar appearance on old ECGs.

Mnemonic for ST elevation

ELEVATION

- E electrolytes
- L left bundle branch block
- E early repolarisation
- V ventricular hypertrophy
- A aneurysm
- T treatment- pericardiocentesis
- I injury (AMI; myocardial contusion)
- O Osborne waves (hypothermia)-a positive deflection at the J point
- N non-occlusive vasospasm

Sgarbossa's criteria for acute myocardial infarction with left bundle branch block

Concordant ST elevation ≥1 mm in leads with a positive QRS complex: 5 points

Concordant ST depression ≥1 mm in V1, V2, V3: 3 points

Excessively discordant ST elevation >= 5 mm in leads with a negative QRS complex: 2 points

3 or more points: 90% specificity for STEMI

(Sgarbossa EB, et al. Electrocardiographic diagnosis of evolving acute myocardial infarction in the presence of left bundle branch block. N Engl J Med. 1996; 334:481–7)

Localisation of ischaemia in the presence of ST elevation

- Anterior wall: V2 toV5
- Antero-septal: V1 toV3
- Lateral: V4 to V6, aVL, I
- Inferior wall: II, III, aVF
- Posterior wall: V7 to V9

Differential diagnosis of ST depression

- **Normal variants or artefacts**

Pseudo-ST depression (wandering baseline due to poor skin-electrode contact)

Physiological J point depression with sinus tachycardia

Hyperventilation induced ST depression

- **Acute coronary ischaemic syndromes**

Sub-endocardial ischaemia

Non-ST segment elevation wave myocardial infarction (NSTEMI)

Reciprocal changes in Q wave myocardial infarction (sub-epicardial ischaemia from distant zone

Acute posterior wall myocardial infarction (anterior leads: V1-V3)

Rate-related ST segment depression (tachycardia)

Repolarisation effects unrelated to ischaemia

- Digoxin effect: coved ST segment depression (reverse tick), flattened T wave, decreased QTc interval
- Secondary ST segment changes with intraventricular conduction abnormalities, eg RBBB, LBBB, WPW
- Right ventricular hypertrophy (right precordial leads) or left ventricular hypetrophy (left precordial leads, I, aVL-repolarisation abnormality ('strain' pattern)

Miscellaneous

- Hypokalaemia
- Mitral valve prolapse
- CNS disease

Seattle criteria for the categorisation of the ECG in athletes

ECG findings which may be normal

Sinus bradycardia: 30 beats per minute or greater

Sinus arrhythmia

Ectopic atrial rhythm

Junctional escape rhythm

1st degree atrio-ventricular block

Mobitz type 1 2nd degree atrio-ventricular block

Incomplete right bundle branch block

Isolated QRS voltage criteria for left ventricular hypertrophy (in absence of left atrial enlargement, left axis deviation, ST segment depression, T wave inversion or pathological Q waves)

Early repolarisation

Convex ST elevation and T wave inversion in leads V1-V4 (in athletes of African origin)

Abnormal ECG findings

- T wave inversion >1 mm in two or more leads V2-V6, II and aVF, or I and aVL (excludes III, aVR and V1)
- ST depression 0.5 mm or greater in two or more leads
- Pathological Q wave: >3 mm in depth or >40 msin duration in two or more leads (except for III and aVR)
- Complete left bundle branch block
- Intraventricular conduction delay: any QRS duration 140 ms or greater
- Left axis deviation: −30° to −90°
- Left atrial enlargement
- Right ventricular hypertrophy pattern
- Ventricular pre-excitation
- Long QT interval (QTc 470 ms or greater-males; QTc 480 msor greater-female)
- Short QT interval (QTc 320 ms or less)
- Brugada-like ECG pattern
- Profound sinus bradycardia: <30 beats per minute; or sinus pauses 3 s or longer
- Atrial tachyarrhythmias: supraventricular tachycardia, atrial fibrillation, atrial flutter
- Ventricular premature beats: 2 or more per 10 s tracing
- Ventricular arrhythmias: couplets, triplets, non-sustained ventricular tachycardia

(Br J Sports Med. 2013;47:122–4)

Causes of sudden cardiac death

- Coronary artery disease: ischaemic heart disease; anomalous coronary artery origin; coronary spasm
- Cardiomyopathies: hypertrophic cardiomyopathy; idiopathic dilated cardiomyopathy; arrhythmogenic right ventricular dysplasia; infiltrative (sarcoid, amyloid); viral myocarditis; commotio cordis
- Valvular heart disease: aortic stenosis; mitral valve prolapse
- Wolff Parkinson White syndrome
- Ion channelopathies: long QT syndrome; short QT syndrome; Brugada syndrome; catecholaminergic polymorphous ventricular tachycardia; idopathic ventricular fibrillation
- High grade atrio-ventricular block
- Sick sinus syndrome

Features associated with sudden arrhythmia death syndrome

- Syncope, especially with exercise or severe stress
- Family history of sudden unexpected death
- Country of origin in the Pacific Rim: South East Asia; Japan; Philippines
- ECG: long QT syndrome; Brugada syndrome; torsade de pointes; ventricular fibrillation

Pacemaker-related presentations

Pacemaker modes (North American Society of Pacing and Electrophysiology/British Pacing and Electrophysiology Group (NASPE/BPEG) five-letter code or NBG code)

- Chamber paced: atrial (A), ventricular (V), or dual (D)
- Chamber sensed: atrial (A), ventricular (V), or dual (D)
- Action that the pacemaker takes when sensing occurs: trigger (T), inhibition (I), dual inhibition and triggering (D), or none (0; pacemaker in asynchronous mode)
- Rate responsiveness to activity (0-none or R-rate modulation)
- Multi-site pacing (A, V, D and 0)

Chest x-ray features of pacemakers

With a **single atrial lead** visible on chest x-ray the pacing mode is almost certainly AAI®

With a **single ventricular lead**, the mode is almost certainly VVI®, although dual-chamber sensing from a single lead is now possible. This is termed VDI.

If **two leads** are attached to the generator the system is dual-chamber, usually DDD®, with one lead in the right atrium and the other in the right ventricle.A biventricular pacemaker (cardiac resynchronization therapy device) has one lead in the right ventricle and one in the left ventricle.

Characteristics of the pacemaker inpulse

Sharp, narrow, vertically oriented spike less than 2 ms in duration

If it appears before a P wave, it is pacing the atrium

If it appears before the QRS complex, it is pacing the ventricle

The QRS complex that follows a pacing spike resembles a LBBB pattern, due to right ventricular stimulation.

There may also be changes in T wave morphology, eg T wave inversion and

QT prolongation

Pacemaker problems

A. **Failure to pace**: no pacing spikes, when there should be

For one or both chambers, either no pacing artefacts will be present on the ECG, or artefacts will be present for one but not the other chamber.

The pacemaker does not fire when it should. The cardiac rhythm is dependent on the patient's native cardiac rhythm.This leads to cerebral hypoperfusion, associated with dizziness, presyncope or syncope, and pulmonary venous hypertension, causing breathlessness

Causes include: lead fracture or disconnection; pulse generator battery depletion; component failure: generator malfunction; over-sensing; external interference (electromagnetic interference)

B. **Failure to sense**: spikes occur inappropriately without sensing

Constant pacemaker spikes despite ongoing intrinsic cardiac electrical activity (native P wave or QRS). Pacemaker spikes occur at inappropriate times, eg in the middle of P waves or shortly after a normal QRS complex. The pacemaker does not detect normal cardiac activity and fires when it does not need to. This is related to

- Low amplitude or slew of intracardiac signals (low intrinsic QRS current)
- Pacing system problems: lead fracture, lead insulation break, lead maturation or dislodgement, fibrosis around the lead tip, inappropriately programmed sensitivity, external interference, pulse generator battery depletion

C. **Failure to capture**: there are pacemaker spikes but no subsequent cardiac activity (no P wave or QRS complex following it); atrial and/or ventricular pacing stimuli are present, with persistent or intermittent failure to capture

- Increase in atrial or ventricular stimulation threshold

Metabolic disturbances: hyperkalaemia, hyperglycaemia, alkalosis or acidosis, hypoxaemia, hypercapnia.

Drugs: quinidine, procainamide, lidocaine, mexiletine, encainide, flecainide.

Myocardial perforation; acute myocardial infarction.

Exit block due to fibrosis around lead tip

- Defective pacing leads: fracture, dislodgement or disconnection, insulation break
- Pulse generator battery depletion

D. **Inappropriate pacemaker rate**

Usually caused by a **pacemaker re-entrant tachycardia** or endless-loop tachycardia (acute termination can be achieved with a magnet over the generator), in which the pacemaker forms the anterograde limb of the circuit, with retrograde conduction via the atrio-ventricular node. Retrograde transmission of a ventricular impulse that is rapidly transmitted to the atrium is sensed by the pacemaker as a native P wave. The ventricular pacemaker awaits the programmed AV interval and then fires, causing ventricular depolarisation. Fast retrograde conduction again occurs, creating a self-sustaining circus movement with a rapid, wide QRS complex rhythm

A **runaway pacemaker** is caused by pulse generator discharge at a rate above its preset upper limit. It is related to battery failure or malfunction, and is resistant to anti-arrhythmic agents, DC shock or magnet application. The definitive treatment is emergency removal of the pulse generator.

Problems with implantable cardioverter defibrillators

- **Inappropriate therapy (shocks)**: oversensing of intra-cardiac signals (T waves or P waves) and extra-cardiac noise such as diaphragmatic myopotentials. Multiple inappropriate ICD shocks in a short period of time are a medical emergency, and may result from recurrent ventricular arrhythmias (ventricular electrical storm), non-sustained ventricular tachycardia, inappropriate shocks caused by supraventricular tachyarrhythmias, oversensing of extra-cardiac signals, or ICD system malfunction (battery depletion, component failure, or under-sensing).
- **Therapy failure (failure of arrhythmia detection):** inadvertent device deactivation-interaction with other implanted device or external environment; under-sensing of fine ventricular fibrillation; delivery of ineffective shocks. Failure to capture results from lead dislodgement or perforation. Failure to pace is caused by premature battery depletion, random component failure, or software error.
- Proarrhythmia: sustained ventricular tachycardia or ventricular fibrillation. External defibrillation is required in cardiac arrest.

Magnet application will temporarily disable the tachyarrhythmia function in all ICD models.

Arterial emergencies

The six Ps of acute arterial ischaemia are:

- Pain
- Pallor
- Paraesthesiae
- Paralysis
- Pulselessness
- Poikilothermia (low skin temperature that does not vary with the environmental temperature)

Acute arterial ischaemia may be difficult to recognize as the presenting features are non-specific. The features may be less obvious in the presence of chronic peripheral arterial disease with collateral vessel formation

Causes of acute upper limb ischaemia

Embolism

- Cardiac: atrial fibrillation; recent myocardial infarction (mural thrombus); left ventricular aneurysm; cardiomyopathies; cardiac masses (thrombus, tumour, vegetation); rheumatic valvular disease; mechanical valve prosthesis
- Aortic arch: atheromatous plaques with thrombosis
- Post-stenotic dilatation of subclavian artery
- Traumatic aneurysm
- Paradoxical embolism (triad of deep vein thrombosis, intra-cardiac communication with a right-to-left shunt, and arterial embolism)

Iatrogenic injury

- Cardiac catheterisation
- Trans-brachial or trans-radial angiography
- Indwelling arterial lines

Inadvertent intra-arterial injection

- Intravenous drug abuse
- Occupational hazard in anaesthetic practice

Trauma

- Shoulder and arm dislocations
- Repetitive external trauma

Medical causes

Arteritis related to collagen vascular disease

- Scleroderma
- Rheumatoid arthritis
- Systemic lupus erythematosus
- Dermatomyositis

Allergic necrotising arteritis

- Takayasu's disease
- Giant cell arteritis

Haematological disorders

- Thrombophilias: deficiency of protein C or S, or of antithrombin III; factor V Leiden; activated protein C resistance, anti-phospholipid syndrome
- Cold agglutinins
- Cryoglobulins
- Polycythaemia vera
- Thrombocytosis

Other syndromes

- Behcet syndrome (triad of recurrent oral and genital ulceration and uveitis; skin lesions)
- Anti-phospholipid syndrome

Mechanisms of acute lower limb ischaemia

- Major arterial occlusion: thrombotic; embolic
- Small vessel occlusion: blue toe syndrome
- Venous occlusion: phlegmasia cerulea dolens

Features suggesting thrombotic arterial occlusion

- Preceding history of intermittent claudication
- Long history (days to weeks)
- Less severe ischaemia
- Signs of chronic ischaemia

Causes of acute arterial ischaemia of the lower limb

Atherosclerosis

- Atherosclerotic peripheral arterial occlusive disease, with acute plaque rupture and thrombosis
- Atheroembolism

Thromboembolism

- Cardiac disease: atrial fibrillation; myocardial infarction; endocarditis; valvular disease (especially mitral)
- Aortic aneurysm
- Peripheral arterial aneurysms
- Proximal critical stenosis

Thrombosed aneurysm with or without embolisation

Thrombosis of an arterial bypass graft, endovascular stent

Hypercoagulable states, with spontaneous thrombosis

- Natural anticoagulant deficiency (antithrombin III, protein C, protein S)
- Procoagulant excess: polycythaemia, thrombocytosis, malignancy, heparin-induced platelet activation

Aortic/arterial dissection

Arterial trauma: blunt; penetrating

Anatomical or developmental anomalies

- Popliteal entrapment syndrome, with thrombosis
- Persistent sciatic artery
- Popliteal adventitial cystic disease, with thrombosis
- Fibromuscular dysplasia

Inflammatory conditions (arteritis)

- Thromboangiitis obliterans (Buerger's disease)
- Vasculitis (collagen vascular disease)

Vasospastic conditions

- Raynaud's phenomenon

- Ergotism
- Recreational drug infusion

Features of critical lower limb ischaemia

- Rest pain for more than 2 weeks
- Ischaemic ulceration/gangrene of feet or toes
- Absent or diminshed pedal pulses
- Ankle systolic blood pressure <50 mm Hg
- Toe systolic blood pressure <30 mm Hg

Features of irreversible ischaemia of the lower limbs

- Fixed skin staining
- Muscle paralysis
- Tense fascial compartments
- Inaudible Doppler arterial and venous signals

Causes of acute aortic occlusion
Aortic occlusive disease

- Thrombosis on pre-existing atherosclerosis (commonest cause)
- Aortic embolus (saddle embolus-lodges at the aortic bifurcation): usually from left ventricle after acute myocardial infarction
- Aortic aneurysm(rare)

Aortic dissection

- Extension of type A or B thoracic aortic dissection
- Isolated infrarenal aortic dissection

Iatrogenic

- Angiography
- Intra-aortic balloon pumping
- Bullet embolus
- Retrograde dissection after extracorporeal bypass

Trauma

- Thrombosis after intimal tear
- Bullet embolus

Features

- Acute lower limb ischaemia, often with neurological dysfunction
- With suprarenal aorta occlusion: gut ischaemia; hypertension; anuria

Arterial injury
Potential causes

- Penetrating trauma: stab wound; gunshot wound; intravenous drug abuse
- Blunt trauma: associated with fracture or dislocation
- Iatrogenic injury: arteriography; cardiac catheterization; balloon angioplasty

Hard signs of arterial injury

Active pulsatile external bleeding
Pulsatile or expanding haematoma
Signs of acute limb ischaemia or signs of acute compartment syndrome
Reduced or absent distal arterial pulses
Audible bruit
Palpable thrill

Soft signs of arterial injury

- History of arterial bleeding at the scene of the injury
- Small stable non-pulsatile haematoma
- Neurological deficit
- Hypotension; shock
- Proximity of wound to a major artery

It is important not to rely on capillary refill or the presence of a Doppler signal to exclude arterial injury

Acute compartment syndrome
Clinical features

- Pain disproportionate in severity with relation to findings on physical examination
- Pain increased by passive stretch of muscles within compartment

- Paraesthesiae
- Pallor
- Paralysis
- Pulselessness
- Poikilothermia (perishingly cold)

Potential causes
Reduced compartment size

- Tight constrictive dressing, bandage or POP cast
- Localised external pressure-prolonged tourniquet use
- Prolonged limb compression (sleep; altered level of consciousness-alcohol, drugs)

Increased compartment contents

- Bleeding:

Arterial injury
Coagulopathy; anticoagulation

- Increased capillary permeability

Trauma: crush injury; fractures (open/closed)
Burns; electrical injury
Severe exertion
Intravenous fluid/medication extravasation (resistance to intravenous injection or infusion; pain, swelling, induration, erythema, venous discoloration and blanching)
High-pressure injection injuries
Intravenous drug abuse
Snake/insect bite
Ischaemic reperfusion post-injury

Heart failure
Acute heart failure has been defined as "a change in heart failure signs and symptoms resulting in the need for urgent therapy"

The patient in acute heart failure can be categorised on the basis of haemodynamic profiles as warm + wet, cold + wet, cold + dry or warm + dry, as defined by peripheral perfusion (warm/cold) and lung auscultation (wet/dry)

European society of cardiology classification of acute heart failure syndromes

- Acute decompensated heart failure (de novo or decompensated chronic heart failure)
- Hypertensive acute heart failure
- Acute heart failure with pulmonary oedema
- Cardiogenic shock
- High output heart failure

Presenting symptoms and signs of heart failure include

- Breathlessness; exercise intolerance; orthopnoea; paroxysmal nocturnal dyspnoea
- Raised jugular venous pressure, peripheral oedema (ankles, sacrum, genitalia); gallop rhythm (S3); lateral displacement of the apex beat; bilateral crackles in the lungs; hepatomegaly; ascites; gain in body weight
- A single measurement in the untreated patient of BNP (B-type natriuretic peptide) <100 ng/L or NT-proBNP (N-terminal pro-BNP) <300 ng/L makes the diagnosis of heart failure unlikely

New York Heart Association Classification of Heart Failure (functional characterisation of patients with chronic heart failure)

Class I
No limitation: ordinary physical exercise does not cause fatigue, dyspnoea or palpitations

Class II
Slight limitation of physical activity: comfortable at rest but ordinary activity results in fatigue, palpitations, dyspnoea or angina

Class III
Marked limitation of physical activity: comfortable at rest but less than ordinary activity results in symptoms

Class IV
Unable to carry out any physical activity without discomfort: symptoms of heart failure are present even at rest with increased discomfort with any physical activity

Causes of Acute Heart Failure
Depressed Ejection Fraction (<40%): Systolic dysfunction (impaired contractility with abnormal emptying)

- Myocardial damage: coronary artery disease with contractile dysfunction: acute coronary syndromes (myocardial infarc-

tion; NSTE-ACS); mechanical complications of acute myocardial infarction; right ventricular infarction
- Systolic pressure overload: hypertension-hypertensive crisis; obstructive valvular disease (aortic stenosis; mitral stenosis)
- Systolic volume overload: regurgitant valvular disease (endocarditis; rupture of chordae tendinae-acute aortic and acute mitral regurgitation); intra-cardiac (left to right) shunting (ventricular septal rupture); extra-cardiac shunting
- Reduced global myocardial function: non-ischaemic dilated cardiomyopathy
- Disorders of rate and rhythm: chronic tachyarrhythmias; chronic bradyarrhythmias

Preserved Ejection Fraction (40–50%): Diastolic dysfunction (limitation in diastolic filling; elevated filling pressures; limitation in forward output due to increased ventricular stiffness):

Primary disorder

- Obstruction to filling: mitral stenosis, left atrial myxoma
- Reduced distensibility: hypertrophic cardiomyopathy; restrictive cardiomyopathies (infiltrative and storage disorders-amyloidosis, sarcoidosis); fibrosis; endomyocardial disorders
- Impaired relaxation: familial hypertrophic cardiomyopathy for HCM, ischaemia
- External compression: constrictive pericarditis, cardiac tamponade, cor pulmonale

Secondary

- Systolic dysfunction

Pulmonary heart disease

- Cor pulmonale (peripheral oedema; raised jugular venous pressure; systolic parasternal heave; loud pulmonary component of second heart sound)
- Pulmonary vascular disorders

High-output states (associated with widening of pulse pressure to greater than 50% of systolic blood pressure)

- Metabolic disorders: thyrotoxic crisis; nutritional disorders: beri beri
- Excessive blood flow requirements: systemic arterio-venous shunting; chronic anaemia; Paget's disease of bone

Causes of pulmonary oedema alone (without hypotension) in acutely ill patients

Non-cardiac:

- Volume overload
- Acute respiratory distress syndrome
- Reduced tissue oncotic pressure

Cardiac:

- Left ventricular systolic failure
- Left ventricular diastolic dysfunction in absence of systolic dysfunction

Causes of pulmonary oedema and hypotension in acutely ill patients

Non-cardiac:

- Septic or neurogenic shock with acute respiratory distress syndrome

Cardiac:

- Left ventricular systolic failure
- Ventricular septal rupture
- Acute mitral regurgitation
- Acute aortic regurgitation

Causes of pulmonary oedema according to aetiology

Non-cardiogenic

- Volume overload: acute kidney injury
- Aspiration of fluid: fresh or salt water near drowning; gastric fluid aspiration (Mendelson syndrome)
- Asphyxia
- Upper airway obstruction
- High altitude
- Acute glomerulonephritis
- Neurogenic pulmonary oedema (related to massive sympathetic discharge with pulmonary and systemic vasoconstriction): suarachnoid haemorrhage; intracranial

haemorrhage; head injury; spinal cord trauma; acute hydrocephalus; seizures; colloid cyst of third ventricle
- Re-expansion pulmonary oedema
- Inhalation of noxious gases: smoke inhalation; nitrous dioxide (silo filler's disease); sulphur dioxide; chlorine
- Drugs: aspirin; valium, Librium; barbiturates; heroin; cocaine; methadone
- Poisons: parathion
- Blood transfusion reaction
- Contrast media reaction
- Adult respiratory distress syndrome

Cardiogenic

- High cardiac output: anaemia; shunts: cardiac; pulmonary; peripheral; hyperthyroidism; beri beri
- Systolic dysfunction (low cardiac output): coronary artery disease; hypertension; arrhythmia-mediated (tachy- or bradyarrhythmia); peri-partum; toxins: eg, alcohol; viral myocarditis; hypothyroidism; idiopathic
- Diastolic dysfunction (normal to high cardiac output): ischaemia; hypertension

Causes of unilateral pulmonary oedema
Ipsilateral

- Rapid removal of large volume of pleural fluid (>1500 ml) by thoracentesis or tube thoracostomy
- Rapid evacuation of a pneumothorax (large pneumothorax; affected lung collapsed more than 3 days)
- Prolonged dependency related to adoption of the lateral decubitus position (eg methadone induced pulmonary oedema)
- Pulmonary contusion
- Postoperative systemic-pulmonary arterial shunts for congenital heart disease
- Bronchial obstruction (drowned lung)
- Relief of endobronchial obstruction following endobronchial stent placement or bronchoscopic removal of mucus plug
- Unilateral veno-occlusive disease
- Unilateral aspiration
- CVP catheter misdirected into a pulmonary artery

Contralateral

- Perfusion defects

Unilateral pulmonary emphysema
Congenital absence/hypoplasia of a pulmonary artery
Swyer-James syndrome
Pulmonary thrombo-embolism involving an entire lung
Lobectomy
- Re-expansion of pneumothorax in a patient with left heart failure

Radiological stages of congestive heart failure

- Redistribution (PCWP 13–18 mm Hg) (pulmonary venous hypertension): redistribution of pulmonary blood flow from lower zones to upper zones (upper lobe diversion); upper zone veins equal in size to, or larger in diameter than, lower zone veins (cephalization)
- Interstitial oedema (PCWP 18–25 mm Hg): peribronchial cuffing; haziness of vessels (perihilar haze); Kerley B lines (septal lines); thickening of interlobar fissures
- Alveolar oedema (PCWP > 25 mm Hg): perihilar batwing pattern of consolidation and air bronchogram; bilateral pleural effusions

Radiological features of cardiogenic pulmonary oedema

- Cardiomegaly
- Upper lobe diversion of blood flow (pulmonary venous hypertension)
- Septal lines
- Pleural effusions
- Peribronchial cuffing

Checklist for factors causing decompensation in chronic congestive heart failure

- Cardiac arrhythmia
- Conduction disorder

- Acute coronary syndrome
- Pulmonary embolism
- Progression of valvular heart disease, including endocarditis
- Systemic infection
- Anaemia
- Renal dysfunction
- Thyroid disorder: hypothyroidism; hyperthyroidism
- Drug therapy: NSAIDs, glucocorticoids, glitazones, excessive beta blockade
- Non-compliance with treatment; inappropriate reduction of maintenance therapy
- Alcohol abuse

Causes of elevated BNP (brain-type natriuretic peptide, which is released in response to volume expansion)

- Congestive heart failure (in the presence of new suspected acute heart failure, a serum BNP level less than 100 ng/L or a serum N-terminal pro-B-type natriuretic peptide (NT-proBNP) level less than 300 ng/L rules out the diagnosis of heart failure
- Left ventricular/right ventricular dysfunction
- Coronary artery disease
- Pulmonary embolism
- COPD with cor pulmonale
- Primary pulmonary hypertension
- Adult respiratory distress syndrome
- Septic shock
- Acute kidney injury
- Cirrhosis of the liver
- Ischaemic/haemorhagic stroke; subarachnoid haemorrhage
- Hyperthyroidism

Causes of acute pulmonary hypertension (presents with refractory systemic arterial hypotension, severe hypoxaemia, and right ventricular dysfunction and failure)

- Mediator induced or hypoxic vasoconstriction: ALI/ARDS; Gram negative sepsis; obstructive sleep apnoea
- Loss of vascular architecture: chronic lung disease (COPD; interstitial pulmonary fibrosis)
- Obstruction of vessels
- Pulmonary arteries: massive pulmonary thromboembolism; vasculitis; mediastinal tumour/fibrosis
- Pulmonary veins: pulmonary veno-occlusive disease

Causes of acute right ventricular failure
Right ventricular pressure overload

- Massive pulmonary embolism
- Pulmonary arterial hypertension
- Positive pressure ventilation

Right ventricular volume overload

- Valvular disease: tricuspid regurgitation; pulmonary regurgitation

Reduced contractility of right ventricle

- Coronary artery disease: right ventricular myocardial ischaemia/infarction
- Arrhythmia
- Sepsis

ECG features of right ventricular strain

- Right axis deviation
- S1Q3T3 pattern
- Right ventricular hypertrophy: dominant R wave in V1 and V2 with prominent S waves in V5 and V6

Causes of chronic cor pulmonale (combination of lung disease and right ventricular failure)
Diseases leading to hypoxic vasoconstriction

- COPD
- Chronic pulmonary hypertension: obesity; neuromuscular disease; chest wall dysfunction
- High altitude living

Diseases causing pulmonary vascular bed occlusion

- Recurrent pulmonary thrombo-embolism (chronic thrombo-embolic pulmonary hypertension)

- Primary pulmonary hypertension
- Veno-occlusive disease
- Collagen vascular disease
- Drug-induced vascular disease

Pulmonary parenchymal disease

- COPD
- Bronchiectasis
- Cystic fibrosis
- Pneumoconiosis
- Sarcoidosis
- Idiopathic pulmonary fibrosis

Causes of cardiac tamponade (compression of the heart due to pericardial accumulation of fluid, pus, blood, clots, or gas. This may be associated in the presence of acute cardiac tamponade with Beck's triad of hypotension, raised jugular venous pressure and diminished heart sounds).

Acute tamponade

- Cardiac trauma
- Iatrogenic: cardiac surgery; cardiac catheterisation; cardiac pacing
- Aortic dissection
- Spontaneous bleeding: anticoagulation; uraemia; thrombocytopenia
- Cardiac rupture post-myocardial infarction

Sub-acute tamponade

- Malignancy
- Idiopathic pericarditis
- Infections: bacterial, tuberculosis
- Radiation
- Hypothyroidism
- Post pericardiotomy
- Systemic lupus erythematosus

Causes of hypotension with raised jugular venous pressure

- Cardiac tamponade (triad of hypotension, jugular venous distension and muffled heart sounds; associated with pulsus paradoxus-an inspiratory fall in systolic blood pressure >10 mm Hg and in pulse wave amplitude)
- Constrictive pericarditis (dyspnoea; peripheral oedema; ascites; hepatomegaly)
- Restrictive pericarditis
- Severe biventricular failure
- Right ventricular infarction
- Pulmonary embolism
- Tension pneumothorax
- Acute severe asthma
- Malignant superior vena caval obstruction

Causes of pericardial effusion (200–250 ml fluid causes a globular appearance of the cardiac silhouette on chest xray)

Serous

- Acute pericarditis
- Hypoalbuminemia
- Myxoedema
- Post-myocardial infarction syndrome (Dressler's syndrome)

Serofibrinous

- Rheumatic fever
- Viral: Coxsackie, Echo
- Tuberculosis
- Chronic kidney disease

Suppurative

- Post-pneumonia
  Pneumococcus
  Staphylococcus

Haemorrhagic

- Aortic root dissection
- Cardiac rupture: post-myocardial infarction
- Trauma
- Metastases

Features of pericardial effusion on bedside ultrasound

- Anechoic pericardial space, separating the bright white highly echogenic parietal pericardium from the heterogeneous grey myocardium.

- A volume greater than 100 ml leads to circumferential fluid filling the entire pericardial space, thereby circumscribing the entire heart
- The collection is larger posterior to the left heart than anterior to the right heart in supine patients
- A haemodynamically significant pericardial effusion causes right ventricular diastolic collapse –persistent inward of the right ventricular free wall during diastole; right atrial systolic collapse; a dilated non-collapsible inferior vena cava without partial collapse with inspiration; and inter-ventricular septal flattening

Superior vena caval obstruction
Clinical features

- Facial oedema and plethora
- Conjunctival congestion
- Venous distension in neck, upper chest and arms
- Upper limb oedema
- Upper airway obstruction: dyspnoea, stridor
- Cerebral oedema: headache, confusion, depressed level of consciousness
- Chest xray typically reveals a right upper thoracic or paratracheal mass

Causes

Malignant mediastinal tumours: bronchogenic carcinoma; non-Hodgkin lymphoma; Hodgkin lymphoma, metastatic tumours; acute lymphoblastic leukaemia
Mediastinal fibrosis
Vascular diseases: aortic aneurysm; vasculitis; arterio-venous fistulas
Infections: tuberculosis, histoplasmosis, syphilis, actonomycosis
Benign mediastinal tumours: thymoma, teratoma
Cardiac causes: pericarditis; atrial myxoma
Thrombosis caused by central vein catheters

Causes of upper limb oedema
Unilateral

Acute deep vein thrombosis of the upper limb: axillary vein thrombosis
Primary

- Spontaneous
- Effort-induced (Paget-Schroetter disease)-associated with strenuous and repetitive activity of the upper limbs, associated with anatomical abnormalities at the thoracic outlet (eg cervical rib, scalenus tendon hypertrophy), eg weightlifting, rowing, wrestling, baseball pitching

Secondary

- Iatrogenic: central venous catheters (PICC; tunneled catheters); implanted vascular access devices-catheters, ports; pacemakers
- Malignancy

Miscellaneous

- Lymphatic obstruction
- Superior vena cava syndrome
- Complex regional pain syndrome

The features of **effort-induced axillary vein thrombosis** include:

- Acute onset of pain and swelling in the shoulder and arm
- A cyanotic appearance of the upper limb with prominent superficial veins
- Tenderness in the deltopectoral groove
- A palpable tender axillary cord
- Normal arterial pulses
- The dominant upper limb is affected

Percutaneously inserted central venous catheter (PICC) line complications presenting in emergency practice

- Infection: fever with chills; malaise; myalgia; swelling, redness, induration, purulent discharge at insertion site; arm swelling
- Phlebitis (mechanical or chemical): redness, pain at insertion site; palpable venous cord

- Blocked line: blood clot; fibrin sheath; malposition; drug precipitation

Potential presentations with groin complications following angiography (bedside ultrasound may be helpful)

- Arterial haematoma
- Pseudoaneurysm: palpable pulsatile mass with bruit
- Arteriovenous fistula
- Femoral artery thrombosis
- Femoral vein thrombosis
- Nerve compression: femoral nerve; lateral femoral cutaneous nerve
- Acute leg ischaemia
- Retroperitoneal bleeding: hypotension; loin pain; falling haemoglobin

Risk factors for complications

- Multiple arterial punctures
- Low puncture site (>2 cm below inguinal ligament)
- Large sheath size
- Hypertension
- Obesity
- Arterial calcification
- Anticoagulation

Causes of unilateral lower limb swelling

- Venous: chronic venous insufficiency; deep vein thrombosis (May-Thurner syndrome: chronic compression of left common iliac vein by the overlying right common iliac artery)
- Lymphatic: lymphatic obstruction
- Infection: cellulitis
- Iliac vein obstruction: abdominal/pelvic tumour; retroperitoneal fibrosis

Causes of bilateral lower limb swelling

Cardiac
  Congestive heart failure
  Constrictive pericarditis
Renal
  Nephrotic syndrome
Hepatic
  Liver failure
  Budd-Chiari syndrome (triad of abdominal pain, ascites and hepatomegaly associated with hepatic vein thrombosis)
Venous
  Chronic venous insufficiency
Hypoalbuminaemia
  Increased protein loss: proteinuria; protein-losing enteropathy; gastrointestinal fistulas
  Reduced liver synthesis: acute or chronic liver disease

Causes of leg ulceration

Venous disease: chronic venous insufficiency (oedema, hyperpigmentation from haemosiderin deposition, eczematous dermatitis, induration with lipodermatosclerosis, recurrent cellulitis and superficial thrombophlebitis, venous claudication); 95% of ulcers are in the gaiter area, around the malleoli
Arterial disease: chronic arterial insufficiency (symptomatic with intermittent claudication; critical leg ischaemia); punched-out ulcers with well demarcated edges and a pale, non-granulating, and sometimes necrotic base, located over the heel or above lateral malleolus; painful at night or in bed with the legs elevated
Infection
Vasculitis: rheumatoid arthritis; polyarteritis nodosa
Skin malignancy: basal cell carcinoma; squamous cell carcinoma; malignant melanoma
Neuropathic: diabetes mellitus

Risk factors for venous ulceration

Chronic venous insufficiency
Varicose veins
Prior deep vein thrombosis, with post-phlebitic syndrome
Thrombophlebitis
Arterio-venous fistulae
Prior leg fracture

Syncope

The characteristic features of syncope include:

- Transient loss of consciousness, with loss of postural tone which can lead to falling
- Rapid onset and short duration
- Spontaneous and complete recovery
- Myoclonic jerks of the limbs can be noted
- Urine incontinence can occur with a full bladder
- Post-ictal confusion and drowsiness are not seen

Pre-syncope is characterized by lightheadedness, dizziness, visual blurring, tinnitus, generalized muscle weakness and gastrointestinal symptoms.

Causes of syncope

Cardiovascular

Neurally mediated or neuro-cardiogenic syncope (exaggerated or overly compensating inherent autonomic reflexes): (the 4 relevant Ps are posture, prodromal symptoms, provoking factors and prompt recovery, associated with post-episode fatigue)

- Vasovagal syncope (triggered by emotional stress, pain, sight of blood, prolonged standing)
- Carotid sinus hypersensitivity (unexplained recurrent syncope, drop attacks and falls; may be precipitated by head turning, circumferential neck compression by tight collar or necktie, or neck tumour or scarring (post-radiation or neck dissection); cardio—inhibitory, vasodepressor or mixed responses within 5–10 s of supine and standing carotid sinus massage)
- Postural hypotension: volume depletion; primary autonomic failure; secondary autonomic failure; drug induced
- Situational syncope: gastrointestinal stimulation (deglutition or swallow, defaecation, post-prandial); post-micturition syncope; post-exercise syncope (following intense exercise); cough syncope
- Hyperventilation and Valsalva manoeuvre
- Others: brass instrument playing, weight-lifting, hair-grooming

Cardiogenic

- **Structural heart disease (obstructive)**
- Valvular heart disease: aortic stenosis; pulmonic stenosis; mitral valve prolapse; prosthetic valve dysfunction
- Cardiomyopathies: hypertrophic cardiomyopathy; dilated cardiomyopathy; arrhythmogenic right ventricular dysplasia
- Ischaemic heart disease: myocardial ischaemia/infarction
- Atrial myxoma
- Massive pulmonary embolism
- Prmary pulmonary hypertension
- Aortopathies: aortic dissection
- Tetralogy of Fallot
- Coronary artery anomalies
- Post-corrective repair of tetralogy of Fallot/ transposition of the great arteries/aortic stenosis
- **Dysrhythmic**:
- Bradyarrhythmias
- Profound sinus bradycardia
- Sick sinus syndrome
- Atrio-ventricular block
- Pacemaker malfunction; pacemaker syndrome
- Tachyarrhythmias: supraventricular tachycardia; ventricular tachycardia
- Channelopathies
  - Long QT syndromes; torsades de pointes
  - Brugada syndrome
  - Familial catecholaminergic polymorphic ventricular tachycardia
  - Congenital short QT syndrome
- Pre-excitation syndromes

Non-cardiovascular

- Neurological: raised ICP (posterior fossa lesion; colloid cyst of 3rd ventricle with intermittent hydrocephalus); subarchnoid hemorrhage; sleep disorders (narcolepsy; cataplexy); basilar artery migraine

- Psychiatric
- Metabolic: hypoglycaemia; hypoxia; hyperventilation
- Unexplained

Warning symptoms in syncope

- Sudden syncope without preceding symptoms
- Syncope in response to loud noise, fright, or extreme emotional stress
- Syncope during exercise
- Syncope while supine
- Syncope with chest pain
- Family history of sudden death in young persons less than 30 years in age
- Syncope with an atypical history

Factors associated with increased risk in syncope

- Age greater than 60 years, and associated co-morbidities
- History of ischaemic heart disease
- Exertional dyspnoea
- Family history of sudden cardiac death
- Systolic blood pressure less than 90 mm Hg
- Anaemia
- Heart failure
- Systolic heart murmur
- Abnormal ECG

Features suggestive of cardiogenic syncope

- Occurrence during exertion
- Associated palpitations
- No prodrome
- Required cardiopulmonary resuscitation
- Resulted in bodily or neurological injury
- Family history of long QT syndrome, drowning, sudden death, or unexplained seizures

ECG abnormalities suggesting an arrhythmic syncope

- Bi-fascicular block: either LBBB, or RBBB combined with left anterior or left posterior fascicular block
- Trifascicular block: alternating complete left and right bundle branch block; new RBBB with prolonged PR interval and left anterior or posterior fascicular block; LBBB and prolonged PR interval;
- Other intra-ventricular conduction abnormalities: QRS duration $\geq$0.12 s
- Mobitz type 2 2nd degree AV block
- Asymptomatic sinus bradycardia (<50 bpm), sino-atrial block, or sinus pause $\geq$3 s in the absence of negatively chronotropic medications (eg beta blockers) or physical training
- Wolff-Parkinson-White syndrome: pre-excited QRS complexes
- Long/short QT interval (corrected QT >450 ms or <350 ms)
- RBBB pattern with ST elevation in leads V1-V3 (Brugada syndrome)
- Incomplete RBBB pattern suggestive of arrhythmogenic right ventricle dysplasia; negative T waves (inversion) in right praecordial leads (V1-V3), epsilon waves, and ventricular late potentials suggestive of arrhythmogenic right ventricular dysplasia
- Q waves suggesting myocardial infarction
- Hypertrophic cardiomyopathy
- Non-sustained VT

Carotid sinus hypersensitivity
Features include:

- Age usually greater than 50 years
- Recurrent pre-syncope or syncope related to turning the head, looking up, or wearing tight collars
- Prodromal symptoms are commoner with vasodepressor syncope
- Recurrent unexplained falls
- There may be retrograde amnesia for the syncopal episode

Diagnosis is achieved by firm steady massage to the right and left carotid sinus separately for 5 s while monitoring ECG and blood pressure. The diagnostic haemodynamic response may be cardio-inhibitory, vasodepressor, or mixed

Cardio-inhibitory response: 3 s or more ventricular asystolic pause

Vasodepressor response: 50 mm Hg or greater fall in systolic blood pressure without significant bradycardia

Disorders commonly misdiagnosed as syncope, including other causes of transient loss of consciousness

- Carotid or vertebro-basilar transient ischaemic attacks
- Hypoglycaemia and other metabolic disorders
- Seizure: generalized clonic-tonic seizures; absence seizures; complex partial seizures
- Alcohol and other intoxication
- Transient increase in intracranial pressure: intermittent hydrocephalus associated with periodic CSF compression (colloid cyst of third ventricle; aqueduct stenosis)
- Hyperventilation with hypocapnia
- Non-epileptic attack disorder
- Concussion following head injury

Causes of exercise associated collapse

- Hypothermia (temperature <35 °C)
- Hyperthermia (temperature >40 °C) and exercise induced heat stroke
- Exertional hyponatraemia (excessive ingestion of hypotonic fluids during after period of exertion, often with slow running speed and longer race time, commoner with female sex and low body mass index; due to dilutional hyponatraemia and excessive vasopressin secretion)
- Cardiogenic syncope

Postural hypotension a fall in systolic blood pressure of at least 20 mm Hg and in diastolic blood pressure of at least 10 mm Hg within 3 min of standing up from the sitting or supine position. Associated symptoms include:

- Dizziness
- Blurred vision
- Distortion or loss of hearing
- Headache
- Fatigue
- Weakness
- Dyspnoea
- Sweating
- Coathanger pain: sub-occipital and paracervical pain in a coathanger distribution
- Syncope or pre-syncope

Causes of postural hypotension

- Intravascular volume depletion: concealed or overt blood loss; dehydration
- Drugs: alpha 1 adrenergic blocking agents, tricyclic antidepressants, monoamine oxidase inhibitors, beta blockers, vasodilators (nitrates)
- Endocrine: adrenocortical insufficiency; diabetes insipidus
- Venous pooling: post-prandial hypotension
- Autonomic disorders:
- Primary: acute/subacute dysautonomias (pure pandysautonomia); chronic autonomic failure syndromes (pure autonomic failure; multiple system atrophy; Parkinson's disease with autonomic failure)
- Secondary: metabolic (diabetes mellitus; chronic renal failure); inflammatory (Gullain-Barre syndrome; transverse myelitis); infections (bacterial-tetanus; viral-HIV infection); neoplasm (brain tumours, especially of posterior fossa); trauma (spinal cord transaction); hereditary (familial dysautonomia)
- Deconditioning and prolonged bed rest
- Post-prandial

Features of postural orthostatic tachycardia syndrome

- An increase in heart rate by at least 30 beats per minute or to greater than 120 beats per minute within the first 10 min of assuming an upright posture, with no associated drop in blood pressure.
- Symptoms of postural intolerance can be cardiac (palpitations, chest discomfort, dyspnoea, presyncope or syncope, effort intolerance) or non-cardiac (nausea, lightheadedness, blurred vision, tremulousness, weakness)

- There may be evidence of dependent acrocyanosis (red-blue discolouration of the legs) with prolonged standing

Causes of hypotension

- Vasodilatory (distributive): anaphylaxis, sepsis, neurogenic shock, adrenocortical insufficiency
- Obstructive (mechanical obstruction impeding venous return): right heart inflow obstruction: cardiac tamponade, tension pneumothorax, constrictive pericarditis, large diaphragmatic hernia with tension gastrothorax; right heart outflow obstruction: massive pulmonary embolism (saddle embolism)
- Hypovolaemic: haemorhage (chest, abdomen, retroperitoneum, gastrointestinal tract, thigh, external); gastrointestinal losses (diarrhoea and vomiting, fistula); diuresis; third space losses (pancreatitis, burns)
- Metabolic: adrenocortical insufficiency; hypo/hyperthyroidism
- Cardiogenic (reduced myocardial contractility): tachyarrhythmia, acute myocardial ischaemia/infarction, valvular heart disease (papillary muscle rupture), cardiomyopathy, myocarditis
- Toxic: beta blockers, calcium channel blockers, opiates, sedatives, tricyclic antidepressants

Causes of hypotension with bradycardia

- Cardiac: inferior ST elevation myocardial infarction with cardiogenic shock
- Metabolic: hyperkalaemia
- Neurological: acute cervical or high thoracic spinal cord injury
- Overdose: beta blocker, calcium channel blocker, digoxin

Checklist for unexplained hypotension

- Sepsis, including toxic shock syndrome
- Painless myocardial infarction
- Occult blood loss (chest; abdomen)
- Anaphylaxis
- Poisoning
- Pulmonary embolism
- Adrenocortical insufficiency
- Cardiac tamponade
- Autonomic dysfunction

Signs of shock

Early

- Tachycardia
- Tachypnoea
- Difference between central and peripheral pulses
- Weak or bounding peripheral pulses
- Reduced skin perfusion: capillary refill time <2 s; pale and cool skin
- Narrowed pulse pressure
- Oliguria
- Lactic acidosis
- Elevated base deficit

Late

- Depressed level of consciousness
- Weak or absent central pulses
- Hypotension

Classes of hypovolaemic shock

Abdominal and cardiac evaluation with sonography in shock (ACES) protocol

- Focused view of the heart
- Inferior vena caval view: diameter and collapse index
- Focused assessment of abdominal aorta by sliding transverse view from diaphragm to bifurcation
- Right and left flank views for peritoneal and pleural fluid
- Pelvic view for bladder size and free fluid

Hypertensive emergencies

A hypertensive crisis is a severe elevation of diastolic blood pressure >120–130 mm Hg, which can be emergent or urgent. A hypertensive emer-

Class	I	II	III	IV
Blood loss	<750 ml	750–1500 ml	1500–2000 ml	>2000 ml
Blood loss as	<15%	15–30%	30–40%	>40%
%age total blood volume				
Pulse rate	<100	>100	>120	>140
Blood pressure	Normal	Normal	Decreased	Decreased
Pulse pressure	Normal or increased	Decreased	Decreased	Decreased
Respiratory rate	14–20	20–30	30–40	>35

gency (see below) warrants immediate blood pressure reduction, to avoid serious end-organ damage, generally by intravenous therapy in an intensive care unit setting

Hypertensive urgency

BP > 180/120 mm Hg without impending or progressive end-organ damage (eg headache, shortness of breath, epistaxis)

Remember to "treat the patient, not the numbers". A hypertensive urgency requires gradual blood pressure reduction over 12–24 h

Hypertensive emergencies

Moderate to severe elevation of arterial pressure which can be associated with impending or progressive end-organ damage

End-organ damage may be:

- Neurological

Hypertensive encephalopathy (seizure, visual disturbance, altered level of consciousness, transient focal neurological deficits; triad of hypertension, altered mental state, and papilloedema)

Acute athero-thrombotic cerebral infarction (ischaemic stroke)

Subarachnoid haemorrhage

Acute intracerebral haemorrhage

- Cardiovascular

Acute coronary syndrome; acute myocardial infarction

Acute pulmonary oedema, including flash pulmonary oedema, secondary to left ventricular failure

Aortic dissection

- Renal

Acute kidney injury

Haematuria

- Retinopathy (Grade 3 or 4)

New flame-shaped haemorrhages, exudates, papilloedema (malignant hypertension)

- Eclampsia
- Microangiopathic haemolytic anaemia
- Severe epistaxis

Causes of hypertensive emergencies

Primary hypertension

Renal: renovascular hypertension (renal artery stenosis), glomerulonephritis

Pregnancy related: pre-eclampsia, eclampsia

Endocrine: Cushing's syndrome; primary hyperaldosteronism; renin-secreting adenomas

Excess circulating catecholamines (adrenergic crisis):

Phaeochromocytoma crisis

Food/drug interactions with monoamine oxidase inhibitors

Sympathomimetic drug use: cocaine; amphetamine

Autonomic hyper-reflexia after spinal cord injury

Rebound hypertension after sudden cessation of antihypertensive therapy (alpha-agonist/beta blocker withdrawal)

Drug induced: amphetamines, cocaine, phencyclidine, oral contraceptive pill

Checklist for evaluation of hypertensive emergencies

- Supine and standing blood pressure (volume depletion)
- Blood pressure in both arms

- Peripheral pulses in all limbs
- Focused neurological examination
- Funduscopy
- Renal bruits

Markers of target organ damage in hypertension

Cardiac

- Clinical, ECG or radiological evidence of coronary artery disease
- Left ventricular hypertrophy or strain on ECG
- Left ventricular hypertrophy on echocardiography
- Left ventricular dysfunction or cardiac failure

Cerebrovascular

- Transient ischaemic attack
- Stroke

Peripheral Vascular

- Absence of one or more major pulses with or without intermittent claudication
- Aortic aneurysm

Renal

- Creatinine > 130 μmol/L.
- Proteinuria
- Microalbuminuria

Retinopathy

- Haemorrhages or exudates
- Papilloedema

Causes of secondary hypertension

- Renal parenchymal disease (raised serum creatinine, abnormal urine sediment; history of urinary tract infections, haematuria, obstructive uropathy, analgesic abuse); glomerulonephritis; chronic pyelonephritis; polycystic kidney disease
- Renal vascular disease: renal artery stenosis; fibromuscular dysplasia
- Endocrine: phaeochromocytoma; Cushing's syndrome; primary aldosteronism (weakness, spontaneous or provoked muscle cramps, hypokalaemia); renin-secreting tumours
- Coarctation of the aorta (hypertension in upper limbs and reduced blood pressure in lower limbs; radio-femoral delay; interscapular systolic murmur)
- Sleep apnoea (obesity, prominent snoring, daytime somnolence)
- Drugs: oral contraception, glucocorticoids and mineralocorticoids, NSAIDs, sympathomimetic agents, interaction of tyramine-containing foods with monoamine oxidase inhibitors
- Pregnancy-induced hypertension: pre-eclampsia and eclampsia

Transient hypertension may be associated with:

- Sympathomimetic toxidromes, including recreational drug use (cocaine, amphetamines)
- Abrupt withdrawal of anti-hypertensive medication
- Alcohol withdrawal

Features suggesting secondary hypertension

- Age of onset <30 years or >60 years
- Hypertensive crisis
- Hypokalaemia
- Renal impairment
- Family history of early onset hypertension
- Treatment-resistant hypertension (three or more anti-hypertensive medications)

Features of phaeochromocytoma

- Triad of episodic headache, sweating and tachycardia
- Sustained or paroxysmal hypertension
- Postural hypotension in the absence of anti-hypertensive medication
- Marked variability of blood pressure

- Weight loss
- Hyperglycaemia
- Abdominal pain (haemorrhage into tumour)
- Positive family history
- Crises: hypertensive crisis; cardiogenic shock

Clues to renovascular hypertension

New onset or drug resistant hypertension under the age of 30 years or over the age of 50 years
Accelerated or malignant hypertension
Progressively worsening renal function in response to therapy with ACE inhibitors or angiotensin II-receptor blockers
Recurrent flash pulmonary oedema with normal left ventricular function
Flank bruit

Causes of hypertension associated with hypokalaemia

- Primary hypertension, when associated with diarrhea and vomiting, diuretic therapy, oral contraceptive or steroid therapy
- Renal disease: renovascular hypertension; potassium-losing nephropathy; renin-secreting renal tumour
- Adrenocortical dysfunction: primary aldosteronism; Cushing's syndrome; exogenous mineralocorticoid administration

Causes of cardiac murmurs

- Continuous: patent ductus arteriosus, coronary arterio-venous fistula, aorto-pulmonary connection, venous hum, ruptured sinus of Valsalva (right ventricle/right atrium)
- Ejection or mid-systolic: aortic stenosis (valvular, supravalvular or subvalvular), pulmonary stenosis, hypertrophic cardiomyopathy, pulmonary flow murmur in atrial septal defect; aortic flow murmur with aortic regurgitation
- Pansystolic: mitral regurgitation, tricuspid regurgitation, ventricular septal defect, aorto-pulmonary shunts
- Late systolic murmur: mitral valve prolapse
- Early diastolic murmur: aortic regurgitation, pulmonary regurgitation (pulmonary hypertension)
- Mid-diastolic murmur: mitral stenosis, tricuspid stenosis, atrial myxoma, Austin Flint murmur (aortic regurgitation), Carey Coombs murmur (acute rheumatic fever)

Characteristics of innocent heart murmurs

- Soft
- Systolic
- Short
- Sounds (S1, S2) normal; no clicks
- Special tests normal (CXR; 12 lead ECG)

2 Respiratory Emergencies

Cough

Causes of cough (a forced expulsive manoeuvre, usually against a closed glottis, and associated with a characteristic sound)

Acute cough (<3 weeks)

- Respiratory tract infections: viral upper respiratory tract infection, viral rhinosinusitis, common cold, acute bacterial sinusitis, acute bronchitis, pneumonia, acute exacerbation of COPD, pertussis
- Inhalation of direct irritants: dust, smoke, ozone, air pollutants
- Inhalation of specific allergen in the asthmatic: pollen, or low concentration of nonspecific irritants: cigarette smoke, perfume; house dust mites
- Allergic rhinitis
- Chemical exposure: chloramines in swimming pools
- Medication: ACE inhibitors

Subacute cough (3–8 weeks)

- Post-infectious cough: prior viral upper respiratory tract infection
- Bordetella pertussis infection
- Subacute bacterial sinusitis
- Asthma
- Neoplasm

Chronic cough (>8 weeks)

- Persistent airway inflammation: COPD, asthma, bronchiectasis
- Smoking
- Neoplasm
- Interstitial lung disease: pulmonary fibrosis
- Persistent infection: tuberculosis; bronchiectasis
- Raised left atrial pressure: mitral stenosis, left ventricular failure
- Inhaled foreign body
- Iatrogenic: ACE inhibitors, radiation pneumonitis, steroid aerosols
- Aspiration syndrome: gastro-oesophageal reflux disease; bulbar dysfunction; oesophageal dysmotility
- Psychogenic
- Post-nasal drip syndrome (posterior nasal discharge and night cough): sinusitis; rhinitis (allergic; non-allergic; vasomotor)
- Primary ciliary dyskinesia

Potential origins of cough

Pharynx

- Post nasal drip

Larynx

- Laryngitis
- Pertussis
- Croup
- Tumour

Trachea

- Tracheitis

A. Banerjee, *Emergency Clinical Diagnosis*, DOI 10.1007/978-3-319-50718-7_2

Bronchi

- Bronchitis: acute and chronic
- Asthma
- Bronchial carcinoma
- Pneumonia
- Bronchiectasis
- Pulmonary oedema
- End-stage interstitial fibrosis

Checklist for cough

- Sudden (foreign body aspiration) or gradual onset
- Duration
- Diurnal variation
- Relation to initial upper respiratory tract infection
- Paroxysms of cough, with or without syncope
- Cough on eating or post-prandial: gastro-oesophageal reflux
- Triggers/aggravating factors: air temperature change; exercise; aerosols
- Production of sputum; haemoptysis
- Smoking
- Occupational history
- Medication history: ACE inhibitors
- Chronic lung disease: COPD, bronchiectasis
- Atopic disease

Possible presenting features of lung cancer

- Cough persisting more than 3 weeks
- Changes in character of smoker's cough
- Unexplained haemoptysis
- Chest, shoulder or arm pain
- Dyspnoea
- Local fixed inspiratory wheeze
- Persistent or recurrent pneumonia or bronchitis
- Lobar collapse
- Pleural effusion
- Voice change (left vocal cord paralysis from recurrent laryngeal nerve involvement)
- Thoracic inlet(Pancoast) syndrome with shoulder and arm pain; Horner's syndrome; brachial plexus lesions
- Phrenic nerve involvement
- Superior vena cava obstruction
- Weight loss; bone pain

Risk factors for lung cancer

- Tobacco smoking (cigarette, cigar, pipe)
- Exposure to asbestos, radon, chemicals (vinyl chloride, nickel chromates, coal products, diesel exhaust), radioactive ores
- Family history of lung cancer
- Passive smoking
- Radiation therapy to the chest (e.g. Hodgkin's lymphoma, breast cancer post-mastectomy)
- Previous lung disease: COPD
- Outdoor air pollution

Chest x-ray patterns of lung cancer

Adenocarcinoma: peripheral solitary nodule
Squamous cell carcinoma: central lesion
Small cell carcinoma: hilar or perihilar mass
Broncholaveolar cell carcinoma: multicentric pneumonic pattern

Possible complications of cough

- Respiratory: subcutaneous emphysema; pneumothorax
- Cardiovascular: syncope; cardiac arrhythmias; subconjunctival haemorrhage
- CNS: headache; cerebral air embolism
- Musculoskeletal: intercostal muscle pain; rib fractures; rectus muscle rupture
- Urine incontinence

Dyspnoea

Dyspnoea is the conscious and unpleasant awareness of increased work done during breathing, and may indicate cardiac, pulmonary, cardiopulmonary or neuromuscular disease. Dypsnoea is not synonymous with respiratory distress. There are a number of underlying mechanisms, which may coexist in the same patient.

Mechanisms of shortness of breath

Increased demand

- Physiological: exercise; high altitude
- Pathological: anaemia; increased metabolism (fever, thyrotoxicosis)

Impaired performance

- Airflow obstruction: upper airway obstruction; obstructive lung disease: asthma, COPD, bronchiectasis; lower airway obstruction: foreign body
- Reduced lung volume (restrictive lung disease): pleural disease/effusion; pneumothorax; kyphoscoliosis; massive obesity; spine or chest wall deformities; interstitial lung disease
- Impaired gas exchange: alveolar lung disease: consolidation (pneumonia); pulmonary oedema
- Loss of lung compliance: interstitial lung disease
- Neuro-muscular diseases: Guillain-Barre syndrome; myasthenia gravis; diaphragmatic paralysis; poliomyelitis; spinal cord injury (cervical cord transection); muscular dystrophies
- Loss of thoracic cage (chest wall) compliance

Hyperventilation resulting from medullary respiratory centre stimulation in response to chemical or neural stimuli

Increased arterial hydrogen ion concentration, e.g. metabolic acidosis producing air hunger (Kussmaul's breathing)
Increased arterial $paCO_2$, e.g. respiratory acidosis
Decreased arterial PaO_2 via aortic, carotid and brain stem chemoreceptors, e.g. pneumonia, impaired oxygen delivery due to anaemia, shock and stroke
Increased central arousal, e.g. exertion, anxiety, thyrotoxicosis, phaeochromocytoma
Pulmonary J receptor discharge, e.g. pulmonary oedema

Auscultation findings in the presence of acute dyspnoea

- Fine end-inspiratory crackles over both lung bases: pulmonary oedema
- Medium end-inspiratory crackles: pulmonary fibrosis
- Localised crackles: pneumonia
- Expiratory wheeze: airways obstruction
- Absent breath sounds: pneumothorax

Symptoms associated with acute dyspnoea

- Chest pain: pleuritic (pulmonary embolism, pneumothorax, pneumonia); cardiac (acute coronary syndrome; mechanical complications: interventricular septal rupture, mitral regurgitation from chordae rupture; cardiac arrhythmia)
- Cough: pneumonia; asthma; COPD
- Orthopnea: congestive heart failure; bilateral diaphragmatic paralysis
- Paroxysmal nocturnal dyspnoea: congestive heart failure
- Severe sore throat: epiglottitis
- Platypnoea (dyspnoea worse on upright posture and relieved on recumbency): hepato-pulmonary syndrome with right-to-left shunt, patent foramen ovale

Clinical evaluation of dyspnoea

- Airway: airway patency
- Breathing
  Respiratory rate
  Oxygen saturation (pulse oximetry)
  Work of breathing
  1. Abnormal airway sounds: altered speech, stridor, expiratory wheeze, grunting
  2. Abnormal positioning: head bobbing; tripod posture (standing or sitting leaning forwards, supporting the upper body with the hands on the knees or another surface)
  3. Use of accessory muscles of respiration

  Retractions: supraclavicular, intercostal and substernal chest wall recession
  Flaring: nasal flaring
  Tracheal tug (abnormal downward movement of trachea during systole)
- Circulation
  Heart rate and rhythm
  Arterial blood pressure

Jugular venous pressure (elevated in congestive heart failure, pericardial tamponade, cor pulmonale)
Pulsus paradoxus (inspiratory fall in systolic blood pressure >10 mm Hg) (cardiac tamponade; severe asthma)

- Exposure
  Barrel chest: COPD
  Kyphoscoliosis: restrictive lung disease
  Central obesity: obstructive sleep apnoea; deconditioning
  Digital clubbing: bronchiectasis; interstitial lung disease; neoplasm; cystic fibrosis
  Oedema/ascites: congestive heart failure

Objective measures of the severity of dyspnoea

- Ability to talk with ease
- Respiratory rate, especially if >30 breaths per minute
- Inability to adopt the supine position (orthopnoea)
- Increased effort of breathing
- Degree of hypoxaemia (oxygen saturation <92%)
- Central cyanosis, which equates to a concentration of deoxygenated haemoglobin greater than 50 g/L
- Peak expiratory flow rate <50% of predicted

Further investigations to be considered in evaluation of acute dyspnoea

- Peak expiratory flow
- Spirometry
- Chest x-ray (including comparison with previous films)
- 12 lead ECG
- Arterial blood gases
- Full blood count
- Inflammatory markers: C-reactive protein
- Renal and liver function tests
- Venous blood lactate
- Cardiac biomarkers
- B-type Natriuretic Peptide
- Bedside transthoracic echocardiography and pulmonary ultrasound

Chest x-ray patterns in the breathless patient
Focal density: consolidation; collapse; effusion; mass

Diffuse infiltrates

- Cardiomegaly: left ventricular failure
- Normal heart size: ARDS; acute coronary syndrome, diastolic failure; interstitial lung disease

Hyperlucency

- Focal: pneumothorax; bulla
- Generalised: airway disease

Normal CXR

- Pulmonary embolism
- Airways disease
- Acidosis; anaemia; hyperventilation
- Neuromuscular disorders

Causes of progressive shortness of breath

Congestive heart failure
Valvular heart disease
Coronary artery disease
Chronic obstructive pulmonary disease
Interstitial lung disease: idiopathic pulmonary fibrosis (age >45 years; persistent dry cough; progressive effort intolerance; dry inspiratory bi-basal "Velcro" crackles, digital clubbing)
Restrictive lung disease: pneumoconiosis, radiation fibrosis
Connective tissue diseases
Chronic thrombo-embolic pulmonary hypertension (caused by obstruction of the pulmonary vascular bed by non-resolving thromboemboli following acute or recurrent pulmonary embolism and leading to severe pulmonary hypertension and right heart failure)

Pulmonary embolism
Risk factors (related to Virchow's triad of hypercoagulability of blood, venous stasis and vascular endothelial injury) may be temporary or reversible (provoked thromboembolism) or persistent.
Major

- Surgery: recent major abdominal or pelvic surgery; hip or knee replacement
- Obstetric: late pregnancy; Casarean section;

puerperium
- Pelvic and lower limb fractures
- Varicose veins
- Malignancy: abdominal or pelvic malignancy; advanced or metastatic malignancy
- Reduced mobility: prolonged bed rest; hospitalization; institutional care
- Previous venous thromboembolism

Minor

- Age >60 years
- Oestrogens: oral contraceptive; oestrogen replacement therapy (HRT)
- Hypercoagulable states
- Chronic indwelling central venous catheters
- Multiple trauma
- Spinal cord injury
- Myeloproliferative disorders (hyperviscosity)
- Chronic heart failure
- Cerebrovascular accident with hemiplegia
- Acute medical illness
- Family history of venous thromboembolism
- Acquired thrombophilic syndromes: antiphospholipid antibody syndrome; paroxysmal nocturnal haemoglobinuria; nephrotic syndrome
- Inherited thrombophilic syndromes: antithrombin III deficiency; protein C and protein S deficiency; factor V Leiden mutation (activated protein C resistance); factor II (prothrombin) gene mutation G20210A causing elevated prothrombin levels; hyperhomocystinaemia
- Mixed thrombophilic syndromes: hyperhomocysteinaemia; elevated factor VIII levels
- Long distance sedentary travel (>4 h in the preceding month)
- Occult malignancy (Trousseau's syndrome of chronic disseminated intravascular coagulation associated with migratory thrombophlebitis, multiple thrombotic events (venous and arterial), bleeding, therapeutic warfarin resistance, and non-bacterial thrombotic endocarditis, is associated with occult cancer). Unprovoked venous thromboembolism may indicate the need for testing for undiagnosed cancer by physical examination, blood tests and chest x-ray.

Syndromes suggestive of pulmonary embolism

It is important to consider the diagnosis in the following circumstances, given the non-specificity of symptoms and signs, aided by the presence of thrombo-embolic risk factors:

- Acute dyspnoea, especially when unexplained
- Cardiovascular collapse, with arterial hypotension (SBP <90 mm Hg for >15 min) and cardiogenic shock related to acute right ventricular failure (massive pulmonary embolism)
- Pleuritic chest pain
- Pulmonary infarction: pleuritic chest pain, dyspnoea and haemoptysis
- Near syncope or syncope
- Chronic progressive dyspnoea (chronic thrombo-embolic pulmonary hypertension)

Atypical presentations of pulmonary embolism

- Pneumonia
- Acute respiratory failure
- Acute abdominal pain
- New onset of atrial fibrillation
- Acute confusional state in the elderly

ECG changes in pulmonary embolism

- Sinus tachycardia
- Atrial arrhythmias, most commonly atrial fibrillation
- New onset incomplete or complete right bundle branch block
- Right axis deviation
- T wave inversion>3 mm in V1 to V3
- ST depression >0.5 mm in V1 to V3
- Q waves in III and aVF
- Right ventricular strain (S1, Q3, T3) (large S wave in I, large Q wave in III, inverted T wave in III)

Two-level Wells Score for likelihood of pulmonary embolism	
Variable	**Points**
History	
Previous DVT/PE	1.5
Surgery under GA or fracture of lower limbs within previous 4 weeks or immobilization >3 days	1.5
Malignancy (receiving treatment, treated in past 6 months or palliative care)	1
Haemoptysis	1
Examination	
Clinical signs of DVT (minimum of leg swelling and pain with palpation of the deep veins)	3
Heart rate > 100 bpm	1.5
Alternative diagnosis less likely than PE (Respiratory disease: pneumothorax; pneumonia; acute exacerbation of COPD; cardiac disease: acute coronary syndrome; acute congestive heart failure, aortic dissection; musculoskeletal chest pain; gastroesophageal reflux disease; any causefor collapse)	3
Clinical probability of pulmonary embolism	**Score**
Likely	4
Unlikely	4 points or less

Wells PS, Anderson DR, Rodger M, et al. Excluding pulmonary embolism at the bedside without diagnostic imaging: management of patients with suspected pulmonary embolism presenting to the emergency department by using a simple clinical model and d-dimer. Ann Intern Med. 2001;135:98–107

PERC (Pulmonary Embolism Rule-Out Criteria)

- Age <50 years
- Heart rate <100 beats per minute
- Oxygen saturation >94% on room air
- No history of DVT/PE
- No recent trauma or surgery
- No haemoptysis
- No exogenous oestrogen
- No clinical signs of DVT

If all eight criteria are met, there is a less than 2% chance of pulmonary embolism

(Kline JA, Mitchell AM, Kabrhel C, et al. Clinical criteria to prevent unnecessary diagnostic testing in emergency department patients with suspected pulmonary embolism. J Thromb Haemostat. 2004;2:1244–55)

Suspect pulmonary embolism in hypotensive patients if

- There is evidence of, or predisposing risk factors for, venous thrombosis
- There is clinical evidence of acute cor pulmonale (acute right ventricular failure) such as distended neck veins, S3 gallop, or a parasternal lift due to right ventricular pressure overload, tachycardia, tachypnoea, and especially if
- There is ECG evidence of acute cor pulmonale manifested by a new S1-Q3-T3 pattern, new incomplete right bundle branch block, or right ventricular ischaemia

Risk stratification in pulmonary embolism

- Stable, no signs of right ventricular dysfunction
- Stable, signs of right ventricular dysfunction
- Shock
- Cardiac arrest

Causes of elevated D-dimer (plasma levels of the degradation product of cross-linked fibrin formed after fibrin lysis by plasmin)

The negative predictive value of D-dimer testing is high, while the positive predictive value is low. A negative D-dimer test measured using a high-sensitivity assay excludes pulmonary embolism when the pre-test probability is low. Causes for an elevated D-dimer include

- Venous thromboembolism
- Acute coronary syndrome
- Acute aortic dissection
- Pregnancy
- Surgery
- Infection
- Cancer
- Trauma

- Liver disease
- Old age (age-adjusted D-dimer cut-off values have been suggested which can be calculated as age in years × 10 mcg/L, replacing a reliance on the conventional 500 mcg/L in patients aged 50 and older).

Causes of haemoptysis (bright red or pink, frothy, mixed in with sputum, alkaline):

Pulmonary
Tracheobronchial
- Tracheobronchitis
- Acute/chronic bronchitis
- Neoplasm: bronchogenic carcinoma; endobronchial metastases; bronchial adenoma; bronchial adenoma
- Bronchiectasis (cystic fibrosis; ciliary dyskinesia; post-lower respiratory tract infection)
- Foreign body aspiration
- Airway trauma

Pulmonary Parenchymal
- Pneumonia (bacterial: Klebsiella, Staphylococcus, Legionella; viral; parasitic)
- Fungal infections: pulmonary mycetoma; aspergilloma (in cavitary lesions)
- Parasitic causes: Paragonimus westermanii; hydatid cyst
- Pulmonary tuberculosis (mycetoma; Rasmussen's aneurysm)
- Lung abscess
- Lung contusion (blunt trauma)
- Pulmonary vasculitis/alveolar haemorrhage syndromes

Vascular
- Pulmonary venous hypertension: congestive heart failure; severe mitral stenosis; left ventricular systolic heart failure; pulmonary embolism
- Pulmonary embolism with infarction
- Eisenmenger's syndrome
- Arterio-venous malformations
- Arterio-bronchial fistula
- Pulmonary artery aneurysms from collagen vascular disease
- Hereditary haemorrhagic telangiectasia (telangiectasia in mouth or nose)

Systemic Coagulopathy
- Oral anticoagulation
- Von Willebrand disease: deficiency or dysfunction of von Willebrand factor characterized by mucocutaneous bleeding
- Haemophilia
- Thrombocytopenia; platelet dysfunction
- Disseminated intravascular coagulation

Non-respiratory Tract Sources (Spurious or Pseudo-haemoptysis)
- Upper airway: nasopharyngeal source of bleeding (epistaxis); oral bleeding
- Upper gastrointestinal bleeding

Miscellaneous
- Pulmonary endometriosis (catamenial haemoptysis)

Causes of pulmonary renal syndromes (pulmonary haemorrhage with acute kidney injury)

Systemic Vasculitis
- Anti-glomerular basement membrane disease (Goodpasture's syndrome)
- ANCA (anti-neutrophil cytoplasmic autoantibody)-positive small vessel vasculitides: granulomatosis with polyangiitis (formerly Wegener's granulomatosis); eosinophilic granulomatosis with polyangiitis (formerly Churg-Strauss syndrome; asthma with eosinophilia and vasculitis); drugs: penicillamine, hydralazine; microscopic polyangiitis
- Other vasculitides: cryoglobulinaemia; associated with systemic lupus erythematosus

Infection: severe bacterial pneumonia (Legionella, Mycoplasma, Leptospirosis); infective endocarditis; post-infectious glomerulonephritis

Pulmonary oedema + acute kidney injury: volume overload; severe left ventricular failure

Multi-organ failure: ARDS + acute kidney injury

Miscellaneous: paraquat poisoning; renal vein or artery thrombosis

Haemoptysis check list

It is important to distinguish between true haemoptysis, pseudo-haemoptysis (coughing of blood that originates from a source other than the lower respiratory tract, namely the upper airway or oral cavity), or haematemesis, based on the history. Haemoptysis is a common symptom, and can vary from streaks of blood in the sputum to massive haemorrhage.

- Post-nasal drip or epistaxis suggest pseudo-haemoptysis
- Smoking history
- Occupational exposure: asbestos; silica
- Weight loss
- Pleuritic chest pain
- Symptoms of congestive heart failure: breathlessness on exertion, orthopnoea, paroxysmal nocturnal dyspnoea
- Productive cough and fever
- Concurrent with menstruation (catamenial haemoptysis related to pulmonary endometriosis)
- History of cancer
- Anticoagulant therapy
- Exposure to tuberculosis
- Travel history
- Coexisting renal disease

Red flags in haemoptysis

- Massive haemoptysis (expectoration of >600 ml blood from below the glottis in 24 h or 150 ml blood in a 1 h period)
- Extensive smoking history
- Back pain
- Malaise, fatigue and weight loss lasting more than 3 weeks
- Dyspnoea at rest

Possible chest x-ray findings in haemoptysis

- Cavitary lesions
- Alveolar infiltrates: diffuse; localized
- Mass lesion
- Bronchiectasis
- Cardiomegaly and increased pulmonary blood flow
- Hilar adenopathy or mass
- Normal

Causes of respiratory failure

Type 1 (hypoxaemia): $paO_2 < 8.9$ kPa (60 mm Hg)

- Low FiO_2: high altitude (reduced barometric pressure); inadvertent hypoxic gas administration; breathing circuit disconnection during mechanical ventilation
- V/Q mismatch (oxygen responsive): COPD exacerbation; pneumonia
- Increased intra-pulmonary shunt (perfusion without ventilation) (oxygen insensitive): No gas exchange but perfused alveoli
  Alveolar filling: oedema, pus, blood (cardiogenic pulmonary oedema, ARDS, pneumonia, lung haemorrhage)
  Atelectasis
- Diffusion impairment: fibrosis (interstitial lung disease); oedema
- Venous admixture
- Anatomical right to left shunts (bypasses pulmonary circuit): pulmonary arteriovenous malformations; intra-cardiac shunts

Type 2 (hypercapnia): $paCO_2 > 6.7$ kPa (50 mm Hg)

- Central respiratory depression causing alveolar hypoventilation
  Drugs: opiates; benzodiazepines; synergistic drug interactions, altered drug metabolism (hepatic or renal failure) and iatrogenic drug overdose are factors to be considered
  Cerebrovascular disease: stroke
  Raised intracranial pressure: space occupying lesion
  Central congenital hypoventilation syndrome (Ondine's curse): results in respiratory arrest during sleep
  Uncontrolled oxygen therapy
  Trauma: head injury
- Chest wall disease: kyphoscoliosis; flail chest; thoracoplasty; ankylosing spondylitis; obesity-hypoventilation syndrome
- Pleural disease: pneumothorax; massive pleural effusion

- Neuromuscular disease affecting respiratory muscles
  Cervical spinal cord injury: trauma; neoplasm
  Neuromuscular disease:
  Neuromuscular junction disorders: myasthenia gravis, organophosphate toxicity, botulism
  Peripheral neuropathies: Gullain Barre syndrome, diphtheritic polyneuropathy, critical illness polyneuropathy
  Amyotrophic lateral sclerosis
  Anterior horn cells in spinal cord: poliomyelitis
  Myopathies: muscular dystrophy
- Upper airway obstruction
- Lung disease
  Obstructive: COPD
  Restrictive

Signs of respiratory failure

- Increased work of breathing: tachypnoea; use of accessory muscles; nasal flaring; recession (intercostal, suprasternal, supraclavicular)
- Sympathetic activation: tachycardia; hypertension; sweating
- End-organ hypoxia: confusion; altered level of consciousness; bradycardia and hypotension (late signs)
- Haemoglobin desaturation: cyanosis

Signs of hypercapnia

- Drowsiness
- Bounding peripheral pulses
- Flapping tremor
- Papilloedema
- Coma

Signs of hypoxaemia

- Confusion
- Agitation
- Altered level of consciousness
- Sweating
- Cyanosis
- Coma

Potential sources of error with pulse oximetry

- Poorly adherent probe
- Dark skin
- Excessive motion: motion artifact
- Low signal-noise ratio with impaired peripheral perfusion: shock; cardiac arrest
- False nails; blue, black or green nail varnish
- Lipaemia: hyperlipidaemia; propofol infusion
- Bright ambient light
- Abnormal haemoglobins: carboxyhaemoglobin; methaemoglobin
- Intravenous dyes: methylene blues
- $SpO_2 < 80\%$
- Venous pulsations: obstructed venous return; severe right heart failure; dependent limb; tourniquet constriction

Causes of hyperventilation
Physiological

- Fever
- Pregnancy
- High altitude

Pathological

- Hypoxaemia: asthma, left ventricular failure, pulmonary embolism, pneumonia
- Severe pain
- Metabolic acidosis: diabetic ketoacidosis
- Drugs: salicylate toxicity; withdrawal syndromes (alcohol; benzodiazepines)

Causes of wheezing in childhood
Intrinsic airway narrowing

- Structural anomalies: tracheobronchomalacia/stenosis; bronchopulmonary dysplasia; α-1-antitrypsin deficiency
- Bronchospasm: anaphylaxis; organophosphate toxicity
- Inflammation: asthma; bronchiolitis; **episodic viral wheeze**, associated with upper respiratory tract infections (in children aged 6 months

to 5 years); smoke inhalation; pulmonary aspiration (gastroesophageal reflux; tracheo-oesophageal fistula)

Intraluminal airway obstruction

- Foreign body aspiration (triad of unilateral monophonic wheeze, cough and unilateral reduction in breath sounds)

Extrinsic airway compression

- Congenital structural anomalies: cystic malformations of lung; vascular ring; cardiovascular enlargement
- Mediastinal tumours
- Enlarged mediastinal lymph nodes

Miscellaneous:

- Congestive heart failure
- Muco-ciliary clearance disorders: cystic fibrosis; bronchiectasis; primary ciliary dyskinesia

Types of wheeze
Polyphonic wheeze

- Asthma
- COPD
- Heart failure
- Extrinsic allergic alveolitis
- Anaphylaxis

Monophonic wheeze

- Foreign body aspiration
- Bronchial carcinoma

Clues to alternative diagnoses in wheezy children

- Symptoms from birth or perinatal period
- Severe upper respiratory tract disease; nasal polpys
- Family history of unusual chest disease
- Chronic wet or productive cough
- Excessive vomiting (gastro-oesophageal reflux, with or without aspiration)
- Dysphagia (with or without aspiration)
- Inspiratory stridor
- Abnormal voice or cry
- Finger clubbing
- Failure to thrive

Features of bronchiolitis

- Affects children aged 2 years or under
- A coryzal period lasting 1–3 days is followed by persistent cough, low grade fever, tachypnoea, chest recession, and either high pitched expiratory wheezing or fine inspiratory crackles on auscultation
- Self-limiting, with symptoms peaking at 3–5 days
- Peak prevalence is in the winter months in temperate climates
- Occurs in association with viral infections (RSV in around 75% cases); also parainfluenza, adenovirus, influenza, rhinovirus, metapneumovirus

Risk factors for severe bronchiolitis

- Age <3 months
- Premature birth, especially 32 weeks or under
- Chronic lung disease (including bronchopulmonary dysplasia, cystic fibrosis)
- Congenital heart disease, which is haemodynamically significant
- Immunodeficiency (congenital or acquired)
- Neuromuscular disease: severe neurological disease

Features suggestive of asthma

- Onset in early life
- Frequent and recurrent episodic wheeze, breathlessness, chest tightness and cough, worse at night and in early mornings (diurnal and day-to-day variability), or in response to exercise, allergen exposure (including exposure to pets), cold air and emotional stress
- History of atopic disease
- Family history of asthma and/or atopic disease
- Widespread wheeze on cardiac auscultation

- Aspirin-induced asthma is associated with the triad of asthma, aspirin intolerance, and sinusitis with nasal polyps

Historical clues which lower the probability of a diagnosis of asthma

- Chronic productive cough in the absence of wheeze or shortness of breath
- Smoking history >20 pack years (pack year= (cigarettes smoked per day/20) × number of years smoking)
- Voice disturbance
- Symptoms with colds only, with no interval symptoms
- Normal physical examination of the chest when symptomatic
- Normal peak expiratory flow when symptomatic
- Cardiac disease

Asthma mimics
"All that wheezes is not asthma"

- Other obstructive lung disease: COPD; bronchiectasis; cystic fibrosis; eosinophilic bronchitis; primary ciliary dyskinesia syndromes
- Respiratory infections: recurrent viral lower respiratory tract infections, pulmonary tuberculosis, allergic bronchopulmonary aspergillosis (fever, malaise, recurrent airway obstruction, cough with expectoration of brownish mucus plugs, haemoptysis and peripheral blood eosinophilia; chest x-ray shows upper lobe infiltrates, atelectasis due to mucoid impaction, and tramline shadowing of central bronchiectasis representing thickened bronchial walls)
- Non-obstructive lung disease: diffuse parenchymal lung disease; pulmonary embolism; chronic eosinophilic pneumonia (with reverse pulmonary oedema appearance on chest x-ray)
- Gastroesophageal reflux
- Vocal cord dysfunction: paroxysmal adduction of the vocal cords on inspiration, expiration or both
- Upper airway obstruction: large airway stenosis
- Foreign body aspiration
- Primary endobronchial tumours
- Adverse drug reactions: ACE inhibitors
- Left ventricular failure ("cardiac asthma")
- Hyperventilation syndrome and panic attacks

Triggers for asthma

- IgE related: allergens (animals and pets; grain; house dust mites; pollen, including trees and grass; moulds and fungi); proteolytic enzymes
- Non IgE related: hardwood dust; colophony fumes (solder); isocyanates; exercise; sex; atmospheric pollution (traffic fumes); emotion; smoking and second-hand smoke; recreational drugs; weather and changes in temperature; viral infections

Categorisation of severity of asthma
Mild:

- PEFR >75% predicted or best

Moderate:

- PEFR 50–75% predicted or best

Severe:

- PEFR <50% predicted or best
- Inability to complete sentences
- Respiratory rate >25/min
- Tachycardia >110/min

Life threatening

Markers of a life threatening attack of asthma

- Unable to talk
- Exhaustion
- Confusion
- Cyanosis of lips and tongue on room air
- Silent chest/feeble respiratory effort
- Saturation <90%
- PFR <33% of predicted or best
- No response to beta 2 agonist therapy
- Bradycardia
- Coma
- Hypotension

Warning signs of asthma exacerbation

- Increased dyspnoea
- A combination of increased wheeze, cough, or mucus secretion
- Nocturnal asthma
- Increased use of short acting sympathomimetics (reliever medication)
- Increased exercise induced asthma
- Decreased morning peak expiratory flow rate

Features suggestive of COPD

- Onset in mid-life: age greater than 35 years
- Exertional breathlessness
- Persistent progressive breathlessness
- Chronic productive cough, with regular sputum production
- Frequent winter 'bronchitis'
- Smoker or ex-smoker

Acute excerbation of COPD (triad of increased dyspnoea, increased sputum volume, and purulent sputum)
Precipitating factors

- Respiratory infection
  Bacteria: Haemophilus influenzae; Streptococcus pneumoniae; Staphylococcus aureus; Moraxella catarrhalis
  Viral: Rhinovirus, influenza virus, parainfluenza virus, coronavirus, adenovirus, picornavirus, parvovirus, respiratory syncytial virus
  Atypical bacteria: mycoplasma pneumoniae; chlamydia pneumoniae; legionella
- Heart failure
- Pulmonary embolism
- Pneumothorax
- Non-pulmonary infections
- Environmental: cold temperature, air pollution, cigarette smoke
- Non-compliance with medication

Causes of spontaneous pneumothorax
Primary: apical sub-pleural bleb or bulla (associated with male gender, tall stature, low body mass index, inhalant use, genetic predisposition and smoking)

Secondary:

Primary airway disease: COPD; acute severe asthma; cystic fibrosis
Lung infections: Pneumocystis jiroveci pneumonia; tuberculosis; necrotizing bacterial pneumonias; fungal pneumonia
Interstitial lung disease: sarcoidosis; idiopathic pulmonary fibrosis; lymphangioleiomyomatosis or LAM (smooth muscle proliferation around bronchioles results in air trapping and characteristic thin-walled lung cysts that are uniform in size; chest x-ray may reveal hyperinflation, chylous pleural effusion and diffuse bilateral reticulo-nodular interstitial pattern)
Connective tissue disease: rheumatoid arthritis; ankylosing spondylitis; polymyositis; dermatomyositis; systemic sclerosis; Marfan's syndrome; Ehlers-Danlos syndrome
Cancer
Catamenial pneumothorax: thoracic endometriosis (within 72 h of menstruation)

Features of pneumothorax on supine chest x-ray
Radiolucency in lower zone

Increased air in anterior and lateral costophrenic sulcus

- Hyper-lucency of upper abdominal quadrants and lower chest
- Deep and sometimes "tongue-like" lateral costophrenic sulcus: deep sulcus sign (deep V)
- Visualization of the anterior costophrenic sulcus: double hemi-diaphragm sign, as the dome and anterior portions of the diaphragm are outlined by lung and pleural air, respectively
- Sharp diaphragmatic or mediastinal contours-increased definition of the mediastinal border (etched mediastinum)

Depression of the ipsilateral diaphragm

Double diaphragm contour

Outline of medial diaphragm under heart silhouette

Presence of a sharply defined pericardial fat pad and a distinct cardiac apex (mediastinal structures sharply outlined by free air)-unusually clear or sharp heart border

Sub-pulmonic air which outlines the visceral pleura of the lung base

Features of pneumothorax on bedside ultrasound

- Absence of dynamic pleural sliding with respiration
- Loss of vertical comet-tail artefacts along the pleural interface
- Stratosphere sign or bar-code sign, where only horizontal lines are seen (continuous ocean pattern) on M-mode. The actual location where the pneumothorax begins can often be detected. This interface between normal lung and pneumothorax is known as the lung point. This can be visualised on the M-mode image, where both the seashore sign and stratosphere sign are seen on the same image

Causes of pseudo-pneumothorax (pneumothorax mimics) on chest x-ray

- Skin fold (straight or minimally curved; dense line sharp on one side and blurred on the other; passes outside chest cavity; does not run parallel to chest wall)
- Medial border of scapula
- Lateral edge of breast tissue
- Calcified pleural plaque
- Post-pleurectomy scarring
- Companion shadow (radiopaque line accompanying inferior rib margin, caused by extrapleural fat or visible subcostal groove, usually on 1st or 2nd rib)
- Folds of blankets or clothing
- Giant bullous emphysema (vanishing lung syndrome) (the compressed lung falls towards trhe costophrenic angle)

Causes of failure of lung re-expansion after chest drain placement

- Blocked drain
- Misplaced drain
- Persistent air leak: bronchopleural fistula

Pleural effusion

Causes of transudative effusion (serous) (<30 g/L)

Right ventricular failure
Congestive heart failure
Constrictive pericarditis
Superior vena caval obstruction
Cirrhosis of the liver
Hypoalbuminaemia: nephrotic syndrome; liver failure
Hypothyroidism
Meigs syndrome
Obstructive uropathy
End-stage chronic kidney disease
Peritoneal dialysis

Causes of exudative effusion

Malignancy: lung; breast; lymphoma; pleural mesothelioma (fixed mediastinum due to pleural encasement; progressive reduction in size of hemithorax associated with pleural thickening); metastases
Infection: para-pneumonic effusions; tuberculosis; fungal; parasitic
Pulmonary infarction
Gastrointestinal: pancreatitis; oesophageal rupture (pleural fluid amylase may be elevated)
Autoimmune: systemic lupus erythematosus
Radiation pleuritis
Post-myocardial infarction
Ovarian hyperstimulation syndrome
Asbestos –related pleural disease
Yellow nail syndrome
Trauma: haemothorax; chylothorax
Fistula (ventriculo-peritoneal; bilio-peritoneal; gastro-peritoneal)
Drugs: nitrofurantoin; methysergide

Exudates can demonstrate on bedside ultrasound the following features:

- Multiple internal echoes from floating debris
- Septations and loculation
- Consolidation of lung
- Pleural thickening

Features of pleural effusion on supine chest x-ray

Asymmetrical, diffuse, hazy opacity that increases in density within the hemithorax in a cephalo-caudad direction, due to layering of the effusion posteriorly

The hemidiaphragm is obscured and the lateral costophrenic angle is blunted

Opacity over lung apex with a concave interface inferiorly (pleural cap): the apex is the most dependent portion of the thorax tangential to the frontal x-ray beam

Absence of air bronchograms and visualization of lung vessels through the density confirms that the increased opacity is extraparenchymal in location

Features of pleural effusion on bedside ultrasound

A pleural effusion appears as an anechoic or hypoechoic zone between the parietal and visceral pleura. The lung sliding sign is absent. A transudate is echo-free. An exudate appears as an echoic collection, with floating echogenic debris, with or without pleural thickening and loculation. Empyema and haemothorax appear homogenous and echoic. The presence of floating fragments within a pleural effusion has been referred to as the plankton sign.

Features of loculated pleural effusion

- Elliptical or oval pleural-based opacities without air bronchograms
- Located along the course of a fissure or between the visceral and parietal pleura when the pleural layers are partly adherent
- Does not shift freely within the pleural space with changing patient position
- Rapid disappearance with diuresis has led to the term vanishing lung tumour

Features of pleural thickening

- Bases: blunting of costophrenic angle, with tenting of diaphragmatic pleura
- Apices: apical pleural cap-curvilinear density at lung apex

Malignant pleural thickening is suggested by:

- Parietal pleural thickening >1 cm
- Nodular pleural thickening >1 cm
- Mediastinal pleural thickening
- Circumferential pleural thickening with lung encasement and volume loss of involved hemithorax
- Chest wall invasion

Risk factors for community-acquired pneumonia

- Age >65 years
- Smoking
- Alcohol abuse
- Poor dental hygiene
- Chronic lung disease: COPD; asthma; cystic fibrosis
- Contact spread: nursing homes; institutions; military barracks; student dormitories
- Chronic kidney disease
- Diabetes mellitus
- Dementia
- Congestive heart failure
- Occupational dust exposure

Clinical features of pneumonia

Although conventionally pneumonia has been classified as typical and atypical, it is now recognized that clinical features correlate poorly with microbial aetiology.

Typical bacteria pneumonia with signs of lobar consolidation

- Sudden onset
- Fever with chills
- Cough with purulent sputum
- Pleuritic chest pain

Atypical pneumonia

Gradual onset, with prodrome of headache and myalgia
Dry cough
Low grade fever
Extra-pulmonary manifestations: abdominal pain, diarrhea, confusion

More protracted course
CXR findings often more severe than clinical presentation

CURB 65 Score

- Confusion (abbreviated mental test score 8 or less, or new disorientation in time, place and person)
- Raised blood urea nitrogen (>7 mmol/L)
- Raised respiratory rate (30 breaths per minute or more)
- Low blood pressure (systolic blood pressure <90 mm Hg, or diastolic blood pressure <60 mm Hg)
- Age 65 years or older

Home-based care can be considered for patients scoring 0 or 1, and hospital-based care for those scoring 2 or more

(Lim W, van der Eerden MM, Laing R, et al. Defining community acquired pneumonia severity on presentation to hospital: an international derivation and validation study. Thorax. 2003;58:377–82)

Pneumonia mimics

- Pulmonary infarction
- Non-infective, inflammatory pneumonia:
- Eosinophilic pneumonia diffuse bilateral alveolar opacities, inter-lobular septal thickening producing Kerley B lines, and bilateral small pleural effusions
- Broncho-pulmonary aspergillosis
- Cryptogenic organising pneumonia (presents with a subacute onset of dry cough, shortness of breath, anorexia, malaise, fever and weight loss; multiple bilateral patchy alveolar opacities with a peripheral sub-pleural and bronchovascular distribution, often migratory as the disease progresses; normal lung volumes; refractory to antibiotic therapy; rapid clinical and radiological improvement with steroid therapy)
- Pulmonary vasculitis: granulomatosis with polyangiitis (Wegener's granulomatosis) (solitary or mutiple pulmonary nodules, with or without cavitation)
- Eosinophilic granuloma
- Acute allergic or toxic pneumonitis

Environmental factors in pulmonary infection

- Water cooling units: Legionella
- Military barracks: Mycoplasma
- Birds: psittacosis, histoplasmosis, aspergillosis
- Dogs, cats, rats, pigs, cattle: leptospirosis
- Goats, pigs, cattle: Q fever
- Abattoirs, veterinary practitioners: brucellosis
- Soil: blastomycosis
- Decaying wood, caves, chicken: histoplasmosis
- Florists, gardeners, plants, straw: sporotrichosis

Radiological features of pneumonia

- Lobar: consolidation, with air bronchogram, no volume loss
- Lobular (bronchopneumonia): multi-focal nodular or reticulonodular opacities which are patchy and/or confluent patchy
- Interstitial: diffuse bilateral reticular, nodular or reticulonodular opacities which are patchy and/or confluent
- Round pneumonia: spherical opacity simulating a parenchymal mass
- Cavitary lesions
- Pneumothorax or pneumatocoele (Pneumocystis jiroveci)

Causes of non-resolving pneumonia

- Complications of pneumonia: empyema; lung abscess; parapneumonic effusion
- Pneumonia mimics: neoplasm (bronchogenic carcinoma, lymphoma, bronchoalveolar carcinoma); inflammatory disorders (cryptogenic organizing pneumonia-failure to improve despite several courses of antibiotics); eosinophilic pneumonia; systemic vasculitis-Wegener's granulomatosis
- Unusual causative organism: tuberculosis; atypical mycobacteria; fungal pneumonia (aspergillosis, cryptococcosis, mucormycosis, histoplasmosis, coccidiodomycosis)
- Resistant organism: drug-resistant Streptococcus pneumoniae; MRSA

Causes of recurrent focal pneumonia

- Causes within the lumen: foreign body; endobronchial tuberculosis; tumour
- Causes affecting the wall: asthma; bronchomalacia
- Causes from external compression: enlarged hilar lymph nodes; enlarged left atrium compressing the left main bronchus
- Infected developmental lung malformations: sequestration; bronchogenic cyst; cystic adenomatoid malformation
- Other causes: bronchiectasis

Risk factors for lung abscess

- Aspiration: alcohol abuse; seizure; dental and periodontal disease; neuromuscular disorders with bulbar dysfunction; gastro-oesophageal reflux; oesophageal dysmotility
- Bronchial obstruction: neoplastic; non-neoplastic
- Immunosuppression

Causes of recurrent respiratory tract infections in children

- Cystic fibrosis
- Ciliary dysfunction: primary ciliary dyskinesia; Kartagener's syndrome; bronchiectasis; immotile cilia syndrome
- Structural lung disease: congenital cystic adenomatoid malformation; pulmonary sequestration
- Immunodeficiency: transient hypogammaglobulinaemia of infancy; X-linked agammaglobulinaemia; combined variable immunodeficiency; hyper-IgM syndrome; secondary IgA deficiency
- Oesophageal disease: achalasia; progressive systemic sclerosis; pharyngeal pouch
- Cardiovascular disease: Left to right shunts: atrial septal defect; ventricular septal defect; heart failure

Causes of cavitating lung lesions

Infection:

- Pulmonary tuberculosis
- Cavitating pneumonia/lung abscess: staphylococcus aureus; Gram negative bacteria, e.g. Klebsiella pneumoniae
- Infected post-pneumonia pneumatocoele
- Fungal infection: aspergillosis; mucormycosis; histoplasmosis; pneumocystis
- Parasitic infections: hydatid cyst

Neoplasia:

- Primary malignancy: bronchogenic carcinoma, lymphoma, Kaposi's sarcoma
- Secondary malignancy: especially squamous cell carcinoma, adenocarcinoma, sarcoma

Vascular:

- Pulmonary embolism with infarction
- Septic pulmonary emboli

Autoimmune:

- Wegener's granulomatosis
- Rheumatoid nodules

Trauma: pulmonary contusion; lung laceration

The mnemonic CAVITY is useful: cancer, autoimmune, vascular, infection, trauma, and youth (pulmonary sequestration, bronchogenic cyst)

Risk factors for aspiration pneumonia and lung abscess

- Oropharyngeal sepsis: periodontal disease; gingivitis; dental abscess; tonsillar abscess
- Impaired level of consciousness: drugs; alcohol; coma; seizure; shock; general anaesthesia
- Impaired cough and gag reflex: vocal cord paralysis; myopathy; myelopathy
- Impaired oesophageal function: achalasia, stricture, diverticula
- Vomiting: ileus, intestinal obstruction

Key diagnoses to be recognized in chest trauma

Primary survey

- Tension pneumothorax
- Dyspnoea; tachypnoea; increasing hypoxaemia; haemodynamic instability, with hypotension and narrowing pulse pressure

- Contralateral tracheal shift
- Hyperexpanded chest
- Hyper-resonance with absent breath sounds
- Jugular venous distension
- Flail chest (anterior or lateral double fractures of three or more adjacent ribs; paradoxical segmental chest wall movement over several respiratory cycles and during coughing)
- Open sucking chest wound
- Massive haemothorax
- Cardiac tamponade

Secondary survey

- Contained rupture of thoracic aorta
- Rupture of tracheo-bronchial tree
- Oesophageal perforation
- Diaphragmatic rupture (asymmetrical chest expansion; absent breath sounds; tracheal deviation; elevated hemidiaphragm with loss of normal contour, and intra-thoracic herniation of a hollow viscus (stomach, colon or small bowel) on chest x-ray)
- Myocardial contusion
- Pulmonary contusion

Features of tracheo-bronchial tree injury

- Cervical trachea injury: hoarseness; stridor; haemoptysis; cervical subcutaneous emphysema
- Intra-thoracic tracheo-bronchial injury: massive subcutaneous emphysema, unilateral or bilateral pneumothorax/haemothorax, pneumomediastinum, mediastinal haematoma, peribronchial air and partial pulmonary atelectasis; fallen lung sign caused by atelectatic lung falling infero-laterally from the hilum in the lower medial pleural space; failure of re-expansion of the lung after chest tube placement, related to massive air leak from bronchopleural fistula; abnormal migration of tip of endotracheal tube; tension pneumothorax with positive pressure ventilation

Radiological features of traumatic aortic injury

- Mediastinal widening, with mediastinal-chest ratio >0.25 and superior mediastinal width >8 cm
- Loss of, or abnormal, aortic knob contour
- Tracheal deviation to the right
- Wide right paratracheal stripe
- Depression of left main stem bronchus
- Oesophageal deviation (nasogastric tube) deviation to the right
- Left apical pleural cap: a curvilinear opacity with mass effect on the lung apex
- Wide left paraspinal line
- Left haemothorax
- Fractures of upper ribs

Causes of mediastinal haematoma

- Aortic injury
- Venous haemorrhage
- Thoracic vertebral body fracture
- Spinal ligamentous injuries

Features of pulmonary contusion

- The commonest injury following blunt chest wall trauma in children
- Caused by alveolar capillary disruption, leading to alveolar haemorrhage and interstitial oedema
- Focal or multi-focal consolidation, crossing fissures and lobes, with sub-pleural sparing (1–2 mm region of non-opaque sub-pleural lung separating the area of consolidation from the adjacent chest wall)
- Chest x-ray signs may take 4–6 h to develop and progress over 24–48 h; resolution within 3–5 days usually

The clinical features of rib fracture include:

- Pleuritic chest pain
- Point tenderness
- Production of pain by anteroposterior or lateral chest wall compression ("springing")
- Local crepitus
- Subcutaneous emphysema
- 1st and 2nd rib fractures may be associated with vascular injury (aorta, subclavian artery) or brachial plexus injury
- 11th and 12th rib fractures may be associated with visceral injury (liver, spleen, kidneys)

Features of sternal fractures

- Caused by direct trauma, such as antero-posterior compression from seat belt or steering wheel injuries, with posterior displacement of the distal sternal fragment, or indirect trauma, such as hyperflexion and axial compression, with posterior displacement of the proximal sternal agent. Manubrio-sternal joint dislocation may also result by these mechanisms.
- Can be associated with myocardial or pulmonary contusion
- Usually diagnosed on a lateral view of the sternum
- Isolated sternal fracture with normal 12 lead ECG and normal chest x-ray carries a very low risk of intrathoracic injury

Causes of subcutaneous emphysema in the chest wall
Air introduced from outside

- Penetrating injury

Air from within

- Pneumothorax
- Acute severe asthma
- Oesophageal perforation
- Tracheo- bronchial disruption (subcutaneous emphysema, persistent air leak, haemoptysis)

Predictors of difficult airway (based on oro-pharyngeal examination, assessment of atlanto-occipital joint mobility and of the space between the horizontal ramus of mandible and the hyoid bone-the potential displacement space)

- Small mouth
- Limited mouth opening (3 cm or less, two fingerbreadths or less); limited temporomandibular joint mobility; trismus
- Protruding upper incisors
- Dental implants
- Short inter-incisor distance
- Large tongue (macroglossia)
- Cleft or high arched narrow palate
- Mandibular hypoplasia (micrognathia)
- Short or muscular neck
- Limited neck mobility
- Obesity

In addition, current airway obstruction, inflammation and haemorrhage are also predictors of a difficult airway

Causes of hypotension with chest trauma
Bleeding

- Massive haemothorax

Reduced venous return

- Tension pneumothorax (increased intra-thoracic pressure)
- Cardiac tamponade (increased intra-pleural pressure)

Direct cardiac injury (cardiogenic shock) (no blood loss)

- Myocardial contusion
- Myocardial infarction
- Conduction abnormalities
- Air embolism

Causes of cardiovascular collapse after rapid sequence induction of anaesthesia and positive-pressure ventilation following chest trauma

- Hypovolaemia
- Unrecognised oesophageal intubation, with hypoxaemia
- Tension pneumothorax
- Pericardial tamponade
- Anaphylaxis
- Systemic air embolism
- Severe blunt cardiac trauma

Causes of bilateral hilar enlargement

- Lymph node enlargement (lobulated)
- Sarcoidosis
- Malignancy: lymphoma; carcinoma

- Infection: tuberculosis; mycoplasma; fungal infection
- Inorganic dust disease: silicosis; berylliosis
- Pulmonary artery enlargement (smooth, with peripheral decreased vascular markings-peripheral pruning)
- Pulmonary arterial hypertension (main pulmonary artery >29 mm in diameter and/or larger than adjacent ascending aorta)
- Left to right intra-cardiac shunt
- High output state
- Cystic fibrosis

Causes of hilar lymphadenopathy
Bilateral asymmetrical and unilateral

- Tuberculosis: primary tuberculosis
- Fungal, atypical mycobacterial, viral, tularaemia, anthrax
- Metastatic or primary hilar tumour (bronchogenic carcinoma)
- Lymphoma
- Sarcoidosis,
- Inorganic dust disease: silicosis, berylliosis
- Angio-immunoblastic lymphadenopathy
- Drug reaction

Bilateral symmetrical

- Sarcoidosis (Garland's sign) (bilateral hilar and right paratracheal node enlargement constitutes the 1–2–3 sign)
- Viral infection (adenovirus, infectious mononucleosis)
- Other causes mentioned can be symmetrical

Causes of diffuse confluent alveolar opacities (widespread pulmonary consolidation) (oedema, exudate, blood, neoplasm)

Pulmonary oedema

- Cardiogenic
- Fluid overload/acute kidney injury
- Non-cardiogenic

Pneumonia

- Pneumocystis jiroveci
- Gram negative bacteria
- Influenza
- Fungi: histoplasmosis; aspergillosis

Pulmonary haemorrhage (Goodpasture's syndrome)

Neoplasm

- Bronchio-alveolar cell carcinoma
- Lymphoproliferative disorder: lymphoma

Alveolar proteinosis
Acute silica inhalation
AIDS
Reaction to drugs
Extrinsic allergic alveolitis

Causes of abnormal chest x-ray in immunocompromised patients

- Infection: bacterial; mycobacterial; fungal; viral
- Neoplasm: lymphoma; leukaemia; metastases/recurrence of primary tumour
- Transfusion reaction
- Graft versus host disease after bone marrow transplantation
- Radiation pneumonitis: acute; chronic
- Adverse drug reaction: early (non-toxic); late (cytotoxic)
- Haemorrhage

Causes of increased transradiancy of one hemithorax
Technical-artifactual

- Rotation of patient (scoliosis; supine position)
- Off-centring of grid (grid cut-off or anode heel effect) (causes diffuse increased haziness of the hemithorax)
- Overexposure; especially in AP view

Chest wall–relative lack of overlying soft tissues

- Loss of soft tissues: mastectomy; Poland's syndrome

Pleura: pneumothorax; especially in supine patient

Lung:

Compensatory over-inflation

- Post-lobectomy
- Overlooked lobar collapse (especially left lower lobe)
- McLeod's syndrome: unilateral emphysema-like condition following early childhood lower respiratory tract infections

Reduced pulmonary perfusion

- Hypoxic vasoconstriction due to hypoventilation caused by inhaled foreign body or endobronchial tumour
- McLeod's syndrome
- Recurrent pulmonary emboli (rarely unilateral)

Causes of asymmetrical lung volumes

Increased ipsilateral density

- Small lung: atelectasis; central airway obstruction; congenital venolobar syndrome (hypoplasia of the lung associated with pulmonary vascular abnormalities); diaphragmatic elevation/paresis
- Large lung

Decreased ipsilateral density

- Small lung: McLeod's syndrome
- Large lung: primary/secondary congenital over-inflation; central airway obstruction with ball-valve effect

Normal density

- Small lung: hypoplasia; interrupted pulmonary artery

Causes of mediastinal masses

Anterior mediastinum (30%) (5Ts: thyroid mass; teratoma; thymic mass; terrible-lymphoma; thoracic aorta)

- Congenital: normal thymus; thymic cyst; thymomegaly; Morgagni hernia
- Inflammatory: mediastinitis; lymphadenopathy; sternal inflammatory disease
- Neoplasm: lymphoma-leukaemia; teratoma and other germ cell tumours; seminoma; thymoma; thyroid or parathyroid tumour; hamartoma; mesenchymal tumour; lipoma
- Traumatic: haematoma; sternal fracture; thymic haemorrhage
- Vascular: aneurysm of sinus of Valsalva; anomalous vessel
- Miscellaneous: histiocytosis; sarcoidosis
- Thyroid (goitre or neoplasm)

Middle mediastinum (30%)

- Congenital: foregut cyst (enteric, respiratory); oesophagus (hiatus hernia, achalasia); extension of normal thymus
- Inflammatory: mediastinitis; lymphadenopathy
- Neoplasm: lymphoma-leukaemia; bronchogenic carcinoma; metastases cardiac tumour or aneurysm
- Traumatic: haematoma; diaphragm rupture
- Vascular (lesions of the aorta and great vessels: aneurysm-aorta; dilated superior or inferior vena cava; anomalies of great vessels)
- Miscellaneous: pancreatic pseudocyst
- Dilated oesophagus and oesophageal masses: tumour: benign, malignant; oesophageal diverticulum; dilated oesophagus

Posterior mediastinum (40%)

- Congenital: foregut cyst; lateral meningocele; Bochdalek hernia; ectopic thymus
- Inflammatory: mediastinitis; spinal inflammatory disease
- Neoplasm: neurogenic (neuroblastoma, ganglioneuroma, ganglioneuroblastoma); nerve root tumours (schwannoma, neurofibroma, malignant schwannoma); paraganglionic cell tumours (chemodectoma, phaeochromocytoma); spinal tumour (metastases, primary bone tumour); lymphoma; mesenchymal

tumour (fibroma, lipoma, leiomyoma, haemangioma, lymphangioma)
- Traumatic: haematoma; pseudo-meningocoele
- Vascular: aneurysm of descending aorta
- Miscellaneous: histiocytosis; extramedullary haematopoiesis

Recognition of abnormal mediastinal widening
Widening of the mediastinum is most often due to technical factors such as patient positioning or the projection used. Rotation, incomplete inspiration, or an AP view, may all exaggerate the width of the mediastinum, as well as heart size.

- Mediastinal width >6 cm in erect PA film
- Mediastinal width >8 cm in supine AP chest film
- Mediastinal width >7.5 cm at aortic knob
- Ratio of mediastinal width to chest width >0.25 at aortic knob

Causes of diffuse mediastinal widening
Smooth

- Mediastinal lipomatosis
- Malignant infiltration: lymphoma; squamous cell carcinoma; adenocarcinoma
- Mediastinal haemorrhage: traumatic arch/great vessel laceration; arterial bleeding; venous bleeding; SVC/right atrial laceration
- Mediastinitis: acute (suppurative); chronic (sclerosing): histoplasmosis, tuberculosis, idiopathic

Lobulated

- Lymph node enlargement
- Thymic mass
- Germ cell neoplasm
- Neurofibromatosis
- Vascular lesions: tortuous great vessels; SVC occlusion

Pneumomediastinum
Pneumomediastinum indicates perforation of some portion of either the respiratory or gastrointestinal tracts

Features of pneumomediastinum

- Free mediastinal air, causing streaky radiolucencies in the mediastinum and outlining the heart borders, the central diaphragm (causing visualisation of the entire disphragm) and the thymus, and extending to the neck
- Subcutaneous emphysema
- Ring shaped radiolucencies around the aorta and pulmonary artery

Causes of pneumomediastinum

- Alveolar rupture: spontaneous; positive pressure ventilation; compressive trauma to the chest; rupture of lung by rib fracture with tracking of air into the mediastinum by way of the chest wall and neck; asthma
- Traumatic laceration of trachea or a central bronchus (associated with double wall sign, caused by intramural air in proximal airways leading to visualisation of both sides of the bronchial wall, and the fallen lung sign of collapse of the inferior lung)
- Spontaneous or iatrogenic perforation of pharynx, oesophagus, duodenum, colon, or rectum, with tracking of air into the mediastinum: Boerhaave syndrome; endoscopic intervention (biopsy, dilatation, sclerotherapy)
- Following placement of an intercostal tube or mediastinoscopy or similar invasive procedures

Defining features of solitary pulmonary nodule

- Single lung lesion
- Less than 3 cm in diameter
- Surrounded on all sides by lung parenchyma
- Benign patterns of calcification: central; diffuse; popcorn; laminated

Causes of solitary pulmonary nodule

- Neoplastic: malignant (bronchogenic carcinoma; solitary metastasis; lymphoma; carcinoid tumour); benign (hamartoma; adenoma; benign connective tissue and neural tumours)

- Inflammatory: granuloma; lung abscess; rheumatoid nodule; inflammatory pseudotumour (plasma cell granuloma)
- Congenital: arteriovenous malformation; lung cyst; broncho-pulmonary sequestration; bronchial atresia with mucoid impaction
- Miscellaneous: pulmonary infarct; intrapulmonary lymph node; mucoid impaction; haematoma; amyloidosis; normal confluence of pulmonary veins; conglomerate mass of silicosis

Mimics of solitary pulmonary nodule

- Nipple shadow
- Cutaneous lesion
- Rib or other bone lesion
- Vanishing pseudotumour of congestive cardiac failure (loculated pleural effusion)

Features suggestive of malignancy

- Clinical: older age; COPD; previous malignancy; environmental exposures; haemoptysis; lung cancer in first degree relatives
- Radiological: speculated appearance; eccentric or speculated calcification; thick walled cavitation

Causes of multiple pulmonary nodules
Neoplastic

- Metastases
- Malignant lymphoma/lymphoproliferative disorders

Inflammatory

- Granulomas
- Fungal and opportunistic infections
- Septic emboli
- Rheumatoid nodules
- Granulomatosis with polyangiitis (Wegener's granulomatosis)
- Sarcoidosis
- Langerhans' cell histiocytosis

Congenital

- Arteriovenous malformations (Osler-Weber-Rendu disease)

Miscellaneous

- Haematomas
- Pulmonary infarcts
- Occupational (silicosis)

Causes of an opaque hemithorax
Ipsilateral pathology

With mediastinum central or same side (ipsilateral volume loss)

- Lung aplasia/agenesis
- Lung hypoplasia
- Collapse/consolidation of lung/lobe
- Complete left lung collapse secondary to central obstructing tumour
- Central mucus plug(postoperative)
- Empyema with collapse/consolidation
- Post-pneumonectomy: elevated gastric bubble; leftward shift of mediastinum; surgical clips in the left hemithorax in the vicinity of the left main stem bronchus

With mediastinum pushed to opposite side

- Pleural fluid: large pleural effusion (often malignant); chylothorax; haemothorax; empyema
- Mesothelioma
- Diaphragmatic hernia (fluid-filled)
- Cystic hygroma
- Thoracic meningocoele
- Tumours

Contralateral pathology with mediastinal shift +/− compression

- Emphysema- congenital lobar; obstructive-secondary to tumour, foreign body
- Cystic adenomatoid malformation
- Tension pneumothorax
- Diaphragmatic hernia(air-filled)

Causes of unilateral elevation of the diaphragm

a. Causes above the diaphragm

Diminished pulmonary volume:
- Atelectasis
- Lobectomy

Phrenic nerve paralysis (paradoxical movement on bedside ultrasound)
Splinting of diaphragm, with rib fractures
Sub-pulmonic effusion
- Blunted posterior costo-phrenic sulcus
- A measurable distance between the stomach bubble and the inferior surface of the lung
- Usually demonstrable on a decubitus film

b. Diaphragmatic causes

Eventration of the diaphragm
Diaphragmatic masses

c. Causes below the diaphragm

Intra-abdominal process:
- Organomegaly
- Gaseous distension of the stomach or splenic flexure
- Subphrenic inflammatory disease: subphrenic abscess; liver or splenic abscess

Causes of focal contour abnormality of the diaphragm

- Hernia (hiatus hernia; foramen of Morgagni; foramen of Bochdalek; traumatic diaphragmatic rupture)
- Partial eventration
- Diaphragmatic tumours
- Basal pleural tumour
- Loculated sub-pulmonic effusion

Patterns of interstitial lung disease on chest x-ray

- Linear (due to thickening of interlobular septa)
- Kerley A lines: 2–6 cm long and <1 mm wide, radiating out from hilum towards pleura
- Kerley B lines: short (1–2 cm long) and 1–2 mm wide, perpendicular to lower lateral pleural edge
- Reticular (mesh-like network appearance): fine, medium, coarse
- Nodular (multiple discrete round opacities): military (1–2 mm), small, medium, large
- Reticulo-nodular

Diagnostic patterns in interstitial lung disease

- Predominantly lower lobe distribution, with reduced lung volumes: idiopathic pulmonary fibrosis, collagen vascular disease, asbestosis, chronic aspiration
- Reticulo-nodular pattern with increased lung volume: lymphangioleiomyomatosis, Langhans cell histiocytosis (multiple upper lobe nodules, many of which cavitate and are replaced by irregular thin-walled cysts of varying sizes)
- Predominantly upper and middle lobe distribution: mycobacterial and fungal disease, silicosis, sarcoidosis, extrinsic allergic alveolitis (hypersensitivity pneumonitis)

Interstitial lung disease checklist

- Natural history: acute (<3 weeks' symptoms), episodic, chronic
- Respiratory risk factors: smoking; family history of respiratory disease; occupational history (asbestos; coal mining); hobbies, travel, environmental exposure to organic antigens at home or work (including birds, pets); HIV risk factors
- Rheumatological symptoms: myalgia; arthralgia; proximal muscle weakness; Raynaud's phenomenon' morning stiffness
- Drug history
- Past medical history

Causes of diffuse interstitial lung disease

- Granulomatous lung disease: sarcoidosis; with vasculitis: eosinophilic granulomatosis with polyangiitis

- Connective tissue disease with lung involvement: rheumatoid arthritis; SLE; scleroderma; dermatomyositis and polymyositis
- Pulmonary infiltration with eosinophilia: allergic bronchopulmonary aspergillosis; tropical pulmonary eosinophilia; helminth infections
- Idiopathic pulmonary fibrosis
- Idiopathic interstitial pneumonias: idiopathic; non-specific; lymphoid; cryptogenic organizing pneumonia
- Drug induced pulmonary disease: antimicrobial agents (nitrofurantoin); cardiovascular drugs (amiodarone; ACE inhibitors; statins); disease-modifying anti-rheumatic drugs (methotrexate; sulphasalazine); cancer chemotherapeutic agents (bleomycin; selective EGFR inhibitors); recreational drugs (heroin; methadone)
- Inhalation secondary to occupational or environmental exposure: inorganic dusts (pneumoconioses-e.g. asbestosis; silicosis; berylliosis; coal dust); animal protein (bird proteins-exotic birds, chickens, pigeons); grain dust (farming); mould (showers; indoor hot tubs)

Causes of rib notching, on Inferior Surface

Arterial obstruction

- Coarctation of the aorta: 4th–8th ribs bilaterally
- Aortic thrombosis
- Subclavian obstruction: after Blalock-Taussig shunt for Tetralogy of Fallot
- Pulmonary oligaemia
- Takayasu's arteritis

Venous obstruction

- Superior vena caval obstruction

Arteriovenous

- Pulmonary arteriovenous malformation
- Chest wall arteriovenous malformation

Neurogenic

- Neurofibromatosis
- Normal variant

Musculoskeletal Emergencies

3

Causes of acute low back pain

Low back pain is usually benign, idiopathic and self-limited. A history of red flags is useful in identifying patients requiring further diagnostic workup, including blood tests and spinal imaging.

Structural

- Mechanical or non-specific musculo-ligamentous pain: usually increased by prolonged sitting or standing and relieved by movement.
- Facet joint arthritis or dysfunction
- Prolapsed intervertebral disc
- Disc degeneration/herniation
- Annular tear
- Spondylolysis or spondylolisthesis (break in the neck of Scottie dog appearance produced by superior facet (ear), pedicle (eye), ipsilateral inferior facet (front leg), ipsilateral transverse process (nose) and contralateral inferior facet (back leg))
- Spinal stenosis (central canal/lateral recess): bilateral neurogenic claudication; unilateral radicular symptoms (foraminal or lateral recess stenosis); cauda equina syndrome
- Fractures: osteoporosis; trauma
- Arachnoiditis: after surgery or injection of intrathecal radiological contrast media

Neoplasm

- Primary; multiple myeloma
- Secondary (metastatic)

Referred pain to spine

- Major viscera: pancreas (pancreatitis, pancreatic tumour); duodenum (peptic ulcer disease); colon; ovaries
- Retroperitoneal structures
- Urogenital system: prostatitis; renal calculi; ovarian cancer; endometrial cancer; pelvic inflammatory disease
- Aorta: Aortic dissection; aortic aneurysm; thrombosis
- Distant musculoskeletal pathology: hip arthropathy; trochanteric bursitis

Infection

- Septic disciitis
- Vertebral osteomyelitis
- Spinal epidural abscess (triad of fever, back pain and neurological deficit)
- Paraspinal abscess
- Tuberculosis of spine
- Herpes zoster (viral radiculopathy)

A. Banerjee, *Emergency Clinical Diagnosis*, DOI 10.1007/978-3-319-50718-7_3

Inflammatory

- Seronegative spondyloarthropathies: ankylosing spondylitis; psoriatic arthritis; Reiter's syndrome; inflammatory bowel disease
- Sacroiliitis or sacro-iliac dysfunction

Metabolic

- Osteoporotic vertebral collapse
- Paget's disease
- Osteomalacia
- Hyperparathyroidism

Vascular

- Epidural haematoma
- Spinal cord infarction
- Spinal arterio-venous malformation
- Spinal dural arterio-venous fistula

Renal

- Renal colic

Gastrointestinal

Pelvic organ pathology

- Prostatitis

Back pain 'red flags'
Age

- Initial onset at age < 16 or > 65 years
- Acute onset in an elderly person

Character and site of pain

- Bilateral or alternating symptoms; radiation of pain into both legs: central disc prolapse; tumour
- Constant or progressive pain
- Night pain; sleep disturbance
- Thoracic pain
- Pain and stiffness worst in morning (morning stiffness > 1 h): ankylosing spondylitis
- Pain worsened by walking and by spine hyperextension: spinal stenosis

Systemic symptoms

- Fever
- Night sweats
- Weight loss

Neurological abnormalities

- Neurological symptoms (bilateral lower limb numbness, saddle region numbness, urinary retention)
- Severe or progressive motor loss
- Radiation of pain into both legs: central disc prolapse; tumour
- Bladder/bowel dysfunction-sphincter disturbance: spinal stenosis; cauda equina syndrome

Past medical history

- History of malignancy
- Immunosuppression
- Current or recent infection
- Tuberculosis
- HIV positive
- Prolonged systemic corticosteroid use: compression fracture
- Intravenous drug use: infection

Red flags indicate the need for further investigation, which may include:

- Venous blood: full blood count, CRP, ESR, metabolic bone screen, myeloma screen
- Plain film radiology
- Specialised imaging: CT/MRI

Patterns of some back disorders
Predominantly back pain

Pain worse with flexion
- Disc prolapse
- Annular tear

Pain worse with extension and rotation
- Facet joint disorder

- Spondylolysis
- Localised buttock pain
- Sacro-iliac disorder

Predominantly leg pain

Claudicant pain eased by flexion, and worse with extension
- Spinal stenosis

Pain worse with flexion
- Disc prolapse

Progressive bilateral neurological deficit and sphincter disturbance
- Central disc prolapse
- Cauda equina compression
- Spinal cord compression
- Spinal vascular accident

Lumbar and sacral nerve root lesions

L2	Hip flexion; adduction
L3	Knee extension; **knee jerk**
L4	Knee extension, ankle dorsiflexion; **knee jerk**
L5	Foot inversion, great toe dorsiflexion, knee flexion
S1	Ankle plantar flexion, knee flexion ankle jerk

Signs of lumbar nerve root irritation

- Femoral nerve stretch test (L2-L4): with the patient in the prone position, the affected knee is maximally flexed (80–100°) passively; then with gentle extension, anterior thigh pain (L2, L3) or medial leg pain (L4) indicate a positive test
- Straight leg raising: with the patient in the supine position, the affected leg is passively lifted off the couch by the foot; when leg pain develops, the leg is lowered slightly and the ankle passively dorsiflexed; a positive test is indicated by the reproduction of radicular leg pain
- Crossed straight leg raising: passive elevation of the unaffected leg causes radicular pain in the affected limb

Features suggesting cauda equina compression (triad of acute bowel or bladder sphincter dysfunction, saddle anaesthesia and motor deficit in the lower limbs; incomplete syndromes, with variable bladder involvement may contribute to diagnostic difficulty)

- Bilateral sciatica
- Severe progressive bilateral lower limb neurological deficit, including major motor weakness (knee extension, ankle dorsiflexion)
- Recent onset of urine retention and/or incontinence, with loss of sensation when passing urine
- Recent onset of faecal incontinence, with loss of sensation of rectal fullness
- Perianal or perineal sensory loss (saddle anaesthesia or paraesthesiae)
- Unexpected laxity of anal sphincter
- Erectile dysfunction

Waddell's signs of non-organic back pain

- Superficial, diffuse and non-anatomical tenderness
- Pain with axial compression or loading and with simulated rotation of the spine
- Negative straight leg raising test with distraction; discrepancy between seated and supine straight leg raising
- Regional weakness or sensory changes
- Overreaction

Yellow flags for delayed recovery after acute low back pain

Avoidance of physical activity

Avoidance of domestic activities and responsibilities

Avoidance of social activities

Work aversion

Causes of sciatica

With radiculopathy, buttock and leg pain predominates over back pain and is worse with sitting, coughing, sneezing and the Valsalva manoeuvre

A discogenic or mechanical mechanism of pain leads to axial back pain, increased by prolonged sitting, standing, coughing, sneezing, and spinal flexion

- Disc prolapse
- Lumbar spinal stenosis (gradual onset of unilateral or bilateral leg pain in dermatomal distribution; neurogenic intermittent claudication)
- Degenerative disc disease
- Spondylolisthesis
- Piriformis syndrome (sciatic nerve compression by piriformis muscle)
- Pregnancy

Features of lumbar disc prolapse
The findings include:

- Loss of lumbar lordosis
- Lumbar scoliosis with the concavity toward the side of the lesion
- Restricted ipsilateral straight leg raising
- Sometimes restricted contralateral straight leg raising (cross-leg pain)
- Distal motor, sensory and reflex deficits dependent on the level of the lesion

Neurological features with disc prolapse
Lesions of the L3-L4 interspace involve the L4 nerve root:

- Reduced sensation in the anteromedial thigh
- Quadriceps weakness
- Reduced knee jerk

Lesions of the L4-L5 interspace involve the L5 nerve root:

- Reduced sensation in the 1st dorsal interdigital web space of the foot and lateral leg
- Weakness of extensor hallucis longus and tibialis anterior

Lesions of the L5-S1 interspace involve the S1 nerve root:

- Reduced sensation in the lateral heel and foot
- Weakness of gastrocnemius and soleus
- Reduction or loss of the ankle jerk

Lumbar disc syndromes

Root	Disc interspace	Reflex	Motor weakness	Sensory changes
L4	L3-L4	knee jerk	knee extension	Anterior thigh
L5	L4-L5	Hamstring jerk	Big toe dorsiflexion	Big toe
S1	L5-S1	Ankle jerk	Foot plantarflexion	Lateral border of foot

L5 dermatome
Lateral lower leg and web space of big toe

S1 dermatome
Back of calf and lateral foot

Myotomes

L2	Hip flexion
L3	Knee extension
L4	Foot dorsiflexion
L5	Big toe dorsiflexion
S1	Foot eversion
S2	Foot plantarflexion

Features of lumbar spinal stenosis

- Age > 50 years
- Back pain
- Cramping and pain in calves after walking short distances (neurogenic claudication)
- Pain eased by leaning forward or sitting or lying down, not by standing still
- Walking uphill is easier than walking downhill
- Bicycle riding, even over long distances, is easy
- Hyper-extension of the back produces pain
- Stiffness of the spine
- Normal straight leg raising
- Normal peripheral pulses
- Late nerve root signs

Features suggesting vertebral osteomyelitis or disciitis, with or without spinal extradural abscess

(the classic triad of fever, back pain and neurological deficit is often not seen in its entirety with early acute spinal infections)

- Focal back pain, of insidious onset and progressively increasing in severity, often worse at night
  - Systemic symptoms: anorexia, vomiting, lethargy, weight loss, variable presence of fever
  - Focal neurological symptoms: limb weakness and paraesthesiae; radicular pain; gait disturbance; bladder and bowel dysfunction
- Plain x-rays of the spine can be normal in the first 2–3 weeks of symptoms; contrast enhanced MRI scanning is required for the diagnosis

Risk factors for acute spinal infections

- Intravenous drug abuse
- Indwelling vascular device
- Recent invasive spinal procedure: epidural catheter
- Alcoholism
- Diabetes mellitus
- HIV/AIDS
- Immunosuppression
- Malignancy
- Adjacent soft tissue infection

Causes of acute inflammatory monoarthritis (red hot joint): septic until proven otherwise. Delayed recognition and treatment of septic arthritis can lead to rapid articular cartilage destruction, leading to loss of joint function.

- Septic arthritis: bacterial infection (Staphylococcus aureus; neisseria gonorrhoeae-triad of tenosynovitis, dermatitis and arthritis; salmonella-sickle cell disease); viral; fungal; spirochaetal (Lyme disease)
- Crystal synovitis: gout, pseudogout (calcium pyrophosphate arthropathy), calcific periarthritis
- Osteoarthritis
- Neuropathic arthropathy (Charcot's joint)
- Haemarthroses
- Reactive arthritis: signs of systemic illness; enthesopathy; conjunctivitis; skin and mucosal lesions; triad of seronegative arthropathy, urethritis and conjunctivitis
- Enteropathic arthritis; systemic autoimmune disease: SLE; sarcoidosis; infective endocarditis
- Traumatic synovitis
- Foreign body synovitis(e.g., plant thorn)
- Synovial disease: pigmented villondular synovitis; synovial osteochondromatosis
- Neuropathic arthropathy (Charcot's joint)
- Monoarticular presentation of polyarthropathy: rheumatoid arthritis; seronegative spondyloarthropathy (psoriatic arthropathy; ankylosing spondylitis)

Differential diagnosis

- Intra-articular fracture
- Bursitis

Organisms that trigger reactive arthritis include:

- Urogenital organisms: Chlamydia trachomatis; ureaplasma urealyticum
- Enterogenic organisms: Shigella flexneri; Salmonella species; Yersinia enterocolitica; Yersinia pseudotuberculosis; Campylobacter jejuni
- Miscellaneous: Clostridium difficile; Chlamydia pneumoniae; Borrelia burgdorferi; Streptococcus; Hepatitis C; Giardia lamblia; Mycoplasma

Risk factors for septic arthritis
Age > 60 years; infancy
Alcohol abuse
Chronic joint disease: degenerative joint disease (osteoarthritis); inflammatory arthritis

(rheumatoid arthritis); neurogenic arthropathy
Corticosteroid therapy
Diabetes mellitus
Intravenous drug abuse
Cytotoxic chemotherapy
Prosthetic joint
Previous intra-articular injection (steroids)
Recent joint surgery
Contiguous spread from skin infection or ulcer
Animal bites; plant thorn injuries

Causes of inflammatory arthropathy
Primary

- Connective tissue disease
  Rheumatoid arthritis
  Systemic lupus erythematous
  Polyarteritis nodosa
  Behcet's syndrome
  Polymyalgia rheumatica
  Progressive systemic sclerosis
- Sero-negative spondyloarthropathies
- Infection associated (reactive, post-infective, post vaccinial, rheumatic fever)
  Ankylosing spondylitis
  Psoriatic arthropathy
  Inflammatory bowel disease

Secondary

Infective: bacterial; viral; fungal
Crystal-induced: monosodium urate; calcium pyrophosphate; hydroxyapatite

Causes of hyperuricaemia (a normal serum urate does not exclude gout; an elevated serum urate does not confirm the diagnosis of gout; serum urate may be normal or low in the presence of an acute attack)

Primary hyperuricaemia
  Increased production of purine
  - Idiopathic
  - Specific enzyme defects: Lesch-Nyhan syndrome, glycogen storage disease

  Decreased renal clearance of uric acid: idiopathic

Secondary hyperuricaemia
  Increased catabolism and turnover of purine:
  - Myeloproliferative disorders
  - Lymphoproliferative disorders
  - Carcinoma and sarcoma (disseminated)
  - Chronic haemolytic anaemias
  - Cytotoxic drugs
  - Psoriasis

  Decreased renal clearance of uric acid:
  - Intrinsic renal disease
  - Functional impairment of tubular transport
    Drug-induced: thiazides, probenecid
    Lactic acidosis
    Ketoacidosis: diabetic ketoacidosis; starvation
    Diabetes insipidus
    Bartter's syndrome

Triggers of acute gout

- Alcohol excess
- High purine diet
- Drugs: thiazides
- Acute medical illness
- Exercise
- Trauma
- Fructose drink ingestion

Causes of polyarthropathy (involvement of more than four joints)

- Viral infections: rubella, mumps, human parvovirus (B19), enterovirus, adenovirus, Coxsackie virus (A9, B2, B3, B4, B6), varicella-zoster virus, HIV, Epstein-Barr virus; acute hepatitis B infection
- Indirect bacterial infections (reactive arthritis): Campylobacter, Chlamydia, Mycoplasma, Salmonella, Shigella, Group A streptococci (acute rheumatic fever), Neisseria gonorrheae, bacterial endocarditis

- Direct bacterial infections: Neisseria gonorrheae (disseminated gonococcal infection-fever, chills, malaise, polyarthropathy, tenosynovitis involving wrists, fingers, ankles and toes; vesiculo-pustular skin rash) ; Staphylococcus aureus; Gram negative bacilli
- Other infections: Borrelia burgdorferi (Lyme disease); Mycobacterium tuberculosis; fungal infections
- Seropositive arthropathies: rheumatoid arthritis
- Osteoarthritis
- Seronegative spondyloarthropathies: psoriatic arthritis; inflammatory bowel disease-enteropathic arthritis; Reiter's syndrome; ankylosing spondylitis
- Adult-onset Still's disease: arthopathy, myalgia, macular or maculo-papular skin rash, non-suppurative pharyngitis
- Crystal-induced synovitis: gout, pseudo-gout
- Connective tissue disease: SLE; PM-DM; scleroderma; MCTD; primary Sjogren's syndrome
- Metabolic bone disease: Paget's disease; osteomalacia
- Endocrine: hyperparathyroidism; hypothyroidism; hyperthyroidism
- Malignancy: metastatic cancer; multiple myeloma; hypertrophic pulmonary osteoarthropathy

Checklist for new onset polyarthropathy

- Symmetrical or asymmetrical distribution
- Pattern of involved joints: axial (spine, centrally located joints: sacroiliac, sternoclavicular, manubriosternal); peripheral (limbs)
- Evolution of joint involvement: migratory; additive; intermittent
- Inflammatory or mechanical arthropathy
- Systemic features
- Extra-articular manifestations: eyes; skin; mucosa; lungs; heart; muscles; central and peripheral nervous systems
- History of recent diarrhea, acute conjunctivitis, urethritis, and fever with or without skin rash (reactive arthritis)
- Family history
- Plain film pattern of joint involvement: synovial disease (soft tissue swelling; bone erosion involving articular cortex); articular cartilage involvement (loss of joint space; calcification of cartilage); enthesopathy (involvement of sites of insertion of capsule, ligament or tendon into bone)

Features of inflammatory arthritis

- Significant morning stiffness (>30 min)
- Pain better with movement
- Local signs of inflammation
- Palpable synovitis
- Systemic features: fever, malaise, weight loss

Plain x-ray signs of arthritis

- Inflammation: acute marginal erosions; juxta-articular osteoporosis; fusiform soft tissue swelling; concentric loss of articular cartilage with symmetrical narrowing of joint space
- Degeneration: osteophytes; subchondral sclerosis; eccentric loss of articular cartilage with asymmetrical narrowing of joint space; chondrocalcinosis (calcification of articular cartilage)
- Metabolic: irregular soft tissue swelling; chronic bony erosions with overhanging edges

Features of acute osteomyelitis

- Risk factors include penetrating trauma; intravenous drug use; sickle cell disease; foreign bodies; spread from adjacent foci of infection, including cellulitis and septic arthritis
- Localised erythema, swelling, warmth and tenderness related to the involved bone;

cellulitis in the metaphyseal region is suggestive of acute haematogenous osteomyelitis
- Effusion in the adjacent joint
- Limp and inability to walk
- Systemic symptoms: fever, lethargy, irritability
- Plain x-rays may show soft tissue swelling, with blurring or loss of normal fat planes, within 24–48 h of onset; periosteal reaction; lytic lesions in the bone may take 7–14 days to appear
- MRI is the best imaging modality for early detection

Diffuse aches and pains
Red flags:

- Age > 50 years: polymyalgia rheumatic; paraneoplastic syndromes
- Systemic symptoms inflammatory disease; vasculitis; sepsis; malignancy
- Weakness: myopathy; endocrine disorder
- New headache: temporal arteritis
- Stiffness after rest (gelling): inflammatory rheumatic disorder

Causes of generalised myalgia

- Inflammatory musculoskeletal disorders: rheumatoid arthritis; systemic lupus erythematosus; polymyalgia rheumatica; polymyositis-dermatomyositis; scleroderma
- Endocrine: thyroid disease; parathyroid disease; diabetes mellitus
- Drug induced: HMG CoA reductase inhibitors (statins); azathioprine; penicillamine
- Generalised soft tissue syndromes: fibromyalgia syndrome (widespread pain in all four quadrants of the body and in the axial skeleton lasting more than 3 months; myofascial trigger points)

Causes of rhabdomyolysis (myalgia, weakness and pigmenturia)

- Exertional rhabdomyolysis: intense physical exercise; status epilepticus; tetanus; delirium tremens
- Trauma with muscle ischaemia: crush syndrome; blast injury; high-voltage electrical injury; deep burns; compartment syndrome
- Metabolic: hyperglycaemic hyperosmolar states; chronic hypokalaemia; myopathies (myophosphorylase deficiency)
- Altered body temperature: hyperthermia; heat stroke; hypothermia
- Drugs and toxins: statins; neuromuscular blocking agents (neuroleptic malignant syndrome); serotonin reuptake inhibitors (serotonin syndrome); heavy metals; cocaine; alcohol
- Infections: bacterial pyomyositis
- Prolonged immobilization: alcohol/drug abuse; fall with prolonged lie (remaining on the ground for more than 1 h after a fall)
- Autoimmune muscle damage: polymyositis; dermatomyositis

Causes of neck pain

- Degenerative

Intervertebral disc and ligaments: cervical spondylosis (varying combinations of neck pain, radiculopathy and myelopathy); cervical disc prolapse (neck pain worsened by flexion; axial compression reproduces or exacerbates pain; associated with occipital headache)

Facet joints; osteoarthritis; osteoporosis

Spinal stenosis

- Infective/post-infective

Intervertebral disc: discitis

Meninges: meningitis; epidural abscess

Mucosal: acute pharyngitis

Nerve: herpes zoster

Soft tissue: acute cervical lymphadenitis; acute suppurative parotitis; Ludwig's angina; retropharyngeal abscess

- Inflammatory

Soft tissue

Facet joints: rheumatoid arthritis (can be complicated by atlantoaxial subluxation, basilar invagination or sub-axial subluxation); ankylosing spondylitis
Metabolic: crystal arthropathy
- Trauma: neck sprain; fracture

Causes of torticollis

- Trauma: muscle spasm; fracture/dislocation; spinal haematoma
- Infection: URTI; otitis media; mastoiditis; cervical lymphadenitis; retropharyngeal abscess
- Atlanto-axial rotary fixation: trauma; pharyngeal infection (Grisel's syndrome of atalanto-axial subluxation related to prevertebral inflammation)
- Inflammation: rheumatoid arthritis
- Neoplasm: CNS tumours; bone tumours
- Dystonic syndromes: drug reactions
- Ocular dysfunction

Causes of upper limb pain

- Cervical radiculopathy: occipital headache, trapezial or inter-scapular pain, neck pain, unilateral arm pain, dermatomal tingling and numbness, and weakness (C5: weak shoulder abduction; C6: weak elbow flexion and wrist extension; C7: weak elbow extension and wrist flexion; C8: weak thumb extension and wrist ulnar deviation)
- Compression syndromes (entrapment neuropathies): carpal tunnel syndrome; thoracic outlet syndrome
- Acute brachial plexitis (neuralgic amyotrophy; Parsonage-Turner syndrome): sudden onset of severe burning pain in the shoulder, neck and/or arm; followed by rapid multi-focal lower motor neurone weakness and atrophy of peri-scapular and peri-glenohumeral muscles as the pain subsides; occurs in the third to seventh decades, with a male preponderance; pain resolves in 1–3 weeks
- Musculo-tendinous syndromes: tendons-rotator cuff tendonitis; joint capsule; ligament attachments
- Myofascial pain syndrome: multiple trigger points

Causes of cervical myelopathy and/or radiculopathy

Extradural: cervical spine degenerative disk (spondylotic myelopathy); vertebral collapse (metastases; tuberculosis); traumatic vertebral fracture-dislocation; cranio-cervical junction anomalies (ankylosing spondylitis; rheumatoid arthritis; Paget's disease)

Intradural, extramedullary: meningioma; neurofibroma; epidural abscess

Intramedullary: tumour (ependymoma, glioma, haemangioblastoma); vascular lesions (spinal arterio-venous malformations, anterior spinal artery occlusion); inflammation (MS; ADEM; SLE; neurosarcoidosis); nutritional (subacute combined degeneration of spinal cord; lathyrism); post-radiation myelopathy; HIV/AIDS vacuolar myelopathy

Features of cervical myelopathy

- Gait disturbance, related to incoordination
- Clumsiness or weakness of the hands, with reduced manual dexterity
- Bladder and/or bowel dysfunction
- Upper motor neuron signs in the upper limbs
- Upper motor neuron signs in the lower limbs
- Lower motor neuron signs in the upper limbs
- Positive Lhermitte's sign: passive neck flexion causes electric shock-like sensations radiating down the spine and into the limbs

Causes of acute shoulder pain

Intrinsic

Peri-articular:

Rotator cuff tear: partial or complete (pain on elevation of arm above the horizontal plane; night pain; loss of power)
Subacromial impingement syndrome: rotator cuff tendinopathy; subacromial bursitis (pain worsened by overhead activity; night pain, causing sleep disturbance and made worse on lying on affected side; painful arc of movement on forward elevation of arm 60–120°)
Acute calcific tendonitis: acute severe shoulder pain worsened by arm elevation or by lying on the affected side; calcific deposits in rotator cuff visible on plain x-ray
Proximal biceps rupture/subluxation
Bicipital tendonitis

Gleno-humeral:
Glenoidal labral tears (pain with overhead activity, often associated with a painful clicking or snapping sensation in the shoulder, and glenohumeral joint line tenderness)
Gleno-humeral arthritis: osteoarthritis; inflammatory arthritis
Adhesive capsulitis: restricted active and passive ranges of movement
Multi-directional gleno-humeral instability (sulcus sign: prominent depression below the lateral aspect of the acromion process with inferior traction applied to the wrist, with the arm extended)
Osteonecrosis

Referred pain

Neck: cervical spondylosis, cervical radiculopathy; cervical disc disease
Chest: myocardial ischaemia; thoracic outlet syndrome; Pancoast tumour
Abdomen: diaphragmatic irritation; splenic trauma; subphrenic abscess; gall bladder disease

Neurological

Brachial plexitis (Parsonage-Turner syndrome)
Suprascapular neuropathy
Remote compression neuropathies: carpal tunnel syndrome; cubital tunnel syndrome

Features of subacromial impingement syndrome (A syndrome of shoulder pain provoked by abduction and elevation of the arm, caused by forced elevation of the humeral head against the coraco-acromial arch, usually the result of chronic repetitive microtrauma to the rotator cuff).

Features include:
Anterior shoulder pain referred to the lateral upper arm, and exacerbated by forward flexion, internal rotation and abduction
Rest pain, including night pain
Reversal of scapulo-humeral rhythm with hunching of the shoulder at the beginning of abduction
A painful arc of movement in the mid-range of abduction (60–120°)
Tenderness beneath the lateral edge of the acromion process

Features of major tear of the rotator cuff

Usually the result of acute trauma superimposed on chronic repetitive trauma

Commoner in males (10:1) over the age of 40

The mechanism is one of lifting or forced external rotation of the shoulder

The features include:

Sudden onset of shoulder pain
Pain on shoulder movement, especially overhead activities
Night pain, interfering with sleep
Pain on lying on the affected shoulder
Irregular scapulohumeral movement with active abduction of the shoulder, with initial hunching of the shoulder (deltoid action)
Point tenderness over the greater tuberosity of humerus
The passive range of glenohumeral abduction is greater than the active range
Incomplete and weak lateral rotation of the shoulder

Abolition of pain by the subacromial injection of local anaesthetic (10 ml of 1% lignocaine) does not improve the active range of movement; if local anaesthetic injection restores voluntary active abduction, a major cuff lesion is unlikely
A palpable gap in the rotator cuff is rarely felt
With chronic injuries, atrophy of the supraspinatus and infraspinatus muscles occurs

Inconsistent clinical features include:

The drop arm sign: the passively abducted arm cannot be held up actively and drops with gravity
The abduction paradox: the arm lifted above 90° can be held up by the action of the deltoid
X-rays may show a reduced acromio-humeral distance (<2 mm); in chronic tears, changes of cuff arthropathy may be seen, with sclerosis, subchondral cysts, osteolysis and notching of the greater tuberosity of the humerus and sclerosis, faceting or concavity in the inferolateral aspect of the acromion

Features of acute calcific tendinitis

- Abrupt onset of well localised shoulder pain
- No preceding trauma
- Severe pain, disrupting all shoulder function and preventing sleep
- Localised point of maximum tenderness in the area of the supraspinatus attachment to the greater tuberosity
- Marked reflex spasm of all muscles around shoulder
- Benign and self-limiting condition
- Calcific deposit on under-penetrated X-ray

Features of clavicle fractures
Caused by a fall on or direct impact to the point of shoulder and clavicle, or by a fall on the outstretched hand

The affected elbow is supported in the opposite hand

Local bruising, swelling, tenderness and crepitus

Palpable step at the fracture site

Anterior, inferior and medial displacement of the shoulder in mid-clavicular fractures

Reduced range of active shoulder movement

Delayed bruising in the supraclavicular and infraclavicular regions of the chest wall 12–36 h post-injury

Pressure necrosis of the skin may occur

Associated injuries to the chest, brachial plexus, and major vessels may be present

Features of fractures of the clavicle requiring early referral for consideration of operative treatment
Open fractures
Neurovascular compromise
Compromise of overlying skin (threatened viability with impending skin necrosis)
Floating shoulder: ipsilateral fracture of the clavicle (or acromio-clavicular separation) associated with an extra-articular fracture of the glenoid neck
Type II distal third fractures (ruptured coracoclavicular ligaments), with superior displacement of the proximal fragment by trapezius and sternomastoid muscles
Scapulo thoracic dissociation

Features of osteolysis of the distal clavicle This can either represent an overuse injury from repetitive microtrauma (in weightlifting or repetitive bench press or push-ups) or can be a sequel of injury to the distal clavicle or acromioclavicular joint

- Activity related local discomfort at the acromio-clavicular joint is associated with tenderness on palpation of the distal clavicle
- Pain is increased by shoulder adduction
- X-rays may show osteoporosis, osteolysis, tapering, cystic changes and osteophyte formation involving the distal clavicle

Checklist for shoulder x-rays after trauma

- The humeral head should be within the glenoid cavity on AP, axillary lateral,

trans-scapular lateral (Y) and apical oblique views. The acromion process and spine of the scapula (posteriorly) and the coracoid process (anteriorly) form the upper arms of a Y shape, with the body of the scapula forming the vertical portion of the Y, in the trans-scapular view, with the humeral head centred to the middle of the Y. The glenoid fossa lies at the intersection of the three limbs of the Y. In anterior dislocations of the shoulder the humeral head lies anterior to the glenoid fossa, and in posterior dislocations it lies posterior to the glenoid fossa.
- The articular surfaces of the humeral head and the glenoid should be parallel, with an even joint space
- Inferior subluxation (pseudo-subluxation) of the humeral head is due to glenohumeral joint capsule distension by haemarthrosis and reflex inhibition of the deltoid muscle

Shoulder dislocations

Acute anterior dislocation of the shoulder

The features include:

- Caused by either direct or indirect trauma, with forced abduction and external rotation of the arm
- Acute severe shoulder pain with functional loss in the upper limb
- The limb is often held supported by the uninjured upper limb
- The arm is held abducted and externally rotated
- There is flattening of the lateral aspect of the shoulder, with loss of deltoid muscle contour
- The acromion process appears prominent
- A subacromial indentation is palpable owing to absence of the humeral head
- Anterior fullness is present, and the humeral head may be palpable anteriorly below the coracoid process

Open reduction is indicated with:

Coexistent fracture of humeral neck

Fracture of the glenoid with over 30% articular surface involvement

Fracture of the greater tuberosity of the humerus with persistent displacement greater than 1 cm after successful relocation of the humeral head

Acute posterior dislocation of the shoulder

The features include:

- Caused by a fall on the outstretched hand with the arm in abduction, direct trauma to the shoulder, or seizures or electric shocks causing violent muscular contraction
- Acute severe shoulder pain
- The arm is held adducted and internally rotated
- External rotation and abduction are grossly impaired and painful
- The coracoid process appears prominent
- Posterior fullness may be noticeable
- The anterior aspect of the shoulder may appear flattened

AP x-rays reveal:

- Cystic(light bulb) sign: Apparent translucency of the humeral head due to marked internal rotation
- Empty glenoid sign: Absence of the elliptical half-moon overlap shadow of the humeral head and glenoid
- Positive rim sign: The space between the anterior glenoid rim and the humeral head is greater than 6 mm.
- Reverse Hill-Sachs lesion: An anteromedial humeral head impaction fracture may be noted.
- Axillary views are confirmatory, but may be difficult to obtain owing to pain.

Features of recurrent gleno-humeral subluxation

- Transient anterior subluxation of the humeral head is associated with transient loss of shoulder function and the sensation of the arm going dead ("paralysing pain" or dead arm syndrome)

- The arm may feel insecure in the cocking phase of the throwing motion(with external rotation and abduction of the shoulder)
- Apprehension is demonstrable with attempted passive external rotation of the abducted arm, the arm being abducted 90° at the shoulder and flexed 90° at the elbow, when posterior pressure is applied to the humeral head.

Recurrent anterior dislocation of the shoulder-predisposing anatomical defects

Capsular lesions

Detachment of the fibrocartilaginous labrum or of the capsule from the anterior glenoid rim (Bankart lesion)

Excessive anterior capsular laxity

Bony lesions

Posterolateral impaction defect of the humeral head (Hill-Sachs lesion)

Glenoid rim fracture

Excessive anterior tilt of the glenoid and excessive retroversion of the humeral head

Features of inferior dislocation of the shoulder (luxatio erecta)

- Caused by hyperabduction of the shoulder or by application of a direct axial force to a fully abducted arm
- The arm is locked in 110–160° of abduction and forward elevation
- The humeral head is palpable on the lateral chest wall and axilla
- On x-rays, the humeral head is subcoracoid in position, with a parallel humeral shaft and a parallel scapular spine

Features of acromio-clavicular joint injuries

- Usually due to direct trauma to the point of the shoulder but can also be caused by indirect trauma from falling on the outstretched hand
- Point tenderness over the acromio-clavicular joint
- Prominence of the lateral end of the clavicle, causing a step deformity at the acromio-clavicular joint, suggests rupture of the acromio-clavicular and coraco-clavicular (conoid and trapezoid) ligaments
- Pain is increased by moving the arm across the body, with overhead activities, lifting, and lying on the involved side

Features of sterno-clavicular joint dislocation

- Anterior: pain localised to joint, tenderness, ecchymosis, and an obvious bony prominence of the clavicular head; no neurovascular compromise; caused by a direct lateral blow to the shoulder with the shoulder extended. On an AP view of the chest there is asymmetry of clavicle length and abnormality of the sterno-clavicular joint
- Posterior: often no obvious deformity, or may be a depression or step deformity between the sternal end of the clavicle and the manubrium of the sternum; dyspnoea, dysphagia, odynophagia, hoarseness; signs of venous congestion, arterial insufficiency or brachial plexopathy involving the ipsilateral upper limb; caused by either indirect trauma to the shoulder girdle region with the shoulder adducted and flexed, or a direct posterior blow to the medial clavicle

Features of scapula fracture

- Shoulder and back pain, swelling, bruising and crepitus
- Arm adducted and protected against motion at the shoulder
- Loss of active abduction and forward extension of the arm (pseudo-paralysis of the rotator cuff) from intramuscular haemorrhage and pain
- Often associated with rib fractures, lung injuries, brachial plexus injuries, vascular injuries

- The fracture can be obscured on x-rays by the ribs and clavicle
- Avulsion fractures can occur at the insertion of the serratus anterior muscle along the inferior angle of the scapula causing winging of the scapula, the insertion of the triceps muscle at the infraglenoid tubercle, the deltoid insertion at the acromion process, the coracoclavicular ligament insertion at the coracoid tubercle, and the insertion of the short head of the biceps and coracobrachialis at the tip of the coracoid process

Features of scapulothoracic dissociation

High-energy trauma

Massive swelling over the shoulder girdle

Associated with brachial plexus, subclavian and axillary artery injuries; may lead to a pulseless and flail upper limb

Closed lateral displacement of the affected shoulder girdle

On AP chest x-ray, increased distance from sternal notch to medial border of scapula. The scapula on the abnormal side is 1–3 cm. farther from the midline than on the normal side (spinous processes of vertebrae to medial border of scapula on a non-rotated chest x-ray with the upper limbs positioned symmetrically). There may be associated with clavicle fracture, grade 3 acromioclavicular joint injury, sternoclavicular dislocation

Features of intrathoracic dislocation of scapula

- Direct blunt trauma to posterior chest wall
- Entrapment of inferior angle of scapula between 3rd and 4th ribs or 4th and 5th intercostal space

Brachial plexus injuries (ventral primary rami of C5-T1; comprising five major components proximal to distal: 5 roots, 3 trunks, 2 divisions, 3 cords and branches)

Causes
- High speed vehicular accidents, especially involving motorcycles
- Hyperabduction of arm
- Traction injuries involving depression of the ipsilateral shoulder with simultaneous contralateral neck deviation
- Hyperextension of the neck during ipsilateral side bending and/or rotation
- Direct blow to the brachial plexus in the supraclavicular region

Features suggesting pre-ganglionic root injury (proximal to dorsal root ganglion)
- Horner's syndrome
- Winged scapula (paralysis of serratus anterior)
- Flail arm
- Paralysis of spinati and latissimus dorsi (parascapular muscles)
- Phrenic nerve paralysis: elevated paralysed hemidiaphragm on chest x-ray
- Absence of Tinel sign (distal tingling on percussion) in neck area

Evaluation of brachial plexus injury includes assessment of

- Back: rhomboids; serratus anterior (scapula winging); latissimus dorsi; trapezius
- Shoulder: deltoid (C5); supraspinatus and infraspinatus (C5)
- Arm: biceps, wrist extensors (C6); triceps, wrist flexors (C7)
- Forearm: forearm extensors (C7)
- Hand (C8,T1)
- Sensory testing: C5 (lateral arm and forearm); C6 (thumb): C7 (middle finger); C8(little finger); T1 (medial forearm)

Checklist for humeral fractures

- Proximal humeral fractures: associated glenohumeral dislocation; axillary nerve paralysis; brachial plexus trauma; axillary artery injury
  - Humeral shaft fractures: radial nerve paralysis

- Distal humeral fractures: radial, median and ulnar nerve paralysis; forearm compartment syndrome

Features of proximal humeral fractures

Commonest in elderly post-menopausal women in association with osteoporosis, caused by a fall from standing height onto the outstretched hand, a direct blow to the lateral aspect of the shoulder or an axial load transmitted through the elbow.

In patients under the age of 40 years, high energy injuries (motor vehicle collisions, athletic injuries, and falls from a height) are causative

The proximal humerus is considered as having four parts for the purposes of fracture classification: humeral head, greater tuberosity, lesser tuberosity and humeral shaft. The majority of fractures are one-part (undisplaced or minimally displaced) fractures.

Pain, swelling and tenderness in the shoulder, associated with marked restriction of shoulder movement. Significant fracture displacement or dislocation may be masked by the deltoid and soft tissue.

Extensive delayed gravitational bruising distally in the arm, elbow and forearm, also spreading to the chest wall and breast area, 24–48 h post-injury

Distal neurovascular deficit may be present, especially in the axillary nerve distribution, as tested by sensation in the lateral aspect of the proximal arm overlying the deltoid. Brachial plexus injury may coexist. An expanding haematoma may indicate axillary artery injury.

Deltoid atony, which resolves within 3–4 weeks of injury, may lead to inferior subluxation of the humeral head on an AP view

In children, proximal humeral epiphyseal injuries are usually Salter-Harris type I or II injuries; Salter I injuries are seen in children less than 5 years old, metaphyseal fractures in children aged 5–11 years, and Salter II injuries in children older than 11 years

Features of subluxation of the tendon of the long head of the biceps

- Caused by resisted abduction and external rotation of the arm
- Pain, a snapping sensation and crepitation in the anterior shoulder
- Point tenderness over the bicipital groove, between the greater and lesser tuberosities of the humerus

Features of humeral shaft fractures

- Presents with arm pain, swelling and deformity
- Direct trauma to the upper arm causes a transverse fracture
- Indirect trauma, from a fall or a twisting injury (e.g. arm wrestling; overhead throwing sports) leads to a spiral or oblique fracture
- Holstein-Lewis fracture is an oblique or spiral fracture of the distal 1/3rd of the humeral shaft, with neurapraxia of the radial nerve, which is injured in the spiral groove of the humerus between the lateral and medial heads of the triceps

Features of rupture of long head of biceps tendon

A sharp snap, followed by pain and bruising

Typical hollowing in the upper arm

The muscle belly retracts to the middle third of the arm on forearm supination and elbow flexion against resistance, producing a lump at mid-biceps level (Popeye sign)

There is little loss of power, as the short head of biceps, brachialis, and forearm flexors produce near normal elbow flexion

Features of supracondylar fractures of the humerus

Most commonly due to a fall on the outstretched non-dominant hand causing elbow hyperextension, leading to fracture of the anterior humeral cortex, with posterior angulation/displacement of the distal humeral fragment

Flexion type fractures are caused by direct impact on the flexed elbow

Can be associated with nerve injury (median, ulnar and/or radial) and vascular injury. The hand may be well perfused even in the absence of a palpable radial and/or ulnar pulse through the extensive collateral circulation around the elbow

There are three main types of displacement with supracondylar fractures of the humerus

Loss of the normal anterior tilt of the distal end of the humerus

Normally the distal end of the humerus forms an angle of 140° with the humeral shaft. A line drawn along the anterior humeral cortex, and extending through the elbow joint in the lateral projection, passes through the middle of the capitellum

Posterior displacement of the distal fragment, with medial or lateral shift, and usually some medial or lateral angulation

Projection of the distal end of the humeral shaft through the deep fascia after buttonholing through the brachialis muscle is associated with bruising in the antecubital fossa, and may indicate difficult reduction from soft tissue interposition

With marked posterior displacement of the distal fragment, the neurovascular bundle is stretched over the distal end of the shaft fragment

Features of fractures of the lateral condyle of the humerus

- Salter-Harris type IV injuries
- Usually occur between the ages of 4 and 10 years
- Caused by a varus force on the extended elbow and supinated forearm, associated with a fall on the outstretched hand, and causing avulsion of the lateral condylar epiphysis via the lateral collateral ligament complex attached to the forearm extensor muscles
- Lateral elbow swelling and tenderness
- The fracture fragments are primarily cartilaginous making fracture visualisation difficult; a small avulsion fragment may represent a large osteochondral avulsion fracture
- Failure of recognition can lead to non-union, late displacement, and malunion with cubitus varus, associated with tardy ulnar palsy

Features of fractures of the medial epicondyle of the humerus

- Avulsion injuries caused by a fall on the outstretched hand causing acute valgus stress to the elbow that produces traction on the medial epicondyle through the flexor muscles
- Usually occur between the ages of 7 and 15 years
- Swelling and bruising along the medial elbow
- Can be associated with posterior elbow dislocation, with interposition of the avulsed medial epicondyle between the distal articular surface of the humerus and the olecranon leading to entrapment in the elbow joint, often following reduction. With intra-articular entrapment there is a mechanical block to elbow extension.
- Visualisation of the medial epicondyle on a lateral x-ray of the elbow indicates entrapment within the joint

Features of trans-physeal fractures of the distal humerus

- Caused by a fall on the outstretched hand or by rotary or shearing force
- Occurs in children under the age of 2 years
- The relationship of the radial head and capitellum is preserved

Features of intercondylar T or Y fractures

- Intra-articular fractures of the distal humerus

- Caused by a fall on the outstretched hand or a direct blow to the flexed elbow
- The coronoid process of the ulna is wedged in the trochlear groove of the humerus. The central vertical intercondylar split extends proximally through both medial and lateral condyles in the form of a T or a Y. Three fragments are formed: the humeral shaft, medial condyle and lateral condyle. Marked comminution is common.
- The normal three point bony relationship between the oleocranon, medial epicondyle and lateral epicondyle is lost

Features of fractures of the capitellum

- Caused by shearing forces transmitted by the radial head after a fall on the outstretched hand
  - The fragment is displaced proximally and typically rotated 90°, with the convex articular surface facing ventrally
  - A bone fragment above the radial head on the lateral view may indicate a capitellar fracture

Evaluation of the elbow x-ray

Checklist for alignment on lateral elbow x-ray

- The anterior humeral line intersects the capitellum; a line along the anterior humeral cortex should intersect the middle third of the capitellum. If the centre of the capitellum is posterior to the line, an extension type supracondylar fracture is likely; if it is anterior to the line, a flexion type supracondylar fracture is likely.
- The radius should point to the capitellum in all views; the radiocapitellar line drawn through the centre of the radial neck should pass through the capitellum in all views, from full flexion to full extension
- The humeral-capitellar angle (Baumann's angle) is in valgus; the angle is formed by a line through the long axis of the humerus, and a line through the coronal axis of the epiphysis of the capitellum
- The distal end of the humeus is tilted anteriorly 30–40°

Checklist for joint effusion/haemarthrosis on lateral elbow x-ray

- The anterior fat pad (comprised of fat in the coronoid and radial fossae) is a small triangular radiolucent shadow anterior to the distal humerus; with an effusion it is displaced superiorly and anteriorly (sail sign)
- The posterior fat pad is not normally seen. With effusion, it is lifted out of the olecranon fossa and is visible as a radiolucent shadow posterior to the distal humerus

Ossification centres around the elbow joint

- Six in number
- The order of appearance is given by the mnemonic CRITOE: capitellum; radial head; internal or medial epicondyle; trochlea; oleocranon; external or lateral epicondyle
- The general guide to appearance of these ossification centres is 1-3-5-7-9-11 years

Injuries that can be missed on a paediatric elbow x-ray (the acronym **TRASH**-The Radiological Appearance Seemed Harmless-has been applied to some of these lesions)

- Minimally displaced supracondylar fracture
- Fracture of the lateral condyle
- Isolated dislocation of the radial head (pseudo-Monteggia lesion; plasticity of the ulna allows transient bowing without progression to fracture)
- Anterior compression fracture of the cartilaginous head leading to posterior suluxation of the radial head
- Medial epicondyle entrapment within the elbow joint
- Displaced medial condyle fractures

- Intra-articular osteochondral fractures of the elbow: oleocranon, radial head, trochlea, capitellum, and trochlea

Causes of elbow pain

Lateral: lateral epicondylitis (point tenderness over lateral epicondyle, pain increased with wrist dorsiflexion, painful grip); radiohumeral joint synovitis; osteochondritis dissecans-capitellum/radius; loose bodies secondary to radio-capitellar overload syndrome; posterior interosseous nerve entrapment (radial tunnel syndrome); radio-humeral bursitis
Medial: medial epicondylitis; flexor-pronator tendonitis (golfer's elbow) or rupture; ulnar neuritis
Posterior: oleocranon bursitis; olecranon stress fracture; traction apophysitis; triceps tendonitis; triceps rupture
Anterior: bicipital tendonitis; biceps rupture; ectopic bone; pronator teres syndrome
Referred: neck (cervical disc disease; cervical radiculopathy); shoulder; distal (carpal tunnel syndrome)

The features of lateral epicondylitis (tennis elbow) include:

- Lateral elbow pain, worsened by resisted wrist dorsiflexion with the elbow extended and the forearm pronated, by passive elbow extension with the wrist palmar flexed and the forearm pronated, and by resisted dorsiflexion of the middle finger
- Impaired grip

Features of radial tunnel syndrome (A syndrome of lateral elbow pain that may present as refractory lateral epicondylitis, which may be produced by repetitive forearm rotation, as in rowing)

- Forearm pain often predominates
- Tenderness 4–5 cm distal to the lateral epicondyle of the humerus.
- Pain is increased by resisted middle finger extension with the elbow extended, by resisted supination of the extended forearm, or by forearm pronation and wrist flexion (arch of Frohse compression)
- Sleep disturbance may be produced by pain

Features of medial epicondylitis (flexor-pronator tendinitis) (golfers' elbow) (An overuse syndrome associated with throwing sports)

Medial elbow pain, increased by resisted wrist palmar flexion with the forearm pronated, and by passive wrist and finger extension causing stretch of the wrist flexors
Tenderness overlying the common flexor origin at the medial epicondyle
A full range of elbow movement
Tenderness of the volar forearm musculature

Features of triceps tendinitis (overuse injury caused by repetitive overhead activity in the presence of full active elbow extension, associated with throwing and racquet sports)

- Posterior elbow pain
- Pain on resisted elbow extension and on passive elbow flexion
- Thickening and tenderness of the triceps tendon in the region of its insertion into the oleocranon process.
- Traction osteophytes or fractures of the tip of the oleocranon may coexist.

Oleocranon bursitis
Causes include:

Chronic repetitive frictional trauma with direct pressure on the oleocranon
Acute blunt trauma with bleeding into the bursa, e.g. from a fall onto the tip of the flexed elbow.

The features include:

A well circumscribed fluctuant swelling overlying the oleocranon process
No effusion in the elbow joint

Full range of elbow movement

If complicated by skin abrasions septic bursitis may ensue, with intense local inflammation and systemic symptoms

X-rays are usually normal or non-contributory but may show a bone spur related to the oleocranon

Sterile aspiration of the bursa yields fluid which can be tested for cells, crystals and cultured if septic bursitis is clinically suspected

Elbow problems secondary to repetitive throwing activities

These can be classified according to the mechanism and site of injury, and are usually the result of valgus stress.

- Medial tension overload leading to extra-articular injury
  - Flexor/pronator tendonitis (medial epicondylitis)
  - Ulnar collateral ligament sprain
  - Recurrent subluxation of the ulnar nerve from the post-condylar groove
  - Ulnar neuritis
  - Avulsion fracture of the medial epicondyle
  - Medial epicondyle apophysitis
- Lateral compression overload leading to intra-articular injury
  - Capitellar osteochondrosis (Panner's disease): flattening, fragmentation and lucency of the capitellar epiphysis; settles with epiphyseal fusion
  - Osteochondritis dissecans of the capitellum, with or without loose bodies
  - Radial head deformity
  - Degenerative joint disease
- Posterior extension and shear overload
  - Osteochondrosis of the oleocranon
- Avulsion of the oleocranon

Elbow dislocation

Mechanisms of posterior or posterolateral dislocation (80–90% of all elbow dislocations)

- Hyperextension injury; fall on to an extended elbow
- Valgus loading, supination and axial forces applied to a slightly flexed elbow from a fall on the outstretched hand

Features

- Pain, swelling and deformity of the elbow, held in partial flexion
- Loss of normal relationship of epicondyles to the oleocranon tip
- Posterior dislocation: apparent shortening of forearm; elbow fixed in 45° of flexion
- Medial and lateral dislocations: elbow appears wider than normal; some active and passive elbow extension may be possible
- Anterior dislocation: elbow fixed in extension; forearm usually supinated; capitellum and trochlea palpable posteriorly
- Spontaneous reduction is common; the x-ray may show signs of antecedent dislocation, such as coronoid process avulsion, medial epicondyle avulsion, or radial epiphyseal fracture.
- Complex dislocations include divergent and convergent dislocations
- Divergent dislocation (posterior dislocation of the elbow, associated with a transverse divergent dislocation of the proximal radius and ulna at the proximal radioulnar joint): forearm appears shortened; elbow fixed in varying degrees of flexion
- Convergent dislocation is associated with translocation of the proximal radius and ulna at the proximal radioulnar joint

Features of pulled elbow (nursemaid's elbow)

- Caused by a pulled arm (longitudinal traction force on the extended, pronated forearm) in pre-school children, under the age of 6 years, with key incidence in the 2–4 year age group
- The radial head subluxes out of the annular ligament, which is interposed in the radio-capitellar joint

- The arm is held with the elbow slightly flexed and the forearm pronated
- No swelling, deformity or tenderness
- There is refusal to use the involved upper limb (pseudo-paralysis) and active supination of the forearm is resisted
- Normal x-rays; x-rays are usually not required
- Rapid forearm supination with the elbow held in flexion is curative; alternatively, hyperpronation of the forearm with the elbow held in extension may be performed

Components of the terrible triad of the elbow: unstable elbow

- Elbow dislocation
- Coronoid process fracture
- Radial head fracture

Features of oleocranon fracture

- Caused by direct trauma or a fall on the outstretched hand with the elbow extended and the forearm rotated; a fall on the point of the elbow or direct trauma can lead to a comminuted fracture
- Posterior elbow pain, bruising and swelling; abrasions over point of elbow
- Palpable gap at fracture site, and loss of active elbow extension against gravity, with displaced fracture causing disruption of triceps mechanism
- The majority of fractures are intra-articular, leading to an elbow effusion
- A fall on the outstretched hand accompanied by sudden contraction of the triceps leads to a transverse or oblique fracture

Features of radial head and neck fractures

- Pain and swelling of the elbow; pain may be referred into the forearm and wrist
- Point tenderness over the radial head
- Lack of full elbow extension
- Restricted forearm supination and pronation
- The injury mechanism is usually a fall forward on the outstretched hand with the elbow extended and forearm pronated, leading to radial head impaction against the capitellum
- X-ray appearances of undisplaced radial head fractures include a vertical radiolucency, cortical disruption, cortical step or abrupt angulation, and a double cortical line.
- Comminuted radial head fractures, caused by axial loading of the forearm from fall from a height or a fall on the outstretched hand, may be associated with subluxation or proximal migration at the distal radioulnar joint and rupture of the interosseous membrane (Essex-Lopresti fracture)

Features of fractures of the radius and ulna

- Caused by a fall on the outstretched hand with axial, rotational and/or bending forces to the radius and ulna
- Pain, swelling, tenderness and deformity of the forearm
- Limited forearm rotation

Radius and ulna x-rays

- True AP and lateral x-rays should be obtained of the forearm, including the elbow and wrist joints
- Both radius and ulna should be visualized along their entire lengths
- The normal ulna is straight and the normal radius is bowed
- On an AP projection, the radial styloid lies 180° opposite the bicipital tuberosity
- On a lateral projection, the ulnar styloid lies 180° opposite the coronoid process

Checklist for radius and ulna fractures

- Perfusion of the fingers
- Signs of forearm compartment syndrome: pain on finger extension; marked swelling
- Status of radial (including posterior interosseous), median (including anterior interosseous), and ulnar nerves
- Monteggia fracture: fracture of proximal ulnar shaft with dislocation of radial

head, which can be anterior (type I), posterior (type II) or lateral (type III); caused by forced pronation of the forearm associated with a fall on the outstretched hand with the elbow flexed, or by direct trauma. An isolated fracture of the ulna with angulation or overriding should draw attention to the possibility of radial head dislocation.
- Galeazzi fracture: fracture of distal radius with distal radio-ulnar joint dislocation; caused by a fall on the outstretched hand, with the forearm forcibly pronated and the wrist in extension
- Essex-Lopresti lesion: radial head fracture, distal radio-ulnar dislocation and disruption of interosseous membrane

Features of plastic deformation (traumatic bowing) of the forearm

- Usually affects children under the age of 10 years
- May involve the ulna and/or radius
- There is little swelling or bruising, but limited forearm rotation with pronation or supination
- No disruption of the cortex or periosteum
- Causes a fixed abnormal curvature of the bone, with localised pain and deformity
- The interosseous space is narrowed

Features of isolated ulnar shaft fractures (nightstick fractures)

- Caused by a direct blow to the forearm
- Localised pain, swelling, tenderness and overlying abrasions
- Associated with radial head fracture or dislocation

Causes of acute wrist pain

Radial

- Trapezio-metacarpal joint arthritis
- Scapho-trapezial-trapezoid arthritis
- Scaphoid pathology: Preiser's avascular scaphoid, non-union, fracture
- De Quervain's stenosing tenovaginitis: pain and swelling at the level of the radial styloid along with crepitus; Finkelstein test (making a fist over the thumb and then moving the wrist into ulnar deviation causes passive tendon sheath and reproduces pain)
- Peritendinitis crepitans (intersection syndrome)
- Flexor carpi radialis tendonitis: pain is increased with resisted active wrist flexion with the wrist in radial deviation, and by passive wrist extension
- Radio-carpal joint arthritis
- Wartenberg's syndrome of radial neuritis

Ulnar

- Extensor carpi ulnaris tendonitis: pain with passive radial deviation in pronation
- Recurrent subluxation of extensor carpi ulnaris
- Flexor carpi ulnaris tendonitis: The pain is increased with resisted active wrist flexion with the wrist in ulnar deviation, and by passive wrist extension; x-rays may show calcification in the tendon.
- Pisi-triquetral arthritis
- Triangular fibrocartilage (TFCC) pathology: tear, detachment, perforation, loose body (ulnar wrist pain and clicking produced by ulnar deviation with the wrist in neutral position or dorsiflexion)
- Distal radio-ulnar joint pathology, with ulnar head dislocation: osteoarthritis may be complicated by attrition rupture of extensor tendons
- Ulnar abutment (impaction) syndrome
- Fracture of hook of hamate: hypothenar pain, pain on grip, pain increased with ulnar deviation and by flexion of little and ring fingers; caused by sports (tennis racquet, baseball bat, or golf club) or fall on outstretched hand
- Fracture of pisiform
- Ulnar neuritis
- Dorsal ulnar nerve branch neuritis
- Ulnar artery thrombosis (hypothenar hammer syndrome)

Central transverse

- Lunatomalacia: Kienbock's avascular necrosis of lunate
- Scapho-lunate pathology
- Ganglion
- Mid-carpal instability
- Arthritis

Features of carpal tunnel syndrome

Entrapment neuropathy of the median nerve in the carpal tunnel at the wrist
Intermittent tingling, burning sensation or numbness in the thumb, index finger, middle finger and radial aspect of ring finger
Symptoms are often worse at night
There may be proximal pain in the forearm, elbow, arm and shoulder
Commoner in postmenopausal women and in the dominant hand
In later presentations, thenar muscle wasting and weakness
Phalen manoeuvre: wrist flexion reproduces symptoms
Tinel sign: percussion on the median nerve at the wrist causes distal paraesthesiae

Causes of carpal tunnel syndrome

- Endocrine: pregnancy; oral contraceptive pill; hypothyroidism; diabetes mellitus; acromegaly
- Mechanical/degenerative: lunate fracture; rheumatoid arthritis
- Oedema: congestive heart failure

Causes of wrist drop (inability to extend wrist, fingers at the metacarpophalangeal joints, and thumb)

Unilateral

- Radial nerve compression in the musculospiral groove (distal or mid-humerus) following sleeping with the arm hanging over armrest of chair (Saturday night paralysis) or in the axilla (proximal humerus) by crutch pressure; trauma related to humeral shaft fracture
- Posterior cord plexopathy (associated with deltoid wasting and sensory loss in the shoulder)
- C7 radiculopathy or middle trunk plexopathy; cervical disc prolapse

Bilateral

- Lead poisoning: occupational exposure
- Myotonic dystrophy

Clinical classification of distal radial fractures

Mechanism: fall on the outstretched hand
With dorsal displacement of distal fragment

- Colles' fracture (dinner fork deformity)
- Dorsal articular rim fracture: dorsal Barton's fracture

With volar displacement of distal fragment

- Smith's fracture (reverse Colles' fracture) (garden spade deformity)
- Volar articular rim fracture (volar Barton's fracture)

Styloid fractures

- Radial styloid: chauffeur's or Hutchinson's fracture-named from causation by back-firing of the crank used to start early model motor vehicles; often associated with inter-carpal ligamentous injuries; either an avulsion injury produced by the radial collateral ligament or caused by a direct blow
- Ulnar styloid: avulsion injury produced by the ulnar collateral ligament or triangular fibrocartilage complex; usually associated with another fracture

Distal radial epiphyseal injuries

Features of Colles' fracture

- Caused by a fall on the outstretched hand with the forearm pronated and wrist dorsiflexed
- Transverse fracture of the distal 2–3 cm of the radius
- The distal fragment shows three characteristic displacements: dorsal shift, dorsal tilt, and radial tilt. There is a varying degree of impaction at the fracture site, and dorsal cortical comminution
- Dinner-fork deformity of wrist, with volar fullness
- Occasionally, signs of median nerve compression. Carpal tunnel compression symptoms may result from fracture fragments, haematoma formation, or increased compartment pressure

Features of Smith's fracture

Caused by a fall on the palmarflexed wrist or by direct impact to the dorsum of the hand and wrist
Transverse fracture of the distal radius
Volar displacement and angulation of the distal fragment; comminution of the volar cortex

Signs of instability in distal radial fractures

- Articular incongruity: >2 mm step in articular surface
- Comminution involving both dorsal and volar radial cortices; one cortex across mid-axial line on lateral x-ray
- Radial shortening 5 mm or more, which predisposes to further collapse, resulting in distal radioulnar instability and ulnocarpal impaction; radial shortening (positive ulnar variance) of more than 10 mm indicates complete disruption of the interosseous membrane
- Angulation of the radial articular surface in the sagittal plane greater than 20°
- Ulnar styloid fracture
- Dislocation of head of ulna (ulna does not overlie radius; ulnar styloid is not aligned with dorsal triquetrum)

Radiological features of distal radio-ulnar dislocation on x-ray

- Dorsal or volar dislocation of the ulnar head
- Widened radio-ulnar distance on the AP view with dorsal dislocation of the ulna
- Ulnar styloid overlies the central portion of the distal ulna on AP view due to abnormal rotation of the ulna

Checklist for hand injuries

- Mechanism of injury: how and where.
- Time of injury: relevant for replants and open fractures
- Potential for foreign bodies
- Position of hand at time of injury
- Hand dominance
- Occupation; recreational hobbies
- With phalangeal and metacarpal fractures, each finger should be oriented towards the scaphoid tubercle with the fingers parallel and actively flexed at the MCP and PIP joints, or on passive wrist extension in uncooperative patients
- Prior hand function
- Prior hand injuries
- Co-morbidity: diabetes mellitus
- Tetanus immunization status

Features of extensor tendon injury

- Abnormal posture of finger from loss of DIP, PIP and MCP joint extension
- Loss of active digital extension of DIP, PIP and MCP joints
- Pain on resisted active digital extension suggests partial tendon transection
- Mallet finger refers to deformity caused by loss of active DIP extension

Features of flexor tendon injury

- Loss in the resting posture of the normal cascade of progressive flexion from the little finger to the index finger

- Loss of active digital flexion
- Pain on resisted active digital flexion indicates partial tendon transaction
- Passive wrist dorsiflexion will not increase flexor tone in fingers (loss of tenodesis effect)
- Loss of active DIP flexion with the middle phalanx stabilized at the PIP joint indicates FDP injury. Jersey finger refers to loss of active DIP flexion with tenderness along the length of the flexor tendon at the site of the proximally retracted stump, due to closed injury
- Loss of active PIP flexion with the adjacent fingers held in full extension to prevent the FDP from flexing the digit indicates FDS injury
- Squeezing the volar forearm at the level of the musculo-tendinous junctions makes the fingers flex in a cascade

Features of digital nerve injury

- Numbness along one side of a finger
- History of profuse bleeding from a volar incised or penetrating wound

Causes of compartment syndrome of the hand

- Crush injury
- Blast injury
- Bleeding after fracture
- Arterial cannulation
- Intravenous injections
- Prolonged pressure on the hand or arm

Features of hand compartment syndrome

- Increasing analgesic requirements
- Pain out of proportion to that expected for the injury
- Severe swelling with loss of normal concavity of the palm
- Digital perfusion and nailbed capillary refill time may be preserved until late

Radiological assessment of the carpus

- Carpal arcs: break in outline of the smooth carpal arcs formed along the radio-carpal and mid-carpal joints, which are roughly parallel, without disruption.

  Carpal arcs (Gilula's lines)

  Arc 1: proximal convex outline of scaphoid, lunate and triquetrum

  Arc 2: distal curve of scaphoid, lunate and triquetrum

  Arc 3: convex proximal surfaces of capitate and hamate

  - Symmetry of inter-carpal joint spaces: abnormal widening; normally all should be equal and less than 3 mm; the normal scapho-lunate joint space is less than 2 mm and usually remains constant within the normal range of radial or ulnar deviation of the wrist
  - Shape of individual bones: bone shapes that do not correspond to a normal AP view; unusual bony overlap. The normal lunate is quadrilateral, but appears triangular when dislocated
  - On a lateral view of the wrist, the distal radius, lunate, capitate and the longitudinal axis of the third metacarpal are aligned
  - The pronator quadratus fat pad is seen on the lateral view as a linear or crescentic radiolucency just anterior to the distal radius and ulna
  - The scaphoid fat pad is seen on the AP view as a radiolucent stripe extending from the radial styloid to the trapezium and almost parallel to the radial aspect of the scaphoid.

Scaphoid fractures comprise 60% of all carpal fractures. The scaphoid is the most commonly fractured carpal bone, most often in young adult males.

Mechanisms:

- Direct: blow on dorsum of forcefully flexed wrist

- Indirect: fall on outstretched hand with hyperextended radially deviated wrist; the scaphoid waist comes into contact in hyperextension with the dorsal rim of the radius when falling on to an outstretched hand

Features

- Pain on radial aspect of wrist, limited mobility, and some swelling
- Tenderness in the anatomical snuff box(bounded by EPL, APB and EPB on the dorsum of the hand): waist fracture
- Tenderness over the scaphoid tubercle (volar-base of thenar eminence)
- Axial or longitudinal compression of thumb and resisted supination of the wrist cause pain
- Soft tissue signs on x-ray include dorsal swelling, and obliteration, distortion or displacement of the scaphoid fat stripe

Assessment of stability of scaphoid fractures

- Stable: undisplaced
- Unstable: >1 mm step or offset; abnormal angulation: >15°; vertical fracture pattern; comminution

Features of fracture of triquetral

- Fall on outstretched hand, with wrist in dorsiflexion
- Pain at ulnar aspect of wrist
- Point tenderness 2 cm distal to ulnar styloid
- Pain on resisted wrist dorsiflexion
- On lateral view, a fleck of avulsed bone is visible dorsal to the proximal carpal row, representing a dorsal shearing injury

Features of fracture of hamate

- Hook of hamate fractures occur in sports that use rackets, clubs or bats and may also follow falls on the outstretched hand with the wrist dorsiflexed
- Body of hamate fractures are caused by direct trauma, such as falling on a dorsiflexed and ulnar-deviated wrist, or associated with posterior dislocation or subluxation of the 4th and/or 5th metacarpal
- Pain in the hypothenar region of the palm, aggravated by grasp and with flexion of the little and ring fingers
- Point tenderness approximately 1.5 cm distal to the pisiform, along a line extending from the pisiform to the third metacarpal head

Radiology of carpal dislocations
Perilunate dislocation of the carpus

- Disruption of the middle carpal arc
- Lunate sits in the concavity of the distal radius, and the concavity of the lunate is empty
- The capitate lies dorsal to the lunate
- Triangular shape of lunate
- Associated with fractures of the scaphoid, radial and/or ulnar styloid process, and dorsal avulsion fracture of the triquetrum

Lunate dislocation

- Proximal arc disruption
- Triangular shape of lunate (spilled teacup sign)
- Median nerve compression may coexist

Scapho-lunate dissociation

- Scapho-lunate gap >2 mm (Terry Thomas sign)
- Signet ring sign caused by end-on visualization of the cortex of the distal pole of the scaphoid due to volar tilt
- Foreshortening of the scaphoid caused by rotation of the distal pole towards the palm

Features of fractures of the base of the 1st metacarpal

- The Bennett fracture-subluxation or dislocation is an intra-articular fracture of the

1st metacarpal base where a triangular fragment consisting of the volar ulnar lip of the proximal fragment continues to articulate with the tubercle of the trapezium, while the distal fragment of the 1st metacarpal shaft is pulled proximally, dorsally and radially. The carpometacarpal joint is disrupted. It is caused by an axial force directed against the partially flexed 1st metacarpal, as in punching with a clenched fist, or by falling on an extended or abducted thumb. There is pain, swelling and bruising related to the base of the thumb and thenar eminence, with weak grip.
- The Rolando fracture is a comminuted, typically T-or Y-shaped, intra-articular fracture of the 1st metacarpal base.
- Extra-articular fractures can be transverse or oblique

Features of fractures of the fifth metacarpal neck (boxer's fracture)

- Caused by axial loading through the long axis of the metacarpal secondary to punching a solid surface with the clenched fist, usually in amateur pugilists
- Swelling and tenderness related to the fifth metacarpal neck, associated with loss of the little finger knuckle prominence
- Pseudo-clawing of the little finger
- A transverse fracture through the metacarpal neck is associated with volar angulation of the distal fragment, i.e. the metacarpal head
- If there is an overlying puncture wound or laceration in the skin, a human bite injury is possible
- Rotational deformity must be assessed

Features of locked metacarpophalangeal joint

- Painful loss of both active and passive extension of the metacarpophalangeal joint without loss of flexion
- Can be caused by osteophyte of the metacarpal head, intra-articular fracture of the metacarpal head, volar plate tear, sesamoid entrapment, or loose bodies

Features of carpo-metacarpal joint dislocations

- The 4th and 5th metacarpals are mobile with a range of 15–25° of flexion and extension at the CMCP joints
- Dorsal displacement of the proximal metacarpal with respect to the distal carpal row
- The dislocation can be overlooked owing to significant swelling
- A true lateral view is required to establish the diagnosis
- Indistinct 4th and 5th CMC joint spaces on AP view

Checklist for finger tip injuries

- Crush or slicing injury
- Presence of tissue loss: skin only; skin and pulp; with pulp loss, is there bone exposure with or without fracture?
- Obliquity of amputation: transverse; dorsal oblique loss; volar oblique loss
- Nail bed involvement
- Tendon involvement

Unstable fractures of phalanges
Distal phalanx

- FDP avulsion fracture (volar DP base)
- Mallet finger with avulsion fracture of dorsal DP base involving more than 30% of articular surface, with or without volar subluxation of the DP

Middle and proximal phalanges

- Long oblique/spiral fractures of the shaft
- Displaced intra-articular fractures involving >30% of the articular surface (volar lip of palmar base of middle phalanx)
- Uni-condylar and bi-condylar fractures
- Comminuted fractures

- Subcondylar fracture of proximal phalanx

Features of volar plate avulsion injury

- Caused by hyperextension of the PIP joint
- May be accompanied by dorsal subluxation or dislocation of the middle phalanx with a larger avulsed volar lip fragment (25–35% of the MP base)
- Maximal tenderness on volar aspect of PIP joint

Features of central extensor slip injury

- Forcible flexion of the extended PIP joint leading to rupture of the central slip of the extensor tendon
- Tenderness at dorsum of PIP joint, with inability to actively extend the PIP joint against resistance
- Small dorsal avulsion fracture at the base of the middle phalanx may be present; if the fragment is large, volar subluxation of the middle phalanx may occur
- The deformity develops 4–6 weeks after the injury

Features of PIP joint dislocation

- PIP joint hyperextension, usually following an axial load to the finger, causes dorsal dislocation of the PIP joint
- The dislocation is often reduced before seeking medical attention
- A small avulsion fracture may be present at the volar lip of the base of the middle phalanx
- Post-reduction, active extension at the PIP joint should be tested to determine the integrity of the central slip of the extensor tendon
- Irreducibility indicates interposition of volar plate and/or flexor tendons between the PP head and MP base
- Open dislocations require referral for joint debridement and primary repair of the volar plate

Metacarpophalangeal joint dislocation
Dorsal dislocation

Simple
- Marked hyperextension (60–80%) of the proximal phalanx
- Articular surface of base of proximal phalanx in contact with dorsum of metacarpal head

Complex
- Volar plate interposition between base of proximal phalanx and metacarpal head
- Modest hyperextension of the proximal phalanx (20–40%)
- Slight flexion of interphalangeal joints
- The metacarpal head is prominent in the palm, where it may cause puckering and blanching of the palmar skin at the level of the joint. It is trapped (button-holed) between the flexor tendons and the lumbrical muscle.
- Sesamoid interposition within widened joint space is pathognomic
- Most commonly involves the index and middle fingers
- Cannot be reduced by closed manipulation

Metacarpal fractures requiring open reduction and internal fixation

- Unacceptable angulation
  - Shaft: index and middle fingers (10–20°); ring finger (30°); little finger (40°)
  - Neck: index and middle fingers (10–15°); ring finger (30–40°); little finger (50°)
- Malrotation: short oblique and spiral fractures
- Comminuted fractures
- Multiple fractures

Features of ulnar collateral ligament avulsion injury of the MCP joint (gamekeeper's or skier's thumb)

- Hyperabduction injury of thumb secondary to a fall on the outstretched hand
- Ligamentous injury or avulsion fracture at UCL insertion into base of proximal phalanx; in children, Salter-Harris III injury of the base of the proximal phalanx

- Retraction of the torn UCL outside the adductor aponeurosis: Stener's lesion
- Pain and tenderness at ulnar aspect of 1st MCP joint in the 1st web space
- Reduced pinch strength
- Valgus (radial) instability with MCP joint in 30° of flexion
- Inadequate treatment leads to persistent pain and instability, early degenerative changes and reduced pinch strength

Features indicating nail bed injury

- Subungual haematoma involving >50% of the nail plate
- Nail plate avulsion from the proximal nail fold
- Transverse fracture of the DP shaft with displacement
- Comminuted DP tuft fracture

Features suggestive of nail bed interposition in the distal phalanx:

- Avulsion of root of nail plate from beneath proximal nail fold
- Widening of fracture site on lateral x-ray

Features of Seymour's fracture

- Salter-Harris II injury of the distal phalangeal epiphysis
- Often an open injury, with avulsion of the proximal end of the nail from the eponychial fold
- The distal fragment is flexed by the unopposed flexor digitorum profundus tendon, leading to a mallet deformity
- Interposition of germinal matrix of nail bed blocks closed reduction

Features of hand infections
Paronychia

- Lateral nail fold infection, usually with cuticle damage, an ingrown nail or a history of trauma, which may extend to involve the proximal nail fold or the opposite lateral nail fold
- Often caused by hangnails, manicuring, and nail biting in adults and finger sucking in children
- Chronic paronychia is related to prolonged repeated water submersion (e.g. dishwashers)
- In severe infections, pus may extend under the nail plate

Distal pulp space infection

- Often related to a puncture wound to the tip of the finger
- Fibrous septa create a closed space within the fingertip
- Severe throbbing pain
- Tense swelling of the distal pulp space
- If untreated can lead to osteomyelitis of the distal phalanx, septic arthritis of the distal interphalangeal joint, or flexor tenosynovitis from proximal extension

Herpetic whitlow

- Caused by type 1 or type 2 herpes simplex virus
- Most often affects the distal pulp space and, occasionally, the proximal and lateral nail folds
- Pain is out of proportion to the clinical findings
- Clear vesicles on an erythematous base
- Typically, only one finger is involved
- The vesicles may coalesce and ulcerate
- The pulp remains soft
- Resolves in 3–4 weeks
- Incision and drainage can lead to secondary bacterial infection

Flexor tenosynovitis

- Commonly caused by a penetrating injury, especially at the distal and proximal flexion creases where the tendon sheaths are more superficial

- Four cardinal signs of Kanavel
  Tenderness over the flexor sheath
  Symmetrical enlargement of the finger
  Flexed position of the finger at rest
  Pain on passive extension of the finger
- Infections of the thumb can spread to the radial bursa and those of the little finger to the ulnar bursa

Web space abscess

- Usually follows an infected palmar blister
- Often has an hourglass (collar button) configuration from spread to the dorsal subcutaneous space and spread deep into the palmar web space
- The fingers adjacent to the affected web space are held abducted at rest

Causes of refusal to use the upper limb in children

Pulled elbow (age 1–5 years; elbow held extended and forearm pronated, with no visible swelling, bruising or deformity)
Infection: septic arthritis; osteomyelitis
Fractures and traumatic periostitis: clavicle, humerus, radius and ulna
Neurological lesions with true paralysis (as opposed to pseudoparalysis from other causes)

Risk factors for pelvic injury

- High energy blunt trauma: motor vehicle collisions; pedestrian versus motor vehicle impacts; falls from a height; industrial accidents
- Osteoporosis: low bone mass
- Age > 60 years
- Low body mass index

Features associated with pelvic ring injuries

- Groin, scrotal, labial, perineal, gluteal and flank haematoma
- Perineal, groin and gluteal open wounds
- Rectal and vaginal lacerations
- Urethral injuries: blood at external meatus, perineal haematoma, high-riding prostate gland on rectal examination
- Lumbosacral plexus injury (L5, S1 roots)
- Pelvic deformity
- Lower limbs: vascular or neurological deficit; rotational deformity (external rotation); leg length discrepancy (shortening); acetabular fractures; hip dislocations
- Hypovolaemic shock, due to retroperitoneal haemorrhage from presacral venous plexus and/or cancellous bone at fracture surfaces, or from arteries
- Neurological injuries: spinal cord injury; cauda equina syndrome

Signs of instability in pelvic fracture

- Pubic symphysis diastasis >2.5 cm, resulting in an externally rotated hemi-pelvis
- Pelvic ring disruption in two or more sites
- Posterior or vertical displacement of hemipelvis >1 cm
- Displacement of posterior sacro-iliac complex >5 mm in any plane
- Displaced sacral fracture, with gap
- Avulsion fractures of ischial spine (sacrospinous ligament), ischial tuberosity, lateral border of sacrum(sacrotuberous ligament) and of L5 transverse process

Stable pelvic fractures

- Isolated pubic or ischial ramus fractures
- Unilateral fractures of both rami
- Iliac wing fracture
- Isolated sacral fracture

Features of pubic ramus fracture

- Caused by low velocity injuries in elderly women, typically a fall from standing height, and associated with osteoporosis

- Unilateral fractures of the pubic rami are considered stable fractures of the anterior pelvic ring, allowing full weight bearing if possible
- Can be associated with occult ligamentous or osseous injuries of the posterior pelvic ring
- Diastasis of the symphysis pubis can occur with fractures of the pubic rami

Causes of gluteal pain

- Hamstring origin tendinopathy
- Referred pain from lumbar spine/sacro-iliac joint
- Ischio-gluteal bursitis
- Piriformis impingement/muscle strain
- Fibrous adhesions around sciatic nerve
- Stress fracture of ischium
- Apophysitis/avulsion fracture of ischial tuberosity
- Spondlyoarthropathies

Hip pain

Causes of anterior hip/groin pain

- Usually indicates intra-articular pathology of the hip joint
- Osteoarthritis; avascular necrosis; tumour; fracture (cortical disruption, impacted hyperlucency, loss of smooth cortical transition from femoral neck to head, disruption of trabeculae)
- Inflammatory or infectious arthritis; osteomyelitis
- Overuse injury: iliopsoas bursitis, labral tear; stress fracture; hip flexor muscle strain/tendonitis

Causes of lateral hip pain

- Usually indicates enthesopathy or trochanteric bursitis
- Greater trochanter pain syndrome: greater trochanteric bursitis (deep trochanteric bursitis causes pain and tenderness localized to the posterior portion of the greater trochanter; superficial trochanteric bursitis causes pain and tenderness over the bursa that is increased with extreme adduction of the hip); gluteus medius pathology
- Iliotibial band friction syndrome (pain worse with downhill running, and with activity after a pain-free start)
- Meralgia paraesthetica: entrapment neuropathy of lateral femoral cutaneous nerve: antero-lateral thigh numbness

Causes of posterior hip pain

- Usually suggests a source outside the hip joint, being referred from the lumbar spine (degenerative disc disease; facet arthropathy; spinal stenosis), sacro-iliac joint, aorto-iliac vascular occlusive disease
- Can also arise from hip extensor/rotator muscle strain
- Ischiogluteal bursitis causes pain and tenderness over the ischial tuberosity, which can radiate down the leg into the hamstrings

Evaluation of hip x-rays

- The femoral heads and joint spaces are symmetrical
- Integrity of acetabular arc
- The width of the symphysis pubis is less than 5 mm
- The width of the sacroiliac joints is less than 2–4 mm
- The pelvic and obturator rings are intact
- Continuity of the four critical lines: iliopectineal, ilioischial, anterior acetabular rim and posterior acetabular rim lines
- Shenton's line, along the superior margin of the obturator ring (inferior edge of superior pubic ramus) and medial edge of femoral neck, should be smooth and continuous
- Disruption of the iliopectineal line (from medial border of iliac wing extending along superior border of superior pubic ramus to pubic symphysis) indicates a fracture of the anterior column
- Disruption of the ilioischial line (from medial border of iliac wing extending along medial order of ischium to the ischial

tuberosity) indicates a fracture of the posterior column. Projection of the acetabular wall medial to the ilioischial line indicates protrusio acetabuli
- Klein's line, along the long axis of the superior aspect of the femoral neck intersects the capital femoral epiphysis in children
- Review of the gluteal, iliopsoas and obturator fat pads

Causes of painful hip after fall

- Femoral neck fracture
- Occult femoral neck fracture (no fracture visible on AP pelvis and lateral hip views, especially when undisplaced and in osteopenic bone): inability to bear weight and the triad of groin tenderness on deep palpation, inability to actively straight leg raise, and painful limitation of passive internal and external rotation of the hip. Pain may be produced in the hip region by percussion on the sole of the foot with the fist.
- Inter-trochanteric or sub-trochanteric fracture
- Pelvic fracture; stress fracture of pubic ramus
- Acetabular fracture
- Isolated fracture of the greater trochanter
- Exacerbation of hip arthritis
- Pathological hip fracture
- Contusion of the hip

Features of femoral neck fractures

Low impact falls in the elderly: fall on to the greater trochanter; lateral rotation with sudden increase in load; spontaneous completion of a stress fracture that causes the fall

High velocity impact in younger patients

Pain in the groin, medial thigh or knee, and inability to bear weight; weight bearing may be possible with an impacted subcapital fracture.

The injured limb is shortened and externally rotated

Plain films should be examined for subtle angulation of the femoral neck, trabecular pattern disruption, cortical defects, a subcapital impaction line, shortening of the femoral neck and loss of the smooth transition from the femoral head to the femoral neck.

Normal plain films do not conclusively exclude a femoral neck fracture

In the presence of inconclusive plain films or negative plain films in a symptomatic patient, MRI or CT is indicated to exclude an occult fracture.

Factors contributing to femoral neck fracture being missed

- Stress fracture
- Impacted fracture (incomplete fracture, with intact medial trabeculae of the inferior femoral neck and valgus angulation at the fracture site due to postero-lateral tilting of the femoral head)
- Coexisting femoral shaft fracture (e.g. dashboard injury)

Features of hip dislocations

- Severe pain in the hip and proximal thigh, with deformity and inability to bear weight
- Posterior: lower limb shortened, hip flexed, internally rotated and adducted; sciatic or common peroneal nerve injury may be associated; fractures of the posterior wall of the acetabulum and of the anterior femoral head (Pipkin fracture), as well as ipsilateral knee injuries, may coexist; usually caused by axial load on femur, with hip flexed and adducted (dashboard injury)
- Anterior: hip minimally flexed, abducted and markedly externally rotated, occasionally associated with a palpable femoral head in the groin; usually an isolated injury; femoral nerve, artery or vein compression may be present
- Central: associated with acetabular fracture

Causes of pain after hip replacement surgery

- Infection (osteomyelitis)
- Stress fracture of pubic ramus
- Aseptic loosening of femoral component-stem (radiolucent zone at cement-bone interface or implant-bone interface with uncemented components; migration of component or cement) (thigh pain) or of acetabular component-cup (groin pain)
- Osteolysis
- Dislocation
- Trochanteric bursitis
- Component malposition
- Psoas tendonitis

Causes of acute groin pain

- Musculoskeletal: osteoarthritis; osteonecrosis (acute groin and gluteal pain; risk factors include high dose corticosteroids, alcohol abuse, pancreatitis, haemoglobinopathies such as sickle cell disease, SLE and myeloproliferative disorders); rheumatoid arthritis (morning pain and stiffness relieved by activity); seronegative spondyloarthropathy; septic arthritis; bone metastases; pathological or stress fracture of femoral neck; bursitis (trachanteric, iliopsoas); muscle tear or avulsion fracture; osteitis pubis; femoroacetabular impingement (activity-related pain aggravated by hip flexion)
- Hernia: inguinal, femoral, obturator (exercise-induced medial thigh pain)
- Nerve entrapment: obturator nerve; lateral femoral cutaneous nerve of the thigh (pain and numbness in lateral thigh); ilio-inguinal nerve
- Neoplasm: metastases in lymph nodes (primary in lower rectum, anal canal, lower vagina, vulva, penis)
- Vascular: femoral artery aneurysm/pseudoaneurysm; femoral vein thrombosis; superficial thrombophlebitis; iliopsoas haemorrhage (sudden onset severe groin and hip pain, radiating to anterior thigh and lumbar region, with iliopsoas muscle spasm-hip held in flexion and external rotation and passive extension is very painful)
- Referred pain: GI tract (appendicitis; diverticulitis); GU (prostatitis; testicular torsion; testicular neoplasm); musculo-skeletal (lumbar disc disease; sacroiliac disease)

Causes of groin pain in the athlete

Musculo-tendinous: strain or tenoperiostitis of the adductor longus/ilipsoas/rectus femoris

Hip joint: labral tear; chondral injury; osteoarthritis; femoroacetabular impingement (deep discomfort in the groin, with provocation of pain during passive hip flexion to 90° with forced internal rotation and adduction)

Bone: stress fracture of the femoral neck/pubic ramus; osteitis pubis; avulsion fractures of the pelvis

Bursae: iliopsoas bursitis; trochanteric bursitis

Herniae: inguinal; femoral

Nerve entrapment: ilioinguinal; genitofemoral; obturator

Fascial insufficiency: Gilmore groin

Intra-abdominal inflammation

Referred pain: Lumbar (L1, L2)

Osteitis pubis

A self-limiting overuse injury seen in association with kicking sports and running

The features include:

A gradual onset of pubic pain, which may radiate to the groin, medial thighs and abdomen

The pain is increased on passive abduction and active resisted addiction of the lower limbs, and on one leg standing.

Symphyseal tenderness along the subcutaneous border of the pubis

Pain is provoked on side to side pelvic compression.

Tightness of the adductor muscles

A waddling gait may result from adductor spasm

Causes of limp in a child

- Pain: antalgic gait
- Structural abnormalities: limb length discrepancy; angular limb deformity; torsional abnormalities; articular surface abnormalities; muscle contractures; shortened tendons
- Neuromuscular problems: weakness; ataxia (cerebellar or sensory)

All ages

- Trauma
- Septic arthritis
- Osteomyelitis
- Cellulitis
- Stress fracture
- Overuse syndromes
- Neuromuscular
- Neoplasm; leukaemia

Toddler (age: 1–3 years)

- Occult fractures: spiral distal tibial fracture
- Transient synovitis of the hip (pain in the groin, hip, thigh or knee; hip held in flexion, external rotation and abduction; recent upper respiratory tract infection; no or minimal fever)
- Septic arthritis
- Developmental dysplasia of the hip
- Leg length discrepancy

Age 4–10 years

- Transient synovitis
- Juvenile rheumatoid arthritis
- Perthes disease

Adolescent (age: 11–16 years)

- Slipped capital femoral epiphysis (posterior and inferior slippage of the capital femoral epiphysis on the femoral neck, causing reduced internal rotation of hip; hip, groin, thigh or knee pain associated with a limp; loss of internal rotation of the leg in flexion is virtually pathognomic. This is often evident in the gait. When lying supine or during gait, the leg is naturally rotated externally. The hip will not flex upwards, but will rotate externally instead. Attempts at internal rotation will cause pain; there is external rotation and abduction of lower limb with passive hip flexion; risk factors include obesity and endocrine disorders such as hypothyroidism, panhypopituitarism, growth hormone deficiency and hypogonadism)
- Avascular necrosis of femoral head
- Overuse syndromes
- Chondromalacia
- Neoplasm
- Gonococcal septic arthritis
- Tarsal coalitions

Evaluation of limping child

- Visualisation of entire lower limb
- Passive and active range of movement in hip, knee and ankle joints
- Bruising
- Focal tenderness
- Cellulitis

X-ray findings in slipped capital femoral epiphysis

- Widening of the proximal femoral epiphysis with metaphyseal irregularity (scalloped irregular metaphysis)
- Double density at the metaphysis due to superimposition of posterior cortical lip on the metaphysis (Steel sign)
- Postero-medial displacement of the femoral epiphysis, seen as failure of a line along the superior margin of the femoral neck (lateral femoral neck) on the AP view, and extended to the acetabulum, to intersect with the femoral epiphysis. Normally, about 1/6th of the epiphysis lies lateral to a line drawn tangentially to the superior margin of the femoral neck (Klein's line).

- On the AP view the entire upper femoral metaphysic lies lateral to the posterior acetabular margin (Capener's sign)
- Epiphysis appears smaller due to posterior slippage: loss of height of femoral epiphysis
- Prominent lesser trochanter due to external rotation of the femoral neck and shaft relative to the head
- Slippage may only be seen on the frog leg view, which makes posterior displacement easier to detect because the displacement of the head is perpendicular to the x-ray beam.
- Loss of articular cartilage width leading to joint space narrowing is seen with chondrolysis
- Late findings include subchondral sclerosis, cyst formation, osteophyte formation, and joint space narrowing

Causes of thigh pain
Anterior

- Quadriceps muscle strain
- Quadriceps muscle contusion
- Myositis ossificans
- Stress fracture of femur; including atypical stress fractures associated with long-term bisphosphonate therapy

Posterior

- Hamstring muscle strain
- Hamstring muscle tear
- Hamstring contusion
- Referred pain from lumbar spine/sacro-iliac joint
- Semimembranosus bursitis
- Chronic compartment syndrome of posterior thigh

Lateral

- Meralgia paraesthetica (entrapment of lateral femoral cutaneous nerve of thigh); associated with paraesthesiae and numbness of the proximal lateral thigh
- Trochanteric bursitis: gluteal and lateral hip and thigh pain associated with point tenderness over the greater trochanter which reproduces the pain
- Iliotibial band syndrome: lateral thigh and knee pain worsened with physical activity such as running or cycling or on walking up and down stairs

Features of femoral shaft fractures

- Caused by high energy trauma in patients aged 40 years or under, as from severe direct trauma or by an axial load to the flexed knee (as in motor vehicle collisions or automobile-pedestrian collisions); more likely to be due to low energy trauma in older patients
- Pathological fractures are associated with osteoporosis, metastases and the presence of hip prostheses or intramedullary fixation devices such as plates and nails (periprosthetic fractures)
- Present with thigh pain, tense swelling, deformity (often with leg shortening) and inability to bear weight
- Deformity depends on the level of the fracture. The proximal fragment is abducted, flexed and externally rotated with sub-trochanteric fractures. The distal fragment is extended by the gastrocnemius in supracondylar fractures, leading to posterior angulation deformity of the femoral shaft.
- Popliteal artery injury may complicate supracondylar fractures
- Hip dislocation may coexist and can be overlooked
- An ipsilateral tibial shaft fracture causes a floating knee injury
- Waddell's triad of femoral shaft fracture, intra-abdominal or intra-thoracic injury, and head injury is seen with high-velocity motor vehicle accidents
- X-rays should show the full length of the femur, including hip and knee joints and should be supplemented by an AP view of the pelvis

Features of femoral condylar fractures

- Caused by axial loading with a varus or valgus force
- The fractures may involve one or both condyles, and may be T- or Y-shaped, with the vertical limb extending into the intercondylar notch
- Impaction, comminution and loss of articular surface congruity are common

Features of quadriceps muscle contusion
A complication of contact sports, it follows blunt trauma to the antero-lateral aspect of the thigh.

Acute severe pain may lead to loss of function, the dead leg syndrome.

Increasing pain and swelling in the thigh, and knee stiffness follow

Active straight leg raising is difficult.

There is often a limited range of passive knee flexion, and delayed onset knee swelling owing to synovial effusion.

Iliotibial tract syndrome
An overuse injury, typically seen in long-distance runners, cyclists and aerobic dancers, the result of repetitive knee movements producing excessive friction along the distal iliotibial band, the underlying bursa, and the lateral femoral condyle.

The features include:

Activity related lateral knee and thigh pain, increased by climbing stairs or walking uphill.
Tenderness is related to the distal iliotibial band and lateral femoral condyle, about 3 cm. proximal to the lateral joint line, associated with a creak palpable on knee flexion and extension

Tightness of the iliotibial band is demonstrable with Ober's test:

The patient lies with the hip flexed on the unaffected side.
The affected knee is flexed and the hip abducted and extended to line up with the trunk.
Attempted passive abduction of the hip is limited by tightness of the band.

Causes of posterior thigh and buttock pain
Musculo-tendinous injury

- Hamstrings
- Gluteals

Neurological

- Piriformis syndrome: sciatic nerve irritation
- Hamstrings syndrome
- Mass compressing sciatic nerve
- Referred pain from lumbar spine

Other

- Referred pain from pelvic viscera
  - Sacro-iliitis/sacro-iliac dysfunction

The features of hamstring tears include:

Sudden onset of posterior thigh pain while engaged in rapid activity, typically sprinting
Localised tenderness
Delayed onset bruising in the posterior thigh
Occasionally a palpable defect in the hamstring tendon
X-rays may reveal avulsion fractures of the ischial tuberosity

Features of anterior knee (patello-femoral) pain

- Worse on ascending or descending stairs/slopes
- Worse on squatting, knelling, running, cycling
- Worse on prolonged sitting with flexed knees (moviegoers' knee)
- Recurrent giving way of the knee

Factors predisposing to patellar instability with lateral subluxation of patella
Abnormalities of bony structure

- Hypoplastic lateral femoral condyle
- Shallow femoral sulcus or trochlea

- Lateral location of tibial tubercle
- Patella alta (small, high riding patella)

Skeletal malalignment

- Rotational malalignment: Increased femoral neck anteversion (internal femoral torsion); increased external tibial torsion
- Alignment of the patella with respect to the tibial tuberosity: increased femoral-tibial Q angle (angle between a line connecting the anterior superior iliac spine and the centre of the patella and a line connecting the tibial tuberosity with the centre of the patella: >15°)
- Genu valgum
- Genu recurvatum
- Excess hindfoot pronation

Soft tissue abnormalities

- Generalized joint laxity
- Abnormal attachment of the iliotibial band
- Weakness of the vastus medialis component of the quadriceps muscle or of the medial retinaculum
- Tight lateral retinaculum

Ottawa knee rules for requesting x-rays after trauma

- Age > 55 years
- Isolated patellar tenderness
- Tenderness at fibula head
- Inability to flex knee to 90°
- Inability to bear weight for four steps immediately after the accident and in the emergency department

Checklist for evaluation of knee x-rays after trauma

- The lateral tibial plateau lies 2–3 mm superior (proximal) to the medial tibial plateau
- The tibia should not extend more than 5 mm beyond a line drawn down the lateral margin of the lateral femoral condyle
- On horizontal beam lateral view a fat-fluid level in the region of the suprapatellar pouch indicates lipohaemarthrosis and may suggest occult intra-articular fracture
- An avulsion fracture of the lateral tibial rim is highly specific for anterior cruciate ligament injury

Features of tibial plateau fractures

- Caused by a combination of valgus or varus stress and a compression force (axial loading on the knee) leading to impaction of the femoral condyles against the tibial plateau. The usual causative factors are falls from a height, and motor vehicle bumper impacts to the lateral aspect of the leg from pedestrian-vehicle collisions
- Lateral plateau fractures are commoner
- Knee haemarthrosis is often present
- There is a risk of compartment syndrome

Features of patellar dislocation

- Caused by a valgus load to the knee and simultaneous quadriceps activation
- Acute pain and disability
- Lateral dislocation of the patella
- Haemarthrosis of the knee
- Tenderness over medial patellar retinaculum

Features of patella fractures

- Acute anterior knee pain following direct impact to the knee (either low velocity, as after a fall from sitting or standing height, or high velocity, as from a dashboard impact following motor vehicle collisions) or indirect injuries caused by forceful quadriceps contraction with the knee flexed associated

with a near fall. High energy impacts lead to comminuted fractures, and are associated with hip dislocation, proximal or distal femoral fractures, and proximal tibial fractures. Indirect injuries lead to transverse fractures, with fracture fragment separation indicating retinacular disruption.
- Haemarthrosis
- Inability to actively extend the knee
- A palpable gap at the fracture site if the fracture is transverse and displaced
- Can be confused with a bipartite patella, which is characteristically smooth edged and corticated on the superolateral aspect of the patella and typically bilateral

Features of patella sleeve fracture

- Chondral or osteochondral avulsion injuries at the inferior pole of the patella caused by forceful quadriceps contraction with the knee flexed, typically in children aged between 8 and 12 years.
- The lower pole of the patella is avulsed along with much or all of the articular surface of the patella
- The avulsed bone fragment adjacent to the inferior pole of the patella appears deceptively small on x-rays because it includes a portion of unossified patella
- High-riding patella
- Tenderness over the lower pole of the patella
- Extensor lag when leg extension is tested

Causes of knee pain

- Articular surface injury: osteoarthritis; inflammatory arthritis; osteochondral defects; osteochondritis dissecans; chondromalacia patellae
- Meniscal tears; meniscal cysts; discoid meniscus
- Bursitis: prepatellar bursitis; infrapatellar bursitis
- Tendinitis: patellar tendinitis; popliteal tendinitis
- Ligament sprains
- Fracture: patella
- Neoplasm
- Infection
- Nerve damage
- Referred pain from hip or spine

Risk factors for osteoarthritis of the knees

- Age > 50 years
- Female gender
- BMI > 25
- Previous knee injury
- Joint laxity or hypermobility syndrome
- Occupational/recreational injury
- Positive family history of osteoarthritis

Knee overuse syndromes causing pain

Anterior

- Patello-femoral stress syndrome (retropatellar or peri-patellar pain, increased on activity, descending steps, and rising from seated position)
- Jumper's knee (patellar tendonitis)
- Osgood-Schlatter disease (localised swelling and tenderness at tibial tuberosity, with pain on extension of the knee against resistance)
- Sinding-Larsen-Johansson syndrome (traction apophysitis of the lower pole of the patella; usually in adolescents aged between 10 and 14 years)
- Stress fracture of patella
- Fat pad syndrome (inflammation of the infrapatellar fat pad from impingement between the patella and femoral condyles during knee extension)

Medial

- Medial meniscal tear
- Synovial plica syndrome (gradual onset of localized or diffuse exercise-induced anterior knee pain, often triggered by prolonged sitting or squatting; symptoms worse on walking downstairs)

- Semimembranosus tendinitis (posteromedial)
- Pes anerinus tendinitis/bursitis
- Breaststrokers' knee
- Medial retinaculitis

Lateral

- Ilio-tibial band friction syndrome
- Lateral meniscal tear
- Popliteus tendinitis (posterolateral)
- Biceps femoris tendonitis
- Biceps bursitis

Posterior

- Fabellitis
- Gastrocnemius muscle strain at distal femoral site

Features of patellar tendinitis (Jumper's knee)
An overuse injury caused by repetitive microtrauma to the ligamentum patellae from eccentric loading while landing from jumps.

The features are:

Pain at the inferior pole of the patella and along the patellar ligament, increased by resisted knee extension. Pain is increased on going downstairs, walking on an inclined surface, and with prolonged sitting with the knee flexed.
Limited hamstring flexibility, demonstrated by limited straight leg raising.
Limited quadriceps flexibility, demonstrated by limited knee flexion in the prone position.
X-rays may show calcification adjacent to the lower pole of the patella on the lateral view.

Knee haemarthrosis
Causes

Traumatic
Anterior cruciate/posterior cruciate ligament injury
Patella fracture; osteochondral fracture
Lateral dislocation of patella
Peripheral meniscal tear
Intra-articular fracture (tibial plateau)
Non-traumatic
Pigmented villonodular synovitis (haemorrhagic joint effusions, subchondral cysts, erosions, with joint space preservation)
Synovial haemangioma
Anticoagulants
Haemophilia
Sickle cell disease

Historical features associated with haemarthrosis

- High velocity impact
- Inability to bear weight immediately and to continue participation in sporting activity
- Audible "pop" with injury
- Rapid joint swelling

Anterior cruciate ligament tears
Causes

Valgus, external rotation movement in a weight-bearing joint
Valgus force in a free-standing limb
Hyperextension

The typical features include:

An audible pop or snap at the time of injury
Immediate loss of function with a fall to the ground
Inability to continue participation in sporting activity
Rapid onset, within 1–2 h, of diffuse tense knee swelling owing to haemarthrosis
Inability to achieve full extension if the knee locks due to an inverted distal ACL stump, displaced bucket handle tear of a meniscus or osteochondral loose fragment
In the acute stage stability testing is painful and uninformative
Pivot shift testing may be possible in subacute presentations. With the knee fully extended, the tibia is internally rotated with simultaneous

valgus stress to the knee. With maintenance of these forces, the knee is flexed. If the ACL is deficient, the tibia subluxes anterior to the femur at 20–40° of flexion.

X-rays may show an avulsed fragment from the anterior tibial intercondylar eminence or a lateral capsular avulsion fracture of the lateral cortex of the lateral tibial condyle, just inferior to the tibial plateau (Segond fracture).

Features of posterior cruciate ligament tear include:

- Posterior knee pain
- Acute onset of mild to moderate knee swelling, due to haemarthrosis
- Abrasions or bruising in the region of the tibial tuberosity
- Ecchymosis in the popliteal fossa
- Positive posterior drawer sign
- Posterior sag sign
- Recurvatum (hyperextension) deformity (unusual)
- X-rays may show an avulsion fracture of the posterior intercondylar eminence.

Features of meniscal tear (triad of joint line pain, swelling, and locking)

- A history of combined axial and rotational forces acting on the knee
- Medial or lateral knee pain, worsened on weight bearing, squatting and hyper-flexion
- Synovial effusion
- True locking (in flexion), with a mechanical block to full extension, associated with a displaced bucket handle tear
- Joint line tenderness
- Quadriceps atrophy
- Sensation of giving way due to reflex inhibition of the quadriceps
- Incomplete flexion
- Tibiofemoral clicking on stairs
- Click reproduction by McMurray test, associated with a posterior horn tear

Causes of locked knee (a better term is blocked knee)

Locking refers to a springy resistance to full passive extension of the knee

- Meniscal bucket-handle tears displaced into the inter-condylar notch
- Loose osteochondral fragments: osteoarthritis; osteochondritis dissecans; synovial chondromatosis
- Patello-femoral joint dysfunction
- Plica syndromes

Features of knee dislocation

- Gross deformity of the knee with swelling
- Usually anterior dislocation of the tibia, caused by hyperextension injury. Posterior dislocation of the tibia is caused by axial loading of the flexed knee (dashboard injury)
- Valgus or varus instability of the knee in full extension if the dislocation has reduced prior to arrival in the emergency department, spontaneous reduction occurring with 50% of knee dislocations
- Co-existing popliteal artery and common peroneal nerve injury
- Buttonholing of the medial femoral condyle through the medial joint capsule causes a dimple sign, indicating irreducibility

Features of quadriceps mechanism rupture

- Caused by unexpected flexion force, resisted by automatic sudden eccentric contraction of the quadriceps
- Usually occurs in persons aged 40 years and above
- This may lead to either avulsion of the quadriceps tendon from the superior pole of the patella, fractured patella, or avulsion at the tibial tubercle
- The presentation is with pain and swelling above the patella
- Extension of the knee may be possible if the patellar retinacula are intact

- X rays reveal a patella baja (inferiorly positioned patella)

Risk factors for quadriceps tendon rupture

- Chronic tendonitis
- Inflammatory arthropathy
- Anabolic steroid use
- Local steroid injection
- Fluoroquinolone therapy
- Chronic kidney disease (secondary hyperparathyroidism)
- Primary hyperparathyroidism

Features of rupture of the patellar ligament

- Usually occurs in persons below the age of 40
- Caused by forceful eccentric quadriceps contraction with the knee flexed, as in jump landing or weight lifting
- Active knee extension against gravity, and the maintenance of passive knee extension, are not possible
- A palpable defect may be felt at the apex of the patella
- X-rays reveal a patella alta (high-riding patella), with the entire patella lying superior to the level of the inter-condylar notch, from unopposed pull of the quadriceps tendon. A small avulsion fracture at the lower pole of the patella may occur

Risk factors for patellar tendon rupture

- Chronic patellar tendonitis (jumper's knee)
- Rheumatoid arthritis
- Diabetes mellitus
- Chronic kidney disease (secondary hyperparathyroidism; haemodialysis)
- Local steroid injection
- Systemic glucocorticoid therapy
- Fluoroquinolone therapy
- Reconstructive knee surgery: total knee replacement; anterior cruciate ligament reconstruction using middle third of patellar tendon

Features of tibial tubercle avulsion

- Avulsion of tibial tubercle apophysis in adolescents
- Follows a discrete jumping incident
- Knee extension limited or impossible
- Joint effusion seldom present

Ottawa knee rules for x-rays with knee injuries

- Age > 55 years
- Tenderness at head of fibula
- Isolated tenderness of the patella
- Inability to flex knee to 90°
- Inability to transfer weight for 4 steps both immediately after injury and in the emergency department

Classification of knee instability

A. Straight
   - Medial (valgus subluxation of tibia on femur): abduction stress test
   - Lateral (varus subluxation of tibia on femur): adduction stress test
   - Posterior: posterior drawer sign
   - Anterior: anterior drawer sign

B. Rotatory
   - Antero-medial (anterior subluxation of medial tibial condyle with external rotation on femur)
     - Abduction stress at 30°
     - Anterior drawer sign in external rotation
     - Antero-lateral (anterior subluxation of lateral tibial condyle with internal rotation on femur)
   - Jerk test
   - Pivot shift test
   - Flexion rotation drawer sign (Noyes)
   - Anterior drawer sign in neutral
   - Postero-lateral (posterior subluxation and internal rotation of lateral tibial condyle)
     - External recurvatum test
     - Reversed pivot shift test
     - Adduction stress at 30°

Causes of exercise-induced lower leg pain

Teno-periosteal: Shin splints (periostitis of the posteromedial border of the tibia-medial tibial stress syndrome): diffuse pain along posteromedial border of the tibia as opposed to local pain from stress fracture

Bony: Stress fracture of the tibia/fibula

Muscular: Compartment syndromes (Anterior: acute/chronic exertional;

Deep posterior); fascial herniae of muscles

Tendinous: Tendinitis of long flexors; tibialis posterior syndrome

Vascular: Popliteal artery entrapment syndrome

Causes of true claudication in the calf

- Atherosclerosis
- Takayasu arteritis
- Thromboangiitis obliterans
- Collagen vascular disease
- Embolism: heart (left ventricular thrombus; paradoxical embolism)
- Cystic adventitial disease
- Popliteal artery entrapment
- Drugs: ergot derivatives

Causes of pseudo-claudication of the calf

- Nocturnal cramps
- Chronic compartment syndrome
- Venous claudication: proximal (ilio-femoral) deep vein thrombosis
- Radiculopathy
- Symptomatic popliteal cyst

Causes of pseudo-claudication of the hip and buttock

- Hip arthritis
- Neurogenic claudication

Features of proximal tibial fractures

- Tibial plateau fractures are caused by varus or valgus injuries associated with axial loading or weight bearing on the knee.
- Cruciate and collateral ligament and meniscal injuries may coexist
- Fractures of the lateral tibial plateau are commoner
- Haemarthrosis of the knee is present
- Compartment syndrome may complicate the injury
- X-rays show a lipohaemarthrosis, with a fat-fluid level on a horizontal beam radiograph

Features of tibial shaft fractures

- Present with acute leg pain and inability to bear weight
- Low energy injuries are usually torsional
- High energy injuries involve direct trauma and are often associated with open injuries, comminution, and the risk of compartment syndrome

Features of toddler's fracture

- Twisting injury in children up to the age of 6
- Undisplaced spiral fracture of middle or distal tibia; the initial x-ray may be normal, with delayed visualisation as a lucent line or periosteal reaction
- Most common in children younger than 2 years' age who are learning to walk
- Often no history of trauma, with presentation with reluctance to bear weight on the leg
- Examine hip, thigh and knee

Features of stress fracture of tibia

- At junction of middle and distal thirds in runners, in middle third in ballet dancers, and in proximal third in military recruits
- Predisposing factors: lower limb malalignment, training errors, poor footwear
- Insidious onset of shin soreness, increased with physical activity
- Point tenderness over fracture site

- Swelling minimal or absent
- X-rays often normal in first 2–4 weeks after the onset of symptoms; localised periosteal thickening (junction of middle and distal thirds); endosteal callus formation (proximal callus)
- Round or fusiform pattern of uptake on triple-phase bone scan
- Eliminate impact loading activity for 4–6 weeks; no immobilization; crutch-assisted ambulation for comfort as required
- Monthly radiographs

Features of fibula shaft fracture

- Caused by a direct blow to the lateral aspect of the leg
- Common peroneal nerve palsy (producing footdrop) may accompany proximal fibular fractures

Causes of calf muscle pain

- Muscle tear: rupture of medial head of gastrocnemius
- Calf cramps
- Deep vein thrombosis
- Popliteal cyst (Baker's cyst)
- Peripheral arterial disease
- Varicose veins
- Nerve entrapment/compression
- Peripheral neuropathy
- Cellulitis
- Achilles tendonitis

Features of rupture of the gastrocnemius (tennis leg)

- An acute overload injury affecting the middle aged and involving the musculotendinous junction of the medial head of the gastrocnemius
    - Acute onset of calf pain with the sensation of being hit from behind
    - Local tenderness and swelling in the medial head of the gastrocnemius
    - Pain is increased on passive ankle dorsiflexion and on active resisted ankle plantarflexion
    - Delayed onset bruising which gravitates to the ankle.
    - Intact Achilles tendon

Two-level Wells' score for deep vein thrombosis

	Points
Previously documented DVT	+1
Paralysis, paresis or recent plaster immobilization of lower extremities	+1
Recently bedridden for 3 days or more or major surgery within 12 weeks requiring general or regional anaesthesia	+ 1
Localized tenderness along the distribution of the deep venous system	+1
Calf swelling 3 cm or > compared to asymptomatic calf, measured 10 cm below tibial tuberosity	+1
Entire leg swollen	+1
Pitting oedema confined to the symptomatic leg	+ 1
Collateral superficial veins (non-varicose)	+1
Alternative diagnosis at least as likely as DVT	−2
Haemoptysis	+1
Active cancer (Treatment ongoing, within 6 months, or palliative)	+1
Clinical probability of DVT Likely 2 points or more Unlikely 1 point or less	

Wells PS. Evaluation of D-dimer in the diagnosis of suspected deep-vein thrombosis. New Engl J Med. 2003;349:1227–35.

Features of acute deep vein thrombosis with bedside ultrasound

Incomplete venous compressibility. If the common femoral and popliteal veins are fully compressible, clinically significant above knee deep vein thrombosis can be excluded

Venous dilatation by echogenic or hypoechoic intraluminal thrombus

(filling defect in normally anechoic lumen)

Colour flow Doppler may show:

- Reduced or absent flow

- Persistent filling defect (colour void) in colour column of vessel lumen
- Reduced or absent respiratory-induced flow phasicity
- Absence of flow augmentation with mechanical calf compression

Further investigation with unprovoked deep vein thrombosis includes

- Investigation for cancer: physical examination; chest x-ray; blood tests: FBC, serum calcium, liver function tests; urinalysis
- Thrombophilia testing; anti-phospholipid antibodies; hereditary thrombophilia screening in patients who have a first degree relative with deep vein thrombosis

Ankle injuries

Ottawa ankle rules for obtaining x-rays after ankle injury

Pain in malleolar or mid-foot zone

Bony tenderness at posterior edge or tip of lateral or medial malleolus (palpate distal 6 cm); 5th metatarsal base or navicular (4 sites for bony tenderness)

Inability to bear weight immediately after the injury and for four steps in the emergency department

These rules are not applicable if:

- Age of patient less than 18 years
- Mental state is altered
- Multi-system trauma
- Subacute injury (>10 days' post-injury)

Evaluation of ankle x-rays following trauma

- Soft tissue swelling; obliteration of fat planes or pre-Achilles fat triangle (Kager fat pad)
- The ankle mortise is a rectangular socket formed by the articular surface of the tibia (plafond), into which the dome of the talus fits
- Look at congruity of articular surface; the joint space should be uniform
- Identify talar shift: lateral talar shift is manifested as an increase in the medial clear space between the talus and medial malleolus, normally <4 mm
- Identify talar tilt (a line parallel with the articular surface of the distal tibia and a line parallel with the articular surface of the talus should be parallel)
- Medial clear space should be uniform and less than 4 mm; lateral clear space should be uniform and less than 5 mm (the clear joint space is formed by the talo-fibular joint and the superior space between the talar dome and tibial plafond)
- The talar dome should be smooth
- The talocrural angle, a line parallel to the articular surface of the distal tibia and the intermalleolar line (connecting the tips of the medial and lateral malleoli) should be 8–15°
- Identify tibio-fibular diastasis (lateral talar displacement or tibiofibular widening): associated with proximal fibular fracture (Maisonneuve fracture)
- The distance between the tibia and fibula 1 cm proximal to the tibial plafond should be less than 6 mm
- Always check the fifth metatarsal base, lateral process of talus, os trigonum or posterior malleolus, anterior process of calcaneus and talar dome (mnemonic FLOAT)
- Be aware of accessory ossicles: os trigonum (posterior to the talus); os subtibiale (distal to the tip of the medial malleolus); and os subfibulare (distal to the tip of the lateral malleolus)

Signs of instability in ankle fractures

- Significant fracture displacement: displacement of medial or lateral malleolus greater than 2–3 mm
- Fracture of the lateral malleolus above the syndesmosis
- Widening of medial joint space >2 mm
- Talar tilt or shift; altered talo-crural angle
- Subluxation or dislocation of the talus under the plafond
- Bimalleolar fracture

- Trimalleolar fracture
- Maisonneuve fracture

Features of pilon fractures of the tibia

- Caused by high energy vertical axial loading injuries secondary to falls from a height or motor vehicle collisions, driving the talus into the tibial plafond
- Present with severe ankle pain and swelling, and inability to bear weight
- Often associated with severe soft tissue injuries
- X-rays show a long oblique distal metaphyseal tibial fracture with comminution, and a fracture of the tibio-talar articular surface

Features of Tillaux fracture

- Salter-Harris type III injury involving the antero-lateral aspect of the distal tibial epiphysis, resulting from an abduction-external rotation mechanism of injury leading to an avulsion of the anterior inferior tibiofibular ligament
- The antero-lateral corner of the distal tibial epiphysis is avulsed
- Occurs usually between the ages of 12 and 15 years

Features of triplanar fracture

- A multiplanar fracture of the distal tibia in adolescence, comprising a vertical (sagittal) distal epiphyseal fracture, a horizontal (axial) distal physeal fracture and a vertical oblique (coronal) distal metaphyseal fracture, resulting from external rotation. The fracture thereby involves the frontal, lateral and transverse planes
- The fracture resembles a Salter-Harris III injury on the AP view and a Salter-Harris II injury on the lateral view
- Susceptibility is related to asymmetrical closure of the distal tibial epiphyseal plate, with closure of the medial epiphyseal plate taking place 12–24 months before closure of the lateral epiphyseal plate

Categorisation of fractures of the lateral malleolus using the Danis-Weber classification

- Type A: distal to the tibio-fibular syndesmosis and below level of talar dome; intact deltoid ligament and tibio-fibular syndesmosis; transverse fracture of lateral malleolus + oblique fracture of medial malleolus
- Type B: at the level of the tibio-fibular syndesmosis, with distal extent at level of talar dome; injury to deltoid ligament or medial malleolus and tibio-fibular syndesmosis may coexist; oblique or spiral fracture of lateral malleolus + avulsion of deltoid ligament +/− avulsion fracture of medial malleolus
- Type C: proximal to level of tibio-fibular syndesmosis; deltoid ligament and tibio-fibular syndesmosis injury coexist

Features of trimalleolar fracture

- Fractures of lateral, medial and posterior malleolus
- Widening of ankle joint space anteriorly and at the distal tibio-fibular syndesmosis
- Posterior and lateral displacement of the talus

Features of calcaneal fracture

- Hindfoot pain, swelling, bruising, broadening and tenderness
- Bruising in sole and along lateral aspect of hindfoot
- Caused by a fall from a height with forced dorsiflexion of the ankle and axial loading of the calcaneus or by a twisting injury (leading to avulsion and extra-articular fractures)
- Can be bilateral in patients with falls from a significant height
- Associated with lumbar spinal compression fractures

- The extent of the injury can be underestimated on plain films and CT is the imaging modality of choice for evaluation of calcaneal fractures
- Sustentaculum tali fracture is indicated by painful passive movement of the great toe (the FHL tendon runs beneath the sustentaculum)
- Avulsion fracture of the tendo Achilles is indicated by weakness of plantar-flexion of the ankle

Bohler's angle (measuring calcaneal height) is measured between a line on the lateral view of the foot from the posterior superior margin of the **calcaneal tuberosity** through the superior tip of the **posterior facet** and a second line from the superior tip of the posterior calcaneal facet through the superior margin of the **anterior articular process** of the calcaneus. The normal angle measures from 20 to 40°. The critical angle of Gissane is formed by lines drawn along the posterior calcaneal facet and the anterior calcaneal process, and the normal range is from 120 to 145°.

Features of talar fracture

- Talar dome fractures result from inversion injury of the ankle and present with either acute ankle pain or with persistent ankle pain or instability (catching, clicking, locking or giving way) following initial non-recognition of the injury. Antero-lateral dome fractures result from inversion of the foot with the ankle dorsiflexed, and postero-medial dome fractures result from inversion of the foot with the ankle plantar flexed.
- Posterior process (Shepherd) fractures result from hyper-plantarflexion of the ankle or avulsion of the posterior talofibular ligament; should be differentiated from os trigonum (a well corticated, smooth, oval or round structure)
- Lateral process (snowboarder's) fractures result from eversion and axial loading injury, with compression of the lateral process between the lateral malleolus and the calcaneus
- Neck fractures are caused by forced dorsiflexion of the foot, leading to impingement of the neck of the talus against the anterior lip of the distal tibia (as with falls from a height or motor vehicle collisions), or inversion of the ankle; there is a high risk of avascular necrosis of the talar dome as most of the arterial blood supply to the talus enters at the neck via capsular attachments
- Head fractures are due to axial compression with a plantar flexed ankle

Features of sub-talar dislocations

- The talus is dislocated at its distal articulations with the calcaneus and navicular at the talocalcaneal and talonavicular joints
- Lateral dislocations are caused by high energy mechanisms leading to forced eversion of the plantar flexed foot, and medial dislocations usually by low energy mechanisms leading to forced inversion of the plantarflexed foot (basketball foot)
- The talar head lies medially with a lateral dislocation (acquired flatfoot), and dorsolaterally, between the EDL and EDH tendons, with a medial dislocation (acquired clubfoot)
- The foot is locked in supination with medial dislocation, and locked in pronation with lateral dislocation
- Urgent closed reduction with the knee flexed 90°, longitudinal traction on the foot with counter-traction, followed by accentuation, then reversal, of the deformity

Causes of heel pain

Beneath or within heel

- Plantar fasciitis: pain in antero-medial heel which is worse in the morning or after rest, including prolonged sitting; association with pes planus/pes cavus; tenderness at calcaneal attachment; pain on toe extension; limited ankle dorsiflexion. Risk factors include obesity, sudden increase in body weight, recent commencement of

running or prolonged walking, recent change in type of running surface, and occupations involving prolonged weight bearing.
- Plantar fascial tear
- Calcaneal spur
- Stress fracture of calcaneus
- Subperiosteal haematoma of calcaneus (heel bruise)
- Tarsal tunnel syndrome
- Heel pad bruising
- Inferior calcaneal bursitis

Behind heel

- Achilles tendonitis
- Delayed diagnosis of rupture of Achilles tendon (partial/complete)
- Retrocalcaneal bursitis (pump bump)
- Posterosuperior calcaneal exostosis (Haglund syndrome)
- Calcaneal apophysis: retrocalcaneal apophysitis (Sever's disease)

Features of posterior tarsal tunnel syndrome (entrapment neuropathy of the posterior tibial nerve produced by the flexor retinaculum behind the medial malleolus of the tibia)

Pain, burning sensation and paraesthesiae on the sole of the forefoot and medial three toes
Pain is increased by activity (walking, running, or prolonged standing)
Night pain may occur.
Intrinsic muscle weakness in the foot
Distal tingling on percussion in the tarsal tunnel, below and behind the medial malleolus (positive Tinel sign)
Peripheral pulses normally palpable

Features of Achilles tendon rupture

- Sudden pain thought to be caused often by an object hitting the back of the leg
- Audible snap
- Visible and palpable defect in the tendon (masked by swelling in late presentation)
- Weakness of plantar-flexion of ankle
- Some active plantar-flexion due to plantaris, flexor hallucis longus and tibialis posterior function
- Calf squeeze with the patient kneeling on a chair does not produce passive plantar-flexion
- Flat-footed gait
- Inability to walk on toes

Features of Achilles tendinitis include:

Activity related pain in the Achilles tendon region
Pain on resisted ankle plantarflexion
Pain on and reduced range of passive ankle dorsiflexion
Tenderness and thickening of the Achilles tendon, and often of the overlying skin and subcutaneous bursa.
No palpable gap in the tendon
Crepitation
Tight posterior ankle structures
Persistent severe pain may indicate impending rupture of the tendon
X-rays may show calcification in the tendon.

Features of sprain of the lateral ligament of the ankle

- Caused by inversion of the ankle, with or without plantar flexion of the foot
- The anterior talofibular ligament is most commonly injured, followed by the calcaneofibular ligament. The posterior talofibular ligament is rarely injured.
- Anterolateral ankle pain, bruising and swelling
- Tenderness over the anterior talofibular ligament (ATFL) and calcaneofibular ligament (CFL)
- There may be an avulsion fracture of the tip of the lateral malleolus
- The anterior drawer test for the ATFL is positive if there is a greater than 3–5 mm

difference in anterior displacement of the talus between the two ankles and no distinct end-point, with the tibia held fixed with one hand

- The talar tilt or varus stress test for the CFL is positive with a greater than 10 degree difference in talar tilt between the two ankles with inversion and no distinct end-point, with the tibia held fixed with one hand

Causes of non-healing ankle sprain

Unrecognised fracture: anterior process of calcaneus in sinus tarsi; lateral process of talus (snowboarder's ankle); avulsion fracture of 5th metatarsal base (at the tubercle at the peroneus brevis tendon insertion); Jones fracture (stress fracture at the metaphyseal-diaphyseal junction) of proximal 5th metatarsal shaft distal to the styloid; fracture of lateral tubercle of posterior process of talus (Shepherd fracture) (distinguished from os trigonum, which is rounded or oval with smooth corticated edges)

Osteochondral injury of talar dome

Peroneal tendon injury (rapid dorsiflexion of inverted foot): tear (pain and swelling inferior and posterior to lateral malleolus); subluxation/dislocation (painful snapping sensation along lateral ankle)

Traction injury to superficial peroneal nerve

High ankle sprain (tibio-fibular syndesmosis): pain on squeezing lower leg at mid-calf level or cross legs with injured leg resting at mid-calf on knee

Antero-lateral ankle impingement: overuse injury caused by repetitive ankle dorsiflexion (ballet dancers, gymnasts); anterior ankle pain is increased by dorsiflexion (e.g. plies in ballet dancers); reduced range of ankle movement; anterior tibial or talar neck osteophytes

Tarsal coalition (most common are talocalcaneal and calcaneonavicular coalition): ankle pain with activity associated with inversion of the foot; rigid hindfoot valgus deformity; no heel varus on standing tiptoe; tightness of peroneal tendons; symptoms develop between the ages of 12 and 15 years

Achilles tendon injury

Salter type I injury of the distal fibular epiphysis ("goose-egg" swelling

over the distal fibula with tenderness over the distal fibular epiphysis)

Causes of chronic ankle pain

Anterior

Anterior tibiotalar exostoses from repetitive forced dorsiflexion (anterior impingement syndrome of ankle (limited ankle dorsiflexion; ankle pain on passive forced dorsiflexion; anterior ankle joint line tenderness; palpable osteophytes)

Anterior tibial tendinitis

Extensor digitorum longus tendinitis

Peroneal neuropathy

Lateral

Lateral impingement syndrome (os subfibulare)

Sinus tarsi syndrome

Recurrent peroneal subluxation

Osteochondral fracture of the talus

Distal fibular stress fracture

Medial

Stress fracture of the medial malleolus

Osteochondral fracture of talar dome

Subluxation of tibialis posterior tendon

Tendinitis of tibialis posterior; flexor hallucis longus

Medial impingement: old medial malleolar tip fracture/old medial talar fracture

Posteromedial

Flexor hallucis longus/flexor digitorum longus tendinitis

Posterolateral

Posterior (talo-tibial) impingement syndrome: posterior tibial spur/os trigonum (posterolateral ankle pain and tenderness, anterior to the Tendo Achilles; pain is provoked by forced passive ankle plantar flexion; reduced range of

ankle plantar flexion; pain occurs on jumping and springing manoeuvres)
Peroneus tendinitis

Causes of foot drop (high steppage gait; inability to dorsiflex and evert foot; sensory loss in entire or distal 1/3 lateral leg and dorsum of foot with sciatic or common peroneal nerve lesions respectively)

Unilateral

- Common peroneal neuropathy: external compression from sitting cross-legged or squatting and associated with recent rapid weight loss; blunt trauma-fibula neck fracture, surgical (total knee replacement); masses near fibular head; anterior compartment syndrome of the leg
- Lumbosacral plexopathy, involving the lumbosacral trunk: prolonged labour; pelvic fracture
- L4–5 radiculopathy: disc prolapse; lumbar spinal stenosis
- Sciatic nerve injury: posterior dislocation of the hip; total hip replacement; intramuscular injection injury; external compression secondary to coma

Bilateral

- Distal myopathy: myotonic dystrophy; facioscapulohumeral muscular dystrophy
- Bilateral peroneal or sciatic neuropathies; bilateral lumbosacral plexopathies
- Cauda equina compression (bilateral L5 radiculopathy)
- Conus medullaris lesion
- Anterior horn cell lesions in spinal cord: poliomyelitis; amyotrophic lateral sclerosis; spinal muscular atrophy; spinal cord injury
- Upper motor neuron lesions: interhemispheric motor cortex in frontal lobes (parasagittal meningioma); stroke-lacunes (internal capsule, cerebral peduncles)

Features of fracture of the navicular

- Cortical avulsion fracture results from twisting of the mid-foot
- Avulsion fracture of the tibialis posterior tendon insertion causes a tuberosity avulsion fracture and should be distinguished from an os naviculare
- Fractures of the body are usually associated with other mid-tarsal joint injuries
- Stress fracture is often seen in runners (repeated foot strike with running on hard surfaces), presenting with the insidious onset of gradually increasing activity-related dorsal mid-foot pain with occasional radiation down the medial longitudinal arch of the foot. There is localised tenderness at the central region of the proximal dorsal navicular. The fracture is often not seen on plain x-rays initially and delayed recognition is common.

Features of fracture of the cuboid

- Avulsion fractures at ligamentous or capsular insertions are the most common type of injury
- Fractures of the body result from direct trauma
- The nutcracker fracture is caused by axial torsional forces (forced forefoot abduction on a fixed plantar flexed hindfoot), leading to compression of the cuboid between the calcaneum and the 4th and 5th metatarsals
- Stress fractures present with mid-foot pain in runners

Causes of forefoot pain
Hallux and 1st MTP joint

- Deformity: hallux valgus (bunion); Morton's toe (short 1st metatarsal)
- No deformity: hallux rigidus (degenerative arthritis); sesamoid disorders: sesamoiditis, osteonecrosis, fracture, arthritis; gout; turf toe; black nail

2nd through 5th (lesser) toes and MTP joints

- Deformities: claw toes; hammer toes; mallet toes
- Instability: long 2nd metatarsal

- Metatarsalgia: Morton's plantar interdigital neuroma (exercise-induced pain or paraesthesiae; pain provoked by squeezing the toes together while holding metatarsals parallel); bunionette (angular deformity of 5th toe); stress fracture; metatarsophalangeal synovitis; inflammatory arthritis; Freiberg's disease: avascular necrosis of 2nd metatarsal head; high-heeled, or tight and restrictive shoes and boots

Features of 1st metatarsal fracture

- Known as the paediatric bunk bed fracture, common in young children
- Caused by plantar flexion and/or abduction
- Salter-Harris II or buckle type fracture at 1st metatarsal base
- The medial cuneiform-1st metatarsal epiphysis is wedged into the 1st metatarsal-2nd metatarsal interspace

Features of metatarsal fractures

- Forefoot pain and swelling
- Point tenderness over fracture site(s)
- Caused by direct trauma (e.g. dropping heavy objects on to the foot), leading to transverse or comminuted fractures
- Stress fractures are seen in athletes, and with long second metatarsals (Morton foot) or after metatarsal shortening procedures in the forefoot altering weight bearing distribution among the metatarsal heads (e.g. hallux valgus surgery). The presentation is with a gradual onset of activity related forefoot pain, relieved on rest, progressing to pain at rest, often preceded by a recent change in activity (prolonged walking or long distance running). The usual sites affected are the neck and shaft of the 2nd and 3rd metatarsal. The fracture is usually at the junction of the proximal shaft and the metaphysis and may not show on conventional x-rays for up to 3–4 weeks. The initial radiographic manifestation is of localized periosteal new bone formation.

Features of puncture wounds of the plantar aspect of the foot

- Most involve the forefoot and are due to penetration by nails, needles, glass and wood
- Organisms common in the soil are often isolated, such as Pseudomonas aeruginosa
- There is a risk of osteomyelitis or septic arthritis

Features of turf toe

- A sprain of the metatarsophalangeal joint of the big toe, affecting the plantar aspect of the joint capsule
- The mechanism of production is forced dorsiflexion of the big toe, or repetitive push-off from the dorsiflexed big toe.
- The lesion is predisposed to with training on synthetic playing surfaces, such as artificial turf
- The features include:
- Swelling and tenderness on the plantar aspect of the 1st metatarsophalangeal joint

Features of interdigital neuroma (Morton's neuroma)

- A syndrome of forefoot pain produced by a fusiform swelling of the plantar nerve or digital nerve just distal to the bifurcation of the plantar nerve
- Narrow tight footwear can help precipitate symptoms.

The features are:

Forefoot pain radiating into the toes

Pain is increased by weight bearing, running and side to side forefoot compression causing metatarsal arch compression

Tenderness to palpation on the plantar aspect of the interdigital web space

The lesion is usually impalpable.

Paraesthesiae and night pain may be associated.

Local anaesthetic infiltration provides temporary relief.

Features of black nail
Due to subungual bleeding caused by repeated shearing of the nail plate on the nail bed, caused especially by running with shoes with a small toe box.

- The features include:
- An initial bluish discolouration of the nail plate
- Later a black discolouration, and loosening and thickening of the nail plate

Features suggesting Lisfranc injury (involving the tarso-metatarsal joint complex, comprised of a medial column (medial cuneiform and 1st metatarsal), a middle column (middle and lateral cuneiforms and 2nd and 3rd metatarsals) and a lateral column (cuboid and 4th and 5th metatarsals))

- Fall forward on a plantar-flexed foot
- Inability to bear weight, with swelling of the dorsum of the midfoot, which may obscure the pedal pulses.
- Plantar arch bruising may be pathognomic
- Inability to walk tiptoes
- Avulsion fracture of the lateral base of the 1st metatarsal or the medial base of the 2nd metatarsal (fleck sign)
- The space between the 1st and 2nd metatarsal bases is widened >2.7 mm (gap sign), especially on weight-bearing views
- Widening of the space between 2nd metatarsal base and middle cuneiform
- Pain with forefoot rotation
- Mid-foot swelling; mid-foot plantar ecchymosis is pathognomic
- Inability to bear weight
- The lateral border of the 1st metatarsal base does not line up with the lateral border of the medial cuneiform
- The medial border of the 2nd metatarsal does not line up with the medial border of the middle cuneiform
- There may be a bony fragment at the base of the 2nd metatarsal or the medial cuneiform

Features of sesamoiditis

- An overuse injury following repetitive jumping with landing on the dorsiflexed 1st metacarpophalangeal joint

The features include:
Pain in the ball of the big toe on running tip-toe or on take off from the stationary start
Pain is increased by dorsiflexion of the big toe with the proximal phalanx either extended or flexed.
Tenderness over the sesamoids under the 1st metacarpal head

Differential diagnosis of acute torticollis

- Atlantoaxial rotary displacement, subluxation, fixation
  Presentation is with torticollis, associated with adoption of the "cock robin" posture (chin rotation to the contralateral side with the neck flexed)
  The open mouth view shows rotation of atlas on axis
  Lateral mass of atlas rotated forward appears wider and closer to the midline (medial offset)
  Lateral mass of atlas rotated backward appears narrower and farther away from the midline (lateral offset)
  On the side where the atlas has rotated backward, the joint between the lateral masses of the atlas and axis may be obscured due to apparent overlapping.
  The spinous process of the axis is not deviated from the midline in the direction opposite that of head rotation until rotation of more than 50% total normal rotation has occurred.
- Neurogenic: spinal cord tumours; cerebellar/posterior fossa tumours
  Arnold-Chiari malformation
  Inflammation:
  - Cervical lymphadenitis
  - Grisel syndrome (atlanto-axial subluxation caused by relaxation of the

transverse ligament of the atlanto-axial joint, not associated with trauma or bone disease, with facet joint asymmetry on AP projection and an increased atlanto-dens interval on the lateral projection)
- Retropharyngeal abscess
- Juvenile rheumatoid arthritis; rheumatoid arthritis

Disc space calcification
Tuberculosis
Neoplasm:
- Osteoid osteoma
- Aneurysmal bone cyst

Sandifer syndrome: spasmodic torsional dystonia with opisthotonus mimicking seizures

Factors increasing risk of cervical spine injury

- High risk injury mechanism
  Fall from height >10 feet
  Motor vehicle collision: speed >50 mph; vehicle rollover; head on collision; ejection; death in same vehicle; collision with large vehicle; motorized recreational vehicle accident; prolonged extrication time; steering wheel or windshield damage; passenger space intrusion
  Axial load to head
  Drowning or diving accident
  Pedestrian collision with vehicle
  Hanging
- Altered mental state (GCS <15) or level of consciousness; drug and alcohol intoxication
- Head or severe facial injury
- Age > 65 years
- Pelvic or multiple limb fractures
- Prior cervical spine trauma/surgery
- Degenerative disease of spine
- Spinal canal stenosis
- Rigid spine disease: ankylosing spondylitis; diffuse idiopathic skeletal hyperostosis
- Down's syndrome
- Rheumatoid arthritis
- Arnold-Chiari malformation; Klippel-Feil syndrome
- Metastatic cancer

Checklist for evaluation of cervical spine x-ray

A: A1: anatomy; adequate film that includes entire extent of cervical spine from occiput toT1 vertebral body

A2: Four parallel and uninterrupted lines of vertebral alignment, with normal dorsal concavity (lordosis):

- Anterior vertebral body line
- Posterior vertebral body line
- Spinolaminar line
- Posterior spinous processes

B: Bone integrity
C: Cartilage or joint space abnormalities
S: Soft tissue abnormalities

X-ray features of the cervical spine that may be normal in children

- C1-C2 widening
- Pseudosubluxation of C2 on C3, or C3 on C4
- Pseudo-Jefferson fracture, related to faster growth of lateral masses of C1 as compared to those of C2
- Increased pre-dental space (5 mm or less)
- Normal posterior angulation of the odontoid
- Os odontoideum
- Loss of the normal lordosis of the cervical spine

X-ray signs of instability after cervical spine trauma

- Widened inter-spinous space (fanning) >2 mm
- Widened apophyseal joint >2 mm
- Anterior listhesis >3.5 mm
- Narrowing or widening of inter-vertebral disk space
- Angulation between vertebrae >10°
- Vertebral compression >25% of height

- Involvement of two or more columns
- Facet joint widening or rotation
- Pedicle widening

Subtle cervical spine injuries
From rostral to caudal, there are only seven cervicocranial injuries that may be radiologically subtle and yet capable of causing an abnormal cervicocranial prevertebral soft tissue shadow:

- Occipitoatlantal subluxation (separation of the occipital condyles from the atlas; significant displacement of the odontoid from the basion; retropharyngeal haematoma; associated with brainstem injury and usually fatal)
- Occipital condylar fracture
- Lateral mass of C1 fracture
- Jefferson bursting fracture
- High dens fracture
- Low dens fracture
- Traumatic spondylolisthesis, type 1

Normal cervical spine measurements

- Lateral atlanto-axial offset on open-mouth view: 2 mm
  - Pre-dental space <3 mm (adult); <5 mm (child)
  - Anterior vertebral height vs. posterior height: 2 mm (except C5)
  - Pre-tracheal space at C6: 22 mm (adult); 14 mm (child)
  - Facet width: 2 mm
  - Listhesis on flexion/extension: 2 mm
  - Retropharyngeal space at C2: 7–8 mm

Clinical clearance of cervical spine

- Awake and alert: GCS 15
  - No neurological symptoms or signs
  - No painful distracting injury
  - No neck pain/midline cervical tenderness
  - Full active range of movement of cervical spine

Types of cervical spine injury according to mechanism
Flexion

- Anterior subluxation (hyper-flexion sprain)
- Wedge compression fracture
- Bilateral inter-facetal dislocation: Anterior displacement of the dislocated vertebra equal to at least one-half the AP diameter of the involved vertebral body; widening of the distance between the spinous processes at the injury site
- Avulsion fracture of spinous processes C6, C7 (clay-shoveller's fracture)
- Flexion teardrop fracture: A large triangular fragment consisting of the antero-inferior aspect of the involved vertebral body; subluxation or dislocation of the interfacetal joints at the level of injury; posterior retropulsion of the cephalad vertebrae; complete disruption of all ligaments and the intervertebral disk at the level of injury; associated with the acute anterior cervical cord syndrome or permanent quadriplegia

Flexion-rotation

- Unilateral inter-facetal dislocation (locked facet): anterior displacement of the dislocated superior vertebra a distance less than one-half of the AP diameter (<50% width) of a cervical vertebral body

Extension-rotation

- Pillar fracture

Vertical compression (axial loading)

- Jefferson fracture of atlas: comminuted fracture of C1 ring involving both anterior and posterior arches; bilateral lateral displacement of the lateral masses of C1 on AP projection, caused by compression between the occipital condyles and the superior articular facets of C2
- Burst fracture: Comminution of the vertebral body; widening of the margins of the vertebral body; loss of height of the vertebral body; varying degrees of retropulsion of the posterior body fragments into the

central canal; posterior arch fracture, usually involving the lamina

Hyperextension

- Hyperextension dislocation (disruption): triad of signs: soft tissue and/or skeletal injury of the mid-face or forehead; acute cervical central cord syndrome; and prominent diffuse pre-vertebral soft tissue swelling and normally aligned cervical vertebrae on the lateral projection; avulsion fracture arising from the anterior aspect of the inferior end plate of the dislocated vertebra
- Fracture anterior arch of atlas
- Fracture of posterior arch of atlas
- Traumatic spondylolisthesis (hangman's fracture): Bilateral fractures of the pars inter-articularis of C2: the relatively thin portion of the articular mass between the superior and inferior articular facets of the axis, sometimes also called the isthmus; anterior dislocation of the body of the axis; anterior rotation of C2; caused by hyperextension with axial loading; usually not associated with neurological deficit
- Extension teardrop fracture: triangular fracture fragment avulsed from the anterior inferior corner of the axis, usually in older patients with osteoporosis and degenerative changes in the spine

Lateral flexion

- Uncinate process fracture

A fracture of the dens must be differentiated from:

- Failure of fusion of the dens with the body of the axis at the sub-dental synchondrosis (os odontoideum): rounded corticated margin around entire surface, more widely separated from the base of the odontoid than a fracture
- Mach bands that result from the overlap of the margins of the anterior and posterior arches of C1 and the teeth on the open-mouth view. The inferior cortex of the posterior arch of the atlas may produce a Mach effect simulating high dens fracture. The Mach effect extends beyond the lateral margin of the dens and is superimposed on the lateral atlanto-dental intervals.

Features of pseudo-subluxation of C2 on C3

- This is a physiological phenomenon due to normal ligamentous laxity
- Anterior subluxation of C2 on C3, less than 4 mm
- The posterior cervical line connecting the anterior cortex of the spinous processes of C1 and C3 passes through the posterior arch of C2 or <2 mm anterior to this (posterior spino-laminar line)

Causes of spino-laminar line displacement

- Anterior or posterior displacement at C1: type II dens fracture with atlanto-axial displacement (anterior or posterior); transverse atlantal ligament injury (anterior)
- Anterior or posterior displacement at C2: hangman's fracture (posterior); C2–3 dislocation (anterior or posterior)

Features of SCIWORA (spinal cord injury without radiological abnormality)

- Traumatic myelopathy, typically seen in children under the age of 8 years
- Acceleration-deceleration or rotational injury, commonly at the cervico-thoracic junction region
- Caused by traumatic deformation of the spinal column without fracture or ligamentous disruption
- Normal plain x-ray, flexion-extension views and CT scan of the cervical spine

Risk factors for persistent symptoms after neck sprain

Accident mechanisms

- Inclined or rotated head position

- Unpreparedness for impact
- Car stationary when hit

Occupant characteristics

- Older age
- Female gender

Symptoms

- Intensity of initial neck pain or headache
- Occipital headache
- Inter-scapular or upper back pain
- Multiple symptoms or paraesthesiae at presentation

Signs

- Reduced range of movement of the cervical spine
- Objective neurological deficit

Radiographic findings

- Pre-existing degenerative osteoarthritic changes
- Abnormal cervical spine curves
- Narrow diameter of cervical spinal canal

Types of thoracolumbar spine injuries
Stable: intact posterior structures

- Pure flexion: wedge compression fracture of body
- Extension: anterior avulsion fracture of body
- Lateral flexion: lateral wedge compression fracture of body
- Vertical compression (axial load): burst injury
- Pure distraction: Chance fracture
- Avulsion: fractures of spinous and transverse processes

Unstable:

- Flexion-rotation: fracture of body
- Shearing
- Flexion-distraction: seat belt injury

Signs of instability in thoraco-lumbar spine fractures

- Loss of >50% in anterior vertebral body height
- Kyphosis >25–30°
- Posterior element injury
- Neurological deficit
- Displacement: dislocation/subluxation >2 mm
- Wide inter-spinous space >2 mm
- Posterior vertebral body line disruption
- Wide inter-pedicular distance
- Wide intervertebral disc space

Factors contributing to spinal stability
Posterior osseo-ligamentous complex (posterior column)

- Pedicles
- Facet joints
- Posterior bony arch
- Inter-spinous and supra-spinous ligament

Middle column

- Posterior 1/3 of vertebral body and annulus fibrosus
- Posterior part of intervertebral disk
- Posterior longitudinal ligament

Anterior column

- Anterior 2/3 of vertebral body and annulus fibrosus
- Anterior part of intervertebral disk
- Anterior longitudinal ligament

Features of sacral fractures

- Low back and buttock pain
- Ecchymosis overlying the sacrum
- Sacral tenderness on rectal examination

- Low lumbar and sacral root neurological deficits

Features of Chance fracture:

Flexion-distraction injury, often caused by lap belt worn without a shoulder restraint
Typically involves L1-L3 levels
Flexion of the spine occurs about an axis at or anterior to the anterior longitudinal ligament
Failure through spinous process, laminae, pars interarticularis, transverse processes, pedicles, vertebral body
Disruption of, and widening of, posterior elements (osseous/ligamentous)
Minimal or no loss of anterior vertebral body height
Minimal or no anterior or lateral displacement of vertebral body on superior vertebral body fragment
Posterior vertebral body height equal to or greater than vertebral body below

Signs of spinal injury in the unconscious patient

- Neurogenic shock (triad of hypotension, bradycardia and peripheral vasodilatation)
- Diaphragmatic breathing
- Flaccid areflexia (spinal shock)
- Flexed upper limbs (loss of C6)
- Response to pain above clavicles only
- Priapism

Features of spinal shock

- Hypotension
- Reflex bradycardia
- Limb paralysis
- Atonic bladder
- Flaccid gastrointestinal tract

Signs of non-accidental injuries in children

- Any bruising to young babies
- Bruising on unusual places, i.e. the cheeks
- Patterned bruising
- Small circular burns
- Scalds to either feet or buttocks
- Red lines to wrists or ankles (from ligatures)
- Isolated tear of upper lip fraenulum
- General neglect
- Failure to thrive without organic causes
- Multiple injuries of different ages
- Injuries to genitalia
- Regression to younger behaviour patterns
- Triad of multi-focal subdural haematoma, retinal haemorrhages and an encephalopathic presentation (shaken baby syndrome)

Fractures suggestive of non-accidental injury

- Rib fractures, especially posterior
- Costo-chondral junction injuries
- Metaphyseal bucket-handle or corner fractures
- Scapular fractures
- Spinous process fractures
- Sternal fractures
- Long bone spiral fractures of the shaft of the femur, humerus and tibia
- Multiple bilateral fractures
- Different stages of healing with multiple fractures
- Complex skull fractures
- Fractures in under 1-year-old

Causes of periosteal reaction on plain x-rays
Trauma

Stress fracture
Non-accidental injury

Infection:

Osteomyelitis: acute; chronic; multi-focal
Syphilis

Metabolic:

- Scurvy
- Healing rickets

Tumour:

- Osteosarcoma
- Ewing's sarcoma
- Neuroblastoma

Miscellaneous:

- Caffey's disease: infantile cortical hyperostosis
- Hypertrophic pulmonary osteoarthropathy

Fracture checklist

- Open versus closed
- Anatomical site within bone (diaphysis, metaphysis, epiphysis)
- Alignment of fragments:
  Displacement: distal fragment displaced anteriorly or posteriorly, medially or lateral
  Rotation: lateral or medial
  Angulation: anterior; posterior; varus; valgus
  Axial: impaction, distraction, overlapped (shortened)
- Direction of fracture line in relation to longitudinal axis of bone: transverse (bending loading); spiral (torsional loading); oblique (bending + axial loading)
- Normal/pathological bone
- Joint involvement

Principles of x-ray diagnosis of fractures

- Examine the bones and joints in at least two planes at 90° to each other
- Consider special views, e.g. for calcaneus, scaphoid
- Consider serial examinations and comparison films (rarely necessary)
- Look at entire length of both bones in assessing fractures of paired bones
- Look for indirect and subtle evidence of bony trauma:
  Widening of soft tissue shadows
  Adjacent joint effusion: fat pad sign (fat pad displacement from oleocranon fossa posteriorly and coronoid and radial fossae anteriorly)
  Air in joint or in surrounding tissues
  Fat-fluid levels with horizontal beam

Describing a fracture

- Open versus closed
- Plane of fracture: transverse; oblique; spiral; avulsion
- Displacement of distal fragment in relation to proximal fragment
- Angulation, described according to direction of apex of fracture angle
- Shortening or over-riding of fragments
- Comminution
- Intra-articular extension
- Associated joint subluxation or dislocation

Radiological signs of fracture
Direct signs

Fracture line: lucent; dense
Cortical step/bulge
Trabecular interruption

Indirect signs

Soft tissue swelling at fracture site
Joint effusion; intra-capsular fat-fluid level; fat pad sign
Fat stripe obliteration or displacement
Periosteal reaction
Air in joint or tissues
Fat fluid level with horizontal beam
- Widening of soft tissue shadows

Salter-Harris classification of epiphyseal injuries
Type

I Complete separation of the epiphysis and metaphysis through the physis, usually by a pure shear mechanism
II A physeal fracture, extending into the metaphysis.
A triangular metaphyseal fragment is created-the 'Thurston-Holland' sign

III A split of the epiphysis, extending into the joint
IV A vertical split through the epiphysis, physis and metaphysis
V Compression of the physis
VI Injury of the perichondrial rim (zone of Ranvier) around the physis

Gustilo and Anderson classification of open (compound) fractures

- Type I: skin wound <1 cm long; inside-out injury caused by sharp bone spike; minimal muscle contamination
- Type II: skin wound 1–10 cm long; minimal contamination; minimal periosteal stripping
- Type III: skin wound >10 cm long; wide periosteal stripping; wide contamination

Causes of pseudo-fractures (fracture mimics)

- Accessory ossicles
- Developmental findings in children: epiphyseal growth plates; ossification centres
- Degenerative changes in the elderly
- Nutrient artery foramina (oblique radiolucency)
- Old fracture
- Mach band (image of two wide bands, one light and one dark, separated by a narrow strip with a light-to-dark component, caused by overlapping bones or soft tissues)
- Irregular mineralization of secondary ossification centres of long bones
- Partial epiphyseal fusion
- Edges of a groove or notch
- Juxta-articular calcification
- Multipartite conditions: bipartite patella; bipartite scaphoid
- Sesamoid bones

Evaluation of bony lesion seen on plain x-ray

- Site within bone: epiphysis; metaphysis; diaphysis; articular surface
- Shape of lesion
- Margins of lesion: sharply/poorly defined
- Behaviour: osteolytic; osteoblastic; mixed
- Bony reaction: periosteal (solid; laminated or onion-skin; speculated; Codman's triangle); sclerosis
- Matrix production: osteoid; chondroid; mixed
- Soft tissue changes
- Joint space preservation or invasion

Features suggesting pathological fractures

- Spontaneous fracture or fracture after minor trauma
- Pain at site preceding fracture
- Multiple recent fractures
- Unusual fracture pattern (banana fracture: transverse fracture after minimal trauma, through an abnormal area of bone)
- History of primary malignancy

Causes of pathological fractures
Systemic skeletal disease

- Osteoporosis; steroid-induced osteoporosis
- Metabolic bone disease: osteomalacia, hyperparathyroidism, renal osteodystrophy
- Paget's disease

Localised bone disease

Benign primary bone tumours: unicameral bone cyst; aneurysmal bone cyst; enchondroma; giant cell tumour
Malignant primary bone tumours
- Metastatic bone tumours from lesions of breast, lung, thyroid, kidney and prostate

X-ray features of stress fracture

- New periosteal bone formation
- Horizontal or oblique patterns of sclerosis
- Endosteal callus
- Radiolucent fracture line

Characteristics of athletic injuries
Tendinitis

- Tender thickened tendon
- Crepitus on passive movement
- Tight tendon
- Pain on passive stretch
- Pain on active resisted motion

Tendon rupture

Complete
  Palpable gap
  Total loss of function
Partial
  Swelling and tenderness of tendon
  Partial loss of function
Muscle tear
  Swelling
  Tenderness
  Partial loss of function
  Pain on passive stretch
  Pain on active resisted motion
  Intramuscular haematoma leads to prolonged pain and delayed recovery
  Intermuscular haematoma is associated with diffuse swelling and superficial bruising.

Muscle rupture

- Visible and palpable gap
- Bulge produced by bunched up proximal end
- Complete loss of function

Ligament sprain

- Tender ligament
- Pain on stress
- Stable unless complete rupture

Enthesopathy

- Tenderness at bone-tendon or bone-ligament junction

Stress fracture

- Localized activity related pain
- Focal bony tenderness

Entrapment neuropathy

- Early sensory symptoms and signs
- Later motor weakness

Dislocation

- Deformity
- Complete loss of joint function
- Mechanical block to joint movement
- Marked periarticular muscle spasm

4 Metabolic and Endocrine Emergencies

Hyponatraemia checklist

- Rate of onset: acute (develops within 48 h following normal serum sodium concentration); chronic (slow development and persisting for greater than 48 h)
- Severity of hyponatraemia: mild (130–135 mmol/L); moderate (125–129 mmol/L); severe (<125 mmol/L)
- Extracellular fluid volume status (hypovolaemic; euvolaemic; hypervolaemic): signs of dehydration; peripheral or pulmonary oedema
- Presence or absence of symptoms attributable to hyponatraemia
- Serum osmolality (2× (Na) + Urea) + (glucose); normal range: 275–295 mOsm/kg (mmol/kg)
- Urine osmolality and sodium
- Review of medications and alcohol intake

Causes of hyponatraemia (based on paired serum and spot urine sodium and osmolality)

a. **Pseudo-hyponatraemia**
   - High plasma osmolality (>295 mOsm/kg) (redistributive; dilutional; hypertonic): hyperglycaemia; mannitol; alcohol administration
   - Normal plasma osmolality (isotonic): laboratory artefact (hypertriglyceridaemia; hyperparaproteinaemia)
b. **True hyponatraemia**

Hypovolaemic hyponatraemia (extracellular fluid volume contraction associated with loss of sodium and water-**depletional hyponatraemia**) (decrease in total body water with a greater decrease in total body sodium)

A. Urine sodium greater than 20 mmol/L (**renal losses**)

Diuretics: thiazide diuretics; loop diuretics; potassium-sparing diuretics; combined diuretics

Mineralocorticoid deficiency: adrenocortical insufficiency

Salt-losing nephropathy

Diuretic phase of acute kidney injury

Osmotic diuresis: diabetic ketoacidosis

Renal tubular acidosis

Cerebral salt wasting (hypovolaemia): neurosurgery; CNS trauma, especially subarachnoid haemorrhage

B. Urine sodium lower than 20 mmol/L (**extra-renal losses**)

Gastrointestinal losses: vomiting; diarrhea; fistula; stoma; bowel purgatives, especially those containing sodium phosphate or magnesium citrate

Third space losses: bowel obstruction; pancreatitis; burns

Hypervolaemic hyponatraemia: increase in total body water greater than rise in total body sodium (**dilutional hyponatraemia**)

A. Banerjee, *Emergency Clinical Diagnosis*, DOI 10.1007/978-3-319-50718-7_4

Signs of volume overload: oedema

A. Urine sodium greater than 20 mmol/L (urine osmolality <100 mOsm/kg): acute kidney injury; chronic kidney disease
B. Urine sodium less than 20 mmol/L (urine osmolality >100 mOsm/Kg): hypoalbuminaemic states (nephrotic syndrome; cirrhosis of the liver); congestive heart failure

Euvolaemic hyponatraemia (dilutional hyponatraemia)

Slight volume excess-total body water increased, but not enough to cause oedema, with normal total body sodium

Urine sodium exceeds 20 mmol/L

a. Urine osmolality >100 mOsm/kg

Glucocorticoid deficiency; secondary adrenocortical insufficiency
Postoperative
ADH analogues
Severe hypothyroidism
Syndrome of inappropriate ADH secretion
Exercise-induced hyponatraemia

b. Urine osmolality <100 mOsm/kg (primary water overload)

Psychogenic polydipsia (water intake >10 l/day; associated with acute psychosis)
Beer potomania
Replacement of isotonic gastrointestinal and third space fluid losses with hypotonic fluids

Features of syndrome of inappropriate ADH secretion

Hyponatremia: <135 mmol/L
Plasma osmolality less than 270 mOsm/kg H_2O (hypo-osmolality)
Urine osmolality greater than 100 mOsm/kg H_2O (inappropriately elevated urine osmolality) in presence of reduced plasma osmolality
Urine sodium >20 mmol/L
Clinical euvolaemia: no signs of dehydration or hypovolemia; overt oedema rarely observed
Normal pituitary, adrenal, and thyroid function
No evidence of renal, hepatic, or cardiac failure
No diuretic use
An incomplete suppression of antidiuretic hormone; a spot urine osmolality <100 mOsm/kg H_2O indicates appropriate complete suppression-seen in psychogenic polydipsia and malnutrition (history of heavy alcohol consumption)

Causes of syndrome of inappropriate ADH secretion

Inappropriate ADH secretion

- Pulmonary disease: pneumonia; tuberculosis
- Cerebral disease: head injury; infection (meningitis, brain abscess); tumour; subarachnoid haemorrhage; stroke
- Drugs: increasing ADH release (carbamazepine; chlorpropamide); potentiating ADH action (NSAIDs; cyclophosphamide; selective serotonin reuptake inhibitors); AVP analogues (vasopressin, desmopressin, oxytocin)
- Metabolic: acute intermittent porphyria
- Miscellaneous: Guillain Barre syndrome; severe hypothyroidism
- Ectopic ADH secretion
- Neoplasm: carcinoma (bronchogenic; pancreatic; prostatic); lymphoma; leukaemia

Causes of acute hyponatraemic encephalopathy

- Psychogenic polydipsia
- Beer potomania (high fluid intake plus minimal food intake)
- Exercise-induced hyponatraemia
- Recreatioanl drugs: ecstasy

Risk factors for osmotic demyelination syndrome (central pontine myelinolysis) caused by rapid over-correction of chronic hyponatraemia (ataxia, cranial nerve palsies, quadriparesis, and the locked-in syndrome)

- Elderly
- Malnutrition
- Liver disease
- Chronic alcoholism
- Chronic severe hyponatraemia (serum sodium <110 mmol/L; duration >48 h)
- Severe hypokalaemia
- Major burns

Causes of polyuria

- Reduced ADH production (central or neurogenic diabetes insipidus): CNS lesions-suprasellar (germinoma; craniopharyngioma) and intrasellar (pituitary adenoma) tumours; traumatic brain injury (basal skull fractures); neurosurgical procedures (pituitary surgery); infections (meningitis, encephalitis); granulomatous disease (sarcoidosis, tuberculosis); haematological disorder (sickle cell disease, histiocytosis); radiation therapy
- Resistance (renal insensitivity) to ADH (nephrogenic diabetes insipidus): congenital (V2 receptor and aquaporin gene defects); acquired: drugs (lithium, demeclocycline), chronic electrolyte abnormalities (hypercalcaemia, hypokalaemia); chronic kidney disease (pyelonephritis; polycystic kidneys)
- Osmotic diuresis: diabetes mellitus
- Polydipsia: psychogenic; anticholinergic agents

Features suggestive of acute adrenocortical insufficiency (Addisonian crisis)

- Long term glucocorticoid therapy (Cushing's syndrome) leading to secondary adrenocortical insufficiency
- Severe refractory septic shock with purpura; unresponsive to massive fluid replacement and vasopressor support
- Severe gastroenteritis with fever, vomiting, dehydration, and cardiovascular collapse
- Glucocorticoid deficiency: hypoglycaemia; hypotension and postural hypotension; refractory to volume replacement and catecholamine-resistant shock
- Mineralocorticoid deficiency: hyponatraemia associated with hyperkalaemia; acidosis; acute kidney injury
- Excess ACTH and MSH secretion: pigmentation of skin (pressure points, extensor surfaces), lips, nipples and skin creases including palmar creases
- Associated hypothalamic-pituitary abnormalities: growth abnormalities; central diabetes insipidus; hypogonadism

Causes of acute adrenocortical insufficiency (Addisonian crisis)

- Infectious adrenalitis (bacterial sepsis; tuberculosis; disseminated fungal infections; viral, eg HIV infection; syphilis)
- Infiltrative/destructive lesions of adrenals: haemorrhage-Waterhouse-Friederichsen syndrome (meningococcal septicaemia) anticoagulants; infiltration: amyloidosis; sarcoidosis; lymphoma; metastases
- Autoimmune disorders of adrenal: autoimmune adrenalitis (Addison's disease); autoimmune polyglandular syndromes
- Inherited disease: congenital adrenal hyperplasia; adrenoleukodystrophy
- Hypothalamic-pituitary lesions: hypothalamic lesions, hypopituitarism, isolated ACTH deficiency; iatrogenic: steroid-induced suppression of hypothalamic-pituitary axis from long term glucocorticoid therapy
- Drugs inhibiting steroid biosynthesis: etomidate; adrenolytic agents (metyrapone, aminoglutethimide); ketoconazole
- ATCH resistance syndromes: familial glucocorticoid deficiencies (types 1 and 2); Allgrove (triple A) syndrome
- Anti-phospholipid antibody syndrome

Precipitating factors in acute adrenocortical insufficiency

- Acute infection (eg pneumonia)
- Diarrhoea and vomiting
- Acute coronary syndrome
- Trauma; burns

- Blood loss; dehydration
- Rapid cessation or reduction of chronic glucocorticoid therapy

Causes of hypernatremia (serum sodium >145 mmol/L) (related to net free water loss or rarely sodium gain; clinical significance depends on severity, rapidity of onset and underlying cause)

Normal Body Sodium-Urine Sodium Variable

a. Reduced water intake: inadequate access to water, eg environmental; altered mental state (critical illness, sedation, unconsciousness); dysphagia
b. Water with solute loss (hypotonic fluid loss-water loss more than solute loss) or pure water loss
    - Skin losses: insensible and sweat losses-fever; heat stroke/exhaustion; exercise; burns
    - Gastrointestinal losses: severe diarrhoea
    - Renal losses: central (pituitary) or nephrogenic diabetes insipidus; renal medullary disease (reflux nephropathy; polycystic disease); drugs: aminoglycosides, amphotericin B; recovery phase of acute tubular necrosis

Low Body Sodium

Urine sodium >20 mmol/L: renal losses: diuretics, renal parenchymal disease

Urine sodium <20 mmol/L: extra-renal losses: diarrhea

High Body Sodium

Solute gain: excess salt intake; infusion of hypertonic sodium solution (iatrogenic salt overlaod)

Increased mineralocorticoid: primary aldosteronism

Increased glucocorticoid: Cushing's syndrome

Features of hypernatremia

- Neurological: headache, irritability, confusion, lethargy, delirium, tremor, ataxia, seizure, coma
- Musculoskeletal: twitching, myoclonic jerks, spasticity, hyperreflexia, weakness
- Signs of volume depletion: reduced skin turgor, dry mucous membranes, postural hypotension, oliguria, weight loss

Risk factors for hypernatraemia

Age >65 years; infants

Dependence on others for water intake: disabled status; immobile; dementia; altered mental state

Diuretic therapy

Uncontrolled solute or osmotic diuresis leading to polyuria (severe uncontrolled diabetes mellitus; hyperosmolar hyperglycaemic state)

Renal disease (obstructive uropathy; sickle cell disease)

Hypertonic infusions

Vasopressin receptor antagonists

Residential care setting

Causes of hypokalaemia

Pseudo-hypokalaemia blood sampling upstream of an infusion of saline or dextrose

Decreased intake inadequate provision of K with prolonged IV fluid administration; eating disorders; nutritional deficiency; oesophageal disease

Increased entry into cells (trans-cellular shift from ECF to ICF compartment)

Elevated extracellular pH: correction of metabolic acidosis; metabolic alkalosis

Insulin treatment

Beta agonists: high dose or prolonged salbutamol treatment for asthma

Theophyllines

Hypokalaemic periodic paralysis

Hypothermia

Increased losses

Extra-renal:

Increased **gastrointestinal** losses

Vomiting

Diarrhoea; laxatives

Intestinal fistula; ileostomy; villous adenoma

Increased **sweat** losses (insensible losses)

Renal: Increased **urinary** losses

With high renin-usually with low or normal blood pressure

Diuretics: loop and thiazide diuretics

Hypomagnesaemia-inducing medications: aminoglycosides; amphotericin

Tubular disease: type 1 renal tubular acidosis

Osmotic diuresis: diabetic ketoacidosis

Diuretic phase of acute kidney injury

Nephrotoxic drugs: cisplatin; amphotericin B

With low renin-may be associated with hypertension

Primary mineralocorticoid excess: Conn's syndrome; Liddle's syndrome; Cushing's syndrome; secondary aldosteronism; liquorice; renin-producing tumour; renovascular hypertension

Increased sweat losses (insensible losses)

Checklist for hypokalaemia

- Severity of hypokalaemia: mild (3.0–3.5 mmol/L); moderate (2.5–3.0 mmol/L); severe (<2.5 mmol/L)
- Presence or absence of symptoms attributable to hypokalaemia: musculoskeletal: weakness, leg cramps; cardiovascular: palpitations; respiratory: dyspnoea; respiratory distress; gastrointestinal: constipation; ileus
- Renal function
- Serum magnesium levels
- Presence of ECG changes
- The risk of cardiac arrhythmia is increased by concomitant metabolic alkalosis, hypercalcaemia, and digoxin therapy

ECG effects of hypokalaemia

Repolarisation changes

- Low voltage
- Flattening of T waves
- Depression of ST segments
- Prominence of U waves
- Fusion of T and U waves (severe)

Conduction abnormalities

- Prolonged QRS duration
- Atrio-ventricular block
- Increased P wave amplitude and direction
- Ventricular arrhythmias, especially torsade de pointes
- Asystole

Causes of hyperkalaemia

(Serum potassium greater than 5.5 mmol/L)

Factitious (pseudo-hyperkalaemia)

Prolonged tourniquet time

Haemolysis of blood sample related to traumatic venipuncture

Delayed processing of blood sample; in vitro haemolysis

Marked leukocytosis; thrombocytosis

Increased potassium load

Excess potassium in diet (dark leafy greens, white beans, fresh and dried fruits, fish)

Parenteral administration

Salt substitutes

Oral potassium supplements

Rapid and massive transfusion of banked blood

Increased release of potassium from cells

(massive release of intracellular potassium, with shift from ICF to ECF)

Metabolic acidosis

Insulin deficiency

Increased tissue catabolism

Hyperosmolar states

Exercise

Digitalis toxicity

Haemolysis

Crush injury; rhabdomyolysis

Hyperkalaemic periodic paralysis

Electrical or thermal burns

Tumour lysis syndrome (hyperkalemia, hyperphosphatemia, hypocalcemia, hyperuricemia)

Reduced urinary excretion of potassium

Acute kidney injury; chronic kidney disease

Mineralocorticoid deficiency: Addison's disease; hyporeninaemic hypoaldosteronism

Distal tubular disease (renal secretory defects): renal tubular acidosis; acute interstitial nephritis, sickle cell nephropathy
Drugs: ACE inhibitors, angiotensin II receptor blockers, cyclosporine, NSAIDs, potassium-sparing diuretics, beta-blockers, lithium toxicity

ECG changes in hyperkalaemia

Tall peaked symmetrical T waves with a narrow base, with normal or short QT interval and short PR interval: 5.5–6.5 mmol/L ("no pot, no T")
Widened QRS complexes with prolonged PR interval: 6.5–7.5 mmol/L
Widened P waves, QT prolongation: 7.0–8.0 mmol/L
Absent P waves with markedly widened QRS (sine wave pattern): >8.0 mmol/L

Causes of hypomagnesaemia (serum magnesium <1.4 mmol/L)

- Reduced intake: starvation; eating disorders (anorexia; bulimia); protein-calorie malnutrition; absence of magnesium in intravenous fluids; alcoholism
- Gastrointestinal losses: nasogastric suction; malabsorption; intestinal fistula; acute haemorrhagic pancreatitis; short bowel syndrome; inflammatory bowel disease; laxative abuse; villous adenoma
- Renal loss: osmotic diuresis (glucose, urea, mannitol)
- Renal disease: chronic pyelonephritis; interstitial nephritis; glomerulonephritis; non-oliguric acute tubular necrosis; post-renal transplant, renal tubular acidosis
- Drugs: loop diuretics; alcohol; aminoglycosides; pentamidine; ciclosporin; cisplatin
- Endocrine and metabolic: diabetes mellitus; primary hyperparathyroidism; hyperthyroidism; hungry bone disease; primary aldosteronism; metabolic acidosis; Bartter syndrome

Features of hypomagnesaemia

- Gastrointestinal: anorexia, nausea, vomiting
- Neuromuscular: weakness; paraesthesiae; tetany; generalized tonic-clonic seizures
- Cardiovascular: ECG changes (non-specific T wave changes; prolonged PR and QT intervals; ST segment depression; ventricular premature beats; monomorphic ventricular tachycardia; torsade de pointes; ventricular fibrillation); enhanced digitalis toxicity
- Metabolic: hypokalaemia; hypocalcaemia

Causes of hypermagnesaemia

- Increased intake: laxatives; antacids
- Reduced elimination:
  Gastrointestinal: chronic constipation; bowel obstruction
  Renal: chronic kidney disease
- Medication: lithium; anticholinergic agents

Changes in urea/creatinine ratio (normally 10: 1 to 20: 1)

Increased

- Old age
- Dehydration
- High-dose glucocorticoids
- Gastrointestinal haemorrhage
- Protein-rich diet
- Severe catabolic state
- Resorption of large haematoma

Decreased

Severe liver dysfunction
Intrinsic renal damage
Malnutrition
Low protein diet
Pregnancy
Rhabdomyolysis
Syndrome of inappropriate ADH secretion

Causes of elevated serum creatine kinase

Exercise
Rhabdomyolysis (triad of myalgia, especially involving proximal muscle groups, weakness and reddish brown urine)
Myopathies; muscular dystrophy
Neuroleptic malignant syndrome
Malignant hyperthermia

Muscle trauma: intramuscular injections; contact sports; seizure; crush injuries; burns; electrocution

Endocrine: hypothyroidism, hypoparathyroidism

Causes of rhabdomyolysis (creatine kinase greater than 5 times the upper limit of normal)

- Compression: prolonged immobilization; fall with long lie; coma from any cause
- Excessive muscular activity: strenuous exercise; seizures; severe dystonia
- Trauma: crush injury
- Burns
- Electrical injury: high-voltage electrical injury; lightning strike; electrical cardioversion
- Compartment syndrome
- Hyperthermia: malignant hyperthermia; neuroleptic malignant syndrome; environmental heat illness (heat stroke)
- Endocrine disorders: diabetic ketoacidosis; hyperosmolar hyperglycaemic state; hypothyroidism
- Drugs: cocaine; heroin; amphetamines; barbiturates
- Medication: statins; anti-psychotics; sedatives; neuroleptics; salicylates
- Toxins: alcohol; toxic alcohols; insect bites (black widow spider); snake bites
- Infection: tetanus

Causes of elevated serum liver enzymes

- Hepatitis: viral (A, B. C); alcoholic; autoimmune; drug induced
- Non-alcoholic fatty liver disease
- Prescription medications: statins; antibiotics; NSAIDs; antiepileptic drugs; polypharmacy; paracetamol overdose
- Non-prescripion medications: herbal remedies; alternative medications
- Haemochromatosis
- α-1 antitrypsin deficiency
- Extrahepatic: skeletal muscle disorders; haemolytic anaemia; hypo- or hyperthyroidism

Hepatocellular pattern: ALT/AST elevated out of proportion to ALP

Cholestatic pattern: ALP elevated out of proportion to ALT/AST

Causes of elevated C reactive protein

- Infection
- Trauma
- Burns
- Inflammation: active inflammatory arthritis; inflammatory bowel disease
- Lymphoma
- Cancer

Causes of raised serum alkaline phosphatase

Physiological
- Infancy
- Puberty
- Third trimester of pregnancy
- Intestinal isoenzyme

Pathological

Bone disease
- Hyperparathyroidism
- Osteomalacia; rickets
- Paget's disease of the bone
- Osteomyelitis

Hepatobiliary diseases
- Bile duct obstruction
- Primary biliary cirrhosis
- Hepatitis
- Primary sclerosing cholangitis
- Drug-induced cholestasis: anabolic steroids

Other
- Carcinoma of the bronchus

Causes of hypoglycemia

Imbalance between insulin and caloric intake

Normal fasting blood glucose: 3.5–5.5 mmol/L

Hypoglycaemia: <2.8 mmol/L

Symptoms of hypoglycaemia

- Neuroglycopenia: confusion, irritability, emotional lability, headache, altered behaviour, blurred vision, slurred speech, seizure, coma
- Autonomic: sweating, hunger, anxiety, tremulousness, palpitations, paraesthesiae (circumoral; finger tips)

Features of nocturnal hypoglycaemia

- Nocturnal hypoglycaemia is often asymptomatic, being commoner in tightly controlled type 1 diabetics
- Waking in the middle of the night, often with damp clothes or sheets as a result of excessive sweating
- Waking with headache, excessive tiredness or a hungover feeling
- Confusion upon waking
- Morning hyperglycaemia (Somogyi rebound phenomenon)
- Tiredness despite a full night's sleep
- Nocturnal seizures
- Nocturnal behavioural disturbance

Causes of hypoglycaemia other than when complicating diabetes mellitus

Fasting

Substrate deficiency (ketonuria present)

- Ketotic hypoglycaemia
- Reduced glucose intake (deficiency); starvation; malnutrition; infancy; late pregnancy
- Liver disease; hepatic failure: hepatitis; cirrhosis
- Hypothermia
- Uraemia
- Toxins: alcohol, insulin, sulphaureas, pentamidine
- Enzyme defects: G6PD deficiency
- Hepatic enzyme deficiencies:
  - Glycogen storage disease
  - Galactosemia
  - Hereditary fructose intolerance
- Metabolic disorders:
  - Reye's syndrome
  - Maple syrup urine disease
  - Tyrosinosis
- Endocrine disorders:
  - Adrenocortical insufficiency
  - Hypopituitarism

Hyperinsulinism (ketones absent)

- Pancreatic nesidioblastosis
- Pancreatic tumours: insulinoma (Whipple's triad: hypoglycaemic symptoms especially after fasting or heavy exercise, low plasma glucose measured at the time of symptoms, and relief of symptoms with treatment of hypoglycaemia)

Reactive (post-prandial)

- Reactive hypoglycaemia (alimentary hyperinsulinism)
- Hereditary fructose intolerance
- Idiopathic

Risk factors for hypoglycaemia in diabetes

Absolute or relative insulin excess

- High dose of insulin, insulin secretagogues and meglitinides, increased insulin absorption from depot
- Increased glucose utilization: vigorous exercise; hypercatabolic state
- Reduced exogenous glucose delivery: missed or delayed meals or snacks; overnight fast; gastroparesis; reduced gastrointestinal absorption
- Reduced endogenous glucose production: alcohol ingestion
- Reduced insulin clearance: progressive renal disease

Insulin excess and compromised glucose counter-regulation

- Hypoglycaemia unawareness
- Tight blood glucose control (low HbA1c)
- Autonomic neuropathy
- Adrenergic blocking drugs

Causes of hyperglycaemia

- Diabetes mellitus: type I and 2
- Exocrine pancreas disease: acute/chronic pancreatitis; trauma; carcinoma; cystic fibrosis; haemochromatosis; pancreatectomy
- Endocrine pancreas or gut tumour: glucagonoma; somatostatinoma; carcinoid syndrome; VIPoma; gatrinoma; multiple endocrine neoplasia syndrome
- Endocrinopathies: GH excess (acromegaly); glucocorticoid excess (Cushing's syndrome); hyperthyroidism
- Drug-induced: glucocorticoids; atypical antipsychotic agents; lithium; thiazide diuretics; protease inhibitors; beta blockers; pentamidine
- Stress-induced hyperglycaemia (critical illness); sepsis; acute coronary syndromes; intracranial disease (encephalitis; meningitis; brain tumour)

Establishing the diagnosis of diabetic ketoacidosis

Confirm hyperglycaemia >11 mmol/L
<10 mmol/L excludes diagnosis
>20 mmol/L is usual

Some patients can present with a 'normal' range glucose (euglycaemic ketoacidosis): liver disease, food deprivation with little carbohydrate intake, excessive vomiting with continued insulin administration

Confirm ketonaemia
Ketonuria: urine ketones ++ or more
Ketonaemia: capillary ketones (beta-hydroxybutyrate) >3 mmol/L

Confirm acidosis
Plasma HCO_3 < 15 mmol/L
pH < 7.3 (venous blood gas)

Presentation:

- Gradual deterioration over 2–3 days
- Polyuria and polydipsia
- Dehydration
- Drowsiness; coma
- Hyperventilation: Kussmaul's breathing
- GI: abdominal pain, nausea, vomiting

Remember the five precipitating is:

- Infection: 30%; urinary tract infection, upper respiratory tract infection, lower respiratory tract infection, skin
- Incidental new diabetes: 25%
- Insufficient insulin: 20%
- Infarction: myocardial infarction, stroke, gastrointestinal tract, peripheral vasculature
- Inter-current illness: diarrhoea and/or vomiting

Precipitating factors for diabetic ketoacidosis

- Non-compliance with medication regimen and/or diet; chaotic lifestyle
- Acute medical illness: infection (pneumonia, urinary tract infection, sepsis), myocardial infarction, stroke, pancreatitis
- Trauma or surgery
- Pregnancy
- Eating disorders: bulimia
- Medication: glucocorticoids; high-dose thiazides; sympathomimetic agents; atypical anti-psychotic agents
- Undiagnosed (new onset) diabetes mellitus
- Drug abuse

Risk factors for cerebral oedema in diabetic ketoacidosis

- Hypocapnia (<2 kPa) at presentation
- Younger age
- First presentation
- Bicarbonate administration
- Rapid fall in corrected sodium
- Elevated serum urea at presentation

Causes of hyperketonaemia

- Diabetic ketoacidosis
- Starvation

- Alcoholic ketoacidosis
- Salicylate toxicity
- Hyperemesis gravidarum

Features of hyperosmolar hyperglycaemic state

- Often undiagnosed type 2 diabetes mellitus
- Marked hyperglycaemia (>30 mmol/L), hyperosmolarity (>320 mOsm/kg), minimal or no acidosis (pH >7.3; HCO_3 > 15 mmol/L) and no ketonaemia
- Signs of hypovolaemia
- Usually signs of acidosis are absent
- Confusion; disorientation
- Coma
- Focal or generalized seizures
- Acute circulatory collapse
- Transient focal neurological signs, including hemiplegia and hemianopia
- Increased risk of venous thrombo-embolism
- Arterial thrombosis, including mesenteric ischaemia

Thyroid storm (undiagnosed or undertreated hyperthyroidism with an acute precipitant)

Clinical features

- Impaired thermoregulation: fever; hyperpyrexia (temperature >40 C); sweating
- Neurological: delirium, apathy, psychosis, emotional lability, hyperkinesis, hyperreflexia, seizure, coma
- Cardiovascular: atrial fibrillation/flutter, profound sinus tachycardia, hypertension, high output congestive heart failure, shock
- Gastrointestinal: nausea and vomiting, diarrhea, abdominal pain, mild jaundice

Acute precipitants

- Infection, including pneumonia
- Withdrawal of anti-thyroid drugs
- Acute medical conditions: myocardial infarction, stroke, pulmonary embolism
- Iodine load: iodinated contrast, radioactive iodine
- Amiodarone cytotoxicity
- Surgery; trauma; childbirth

Myxoedema coma (undiagnosed or undertreated hypothyroidism with acute precipitant).

Features

- Hypothermia
- Lethargy; confusion; areflexia; seizure; coma
- Hypoventilation with type 2 respiratory failure
- Hypotension; bradycardia
- Hypoglycaemia; hyponatraemia
- Pericardial effusion
- Signs of hypothyroidism
- Elevated serum creatine kinase

Acute precipitants

- Cold exposure
- Infection, including pneumonia
- Acute medical conditions: stroke, acute coronary syndrome
- Trauma
- CNS depression: narcotics, barbiturates, sedatives

Causes of metabolic alkalosis

a. **Reduction (loss) of anion (acid)**
   Hypochloremic (loss of chloride):
   Gastro-intestinal: vomiting; chloridorrhea (villous adenoma; some chloride-secreting diarrhoeas); pyloric obstruction
   Renal: chloruretic agents (loop diuretics, thiazides); chloride channelopathies (Bartter syndrome; Gitelman syndrome)
   Sweat: cystic fibrosis
b. **Increase (gain) of cation (alkali)**: sodium citrate (massive blood transfusion), sodium lactate, sodium bicarbonate, sodium acetate

Hypernatraemic: hyperaldosteronism-primary, secondary
Hypercalcaemic: milk-alkali syndrome, calcium carbonate
Alkaline overshoot during treatment of diabetic ketoacidosis

c. Contraction alkalosis: rapid diuresis

Factors that maintain metabolic alkalosis

- Chloride depletion: loss of gastric acid; diuretics
- Potassium depletion: mineralocorticoid excess (hyperaldosteronism; Cushing's syndrome); kaliuretic diuretics
- Reduced glomerular filtration rate
- Extracellular fluid volume contraction (depletion): stimulates tubular bicarbonate reabsorption
- Continued acid loss
- Continued addition of base

Causes of metabolic acidosis

- Increase (gain) of anion
  Hyperchloremic (addition of chloride) (potassium chloride, calcium chloride, hydrochloric acid, sodium chloride, arginine hydrochloride, lysine hydrochloride, ammonium chloride)
  Anion-gap acidosis: lactic acidosis, ketoacidosis (diabetic, alcoholic, starvation), other unmeasured anions-toxic alcohols (ethylene glycol, propylene glycol, methanol), thiosulphate; renal failure (reduced excretion of organic anions: urea, phosphates, sulphates)
  Hyperphosphataemic
- Reduction (loss) of cation (Na and K)
  Renal (reduced hydrogen ion excretion): distal renal tubular acidosis; natriuretic agents (amiloride, triamterene); sodium with anions in urine (ketoacids; D-lactate; hippurate)
  Gastrointestinal (bicarbonate loss): diarrhoea with bicarbonate or bacterial organic anions in stool; vomiting pancreatic secretions, pancreatic fistula, small bowel fistula, obstructed ileal conduit

Causes of increased anion gap

- Increased unmeasured anions: organic acids (lactate; ketoacids); inorganic acids (phosphate, sulphate); exogenous (salicylates, nitrates); toxic alcohols (ethanol, methanol, ethylene glycol, propylene glycol)
- Increased measured cations: hypernatraemia
- Reduced unmeasured cations
- Alkalosis
- Laboratory error

Causes of metabolic acidosis with increased anion gap

- Organic acidaemia
- Lactic acidosis
  Type A (impaired perfusion): hypoxia and/or tissue hypoperfusion
  Type B (impaired carbohydrate metabolism): metabolic disease; aspirin poisoning; ethanol; ethylene glycol; methanol; cyanide; hepatic failure; metformin; isoniazid
- Ketoacidosis: diabetic ketoacidosis; alcoholic ketoacidosis; starvation ketoacidosis
- Acute kidney injury
- Toluene and other toxins

Causes of normal anion gap acidosis

- Renal causes (bicarbonate loss): renal tubular acidosis; carbonic anhydrase inhibitors (acetazolamide); aldosterone inhibitors
- GI tract causes (bicarbonate loss): severe diarrhoea; uretero-enterostomy or obstructed ileal conduit; drainage of pancreatic or biliary secretions; small bowel fistula
- Other causes: recovery from ketoacidosis; addition of HCl, NH_4Cl

Lactic acidosis

Features
- Metabolic acidosis (pH < 7.35)
- Anion gap >16 mmol/L
- Arterial lactate >4 mmol/L (normal <1.5 mmol/L)

Type A: Clinical evidence of inadequate tissue oxygen delivery

- Anaerobic muscular activity: sprinting, generalised convulsions
- Tissue hypoperfusion: shock-septic, cardiogenic or hypovolaemic; cardiac arrest; acute heart failure; regional hypoperfusion, especially mesenteric ischaemia; malaria
- Reduced tissue oxygen delivery or utilization with increased oxygen demands: hypoxaemia; carbon monoxide poisoning; severe anaemia; hypercatabolic states

Type B (metabolic): No clinical evidence of inadequate tissue oxygen delivery

- Type B1: associated with underlying diseases (eg diabetic ketoacidosis, leukaemia, lymphoma, AIDS)
- Type B2: associated with drugs and toxins: biguanides, cyanide, beta agonists, methanol, nitroprusside infusion, ethanol intoxication in chronic alcoholics, anti-retroviral drugs
- Type B3: associated with inborn errors of metabolism: eg congenital forms of lactic acidosis with various enzyme defects, eg pyruvate dehydrogenase deficiency, glucose-6-phosphatase deficiency (type 1 glycogen storage disease); fructose-1,6-diphosphatase deficiency; pyruvate carboxylase deficiency

Causes of respiratory alkalosis

Central causes (direct action via respiratory centres causing increased respiratoy drive)
- Head injury
- Stroke
- Anxiety-hyperventilation syndrome (psychogenic)
- Other supra-tentorial causes: pain, fear, stress, voluntary
- Various drugs: theophyllines, propanidid, salicylate toxicity
- Various endogenous compounds: progesterone during pregnancy, cytokines during sepsis, toxins in patients with chronic liver disease

Hypoxaemia (acting via peripheral chemoreceptors)
- Respiratory stimulation via peripheral chemoreceptors: low inspired oxygen concentration (eg high altitude)

Pulmonary causes (act via stimulation of intrapulmonary receptors)
- Pulmonary embolism
- Pneumonia
- Asthma
- Pulmonary oedema (all types)

Iatrogenic (act directly on ventilation)
- Excessive controlled ventilation

Features associated with respiratory alkalosis

- Central nervous system: lightheadedness, confusion, generalised seizures
- Cardiovascular system: angina; cardiac arrhythmias
- Neuromuscular: circumoral and limb paraesthesiae; tetany, withmuscle cramps and carpopedal spasm; laryngospasm

Causes of respiratory acidosis

A. Inadequate alveolar ventilation

Central respiratory depression and other CNS problems: drug depression of respiratory centre (eg opiates, sedatives, anaesthetics)

CNS trauma, infarct, haemorrhage or tumour

Hypoventilation of obesity (Pickwickian syndrome)
Cervical cord trauma or lesions (at or above C4 level)
High central neural blockade
Poliomyelitis; tetanus
High Flow oxygen administration in the presence of chronic hypercapnia
Cardiac arrest with cerebral hypoxia
Nerve or muscle disorders: neuropathies (Guillain Barre syndrome); myopathies (myasthenia gravis; myotonic dystrophy); muscle relaxant drugs; toxins-eg organophosphates, snake venom
Lung or chest wall defects: kyphoscoliosis; obstructive lung disease: acute exacerbation of COPD; chest trauma (flail chest; multiple rib fractures); pneumothorax; diaphragmatic paralysis or splinting; pulmonary oedema; ARDS; restrictive lung disease; aspiration
Airway disorders: upper airway obstruction; laryngospasm; severe asthma
External factors: inadequate mechanical ventilation
Over-production of carbon dioxide: hypercatabolic disorders: malignant hyperthermia
Increased intake of carbon dioxide: rebreathing of CO_2-containing expired gas; addition of CO_2 to inspired gas

Causes of mixed acid-base disorders
Additive

- Metabolic acidosis + respiratory acidosis:
  Respiratory failure
  Sepsis
  Cardiac arrest
  Poisoning: eg ethanol; methanol
- Metabolic alkalosis + respiratory alkalosis:
  Vomiting and congestive heart failure
  Diuretic therapy and liver failure or pneumonia
- Metabolic alkalosis + respiratory acidosis:
  Diuretic therapy + COPD
  Vomiting + COPD
  Severe potassium depletion
- Metabolic acidosis + metabolic alkalosis:
  Vomiting and renal failure
  Diuretic therapy and ketoacidosis
  Severe vomiting in ketoacidosis
- Chronic respiratory acidosis with superimposed acute respiratory acidosis
  Acute exacerbation of COPD
  COPD with worsening hypoventilation secondary to oxygen therapy or sedative action
- Chronic respiratory acidosis and anion gap metabolic acidosis
  COPD with shock and lactic acidosis
  Respiratory alkalosis and metabolic acidosis
  Salicylate intoxication
  Gram negative sepsis
  Severe pulmonary oedema
  Acute cardio-pulmonary arrest

Mixed acid-base disorders should be suspected when

- The expected compensatory response does not occur (normally changes in bicarbonate parallel changes in pCO_2 and vice versa-ie they move in the same direction, increase in one component leading to a compensatory increase in the other; overcompensation or return to a normal pH do not occur). A normal pH in the presence of an acid-base disorder suggests a mixed disorder.
- The level of compensation is higher or lower than expected
- Whenever pCO_2 and HCO_3 become abnormal in opposite directions (one is elevated whilst the other is reduced)
- The pH is normal but pCO_2 or HCO_3 is abnormal
- In anion gap metabolic acidosis if the change in HCO_3 level is not proportional to change in the anion gap

Hypercalcaemia

Normal serum calcium: 2.2–2.5 mmol/L
Mild: 2.6–3.0 mmol/L
Moderate: 3.0–3.4 mmol/L
Severe: >3.4 mmol/L

Causes of hypercalcaemia (involve increased bone resorption, increased gastrointestinal absorption, and reduced excretion)

Low or normal phosphate

Increased **bone resorption**

- Primary hyperparathyroidism; tertiary hyperparathyroidism
- Neoplasia (tumours producing PTH-related proteins): osteolytic metastases (ovary, kidney, lung cancer)
- Malignant melanoma (osteoclast activating factor)
- Immobilisation
- Thyroid disease: hyperthyroidism

Reduced excretion of calcium

- Paget's disease of bone
- Drugs: thiazide diuretics, lithium
- Acute kidney injury with rhabdomyolysis
- Familial hypocalciuric hypercalcaemia (hypercalcaemia; normal or elevated plasma PTH; normal renal function; hypocalciuria; hypermagnesaemia; most cases are asymptomatic)

High phosphate **(increased gastrointestinal absorption of calcium)**

- **Excess vitamin D**: granulomatous disorders associated with increased production of active vitamin D metabolites: sarcoidosis, tuberculosis, granulomatous reaction to silicone injections; neoplasia: 1,25-dihydroxyvitamin D3 production, especially Hodgkin's lymphoma; vitamin D intoxication
- **Excess calcium intake**: milk alkali syndrome (calcium carbonate ingestion; excess ingestion of calcium-containing antacids)

Causes of malignant hypercalcaemia

- Osteolytic bone metastases (breast cancer)
- Secretion of PTH-related peptides (solid tumours-lung; head and neck; renal cell)
- Osteoclastic activating factors: multiple myeloma; lymphoma
- Renal impairment
- Excess vitamin D activity: some lymphomas produce active metabolites of vitamin D

Features of hypercalcaemia

- Gastrointestinal presentations: nausea, vomiting, abdominal pain, constipation, pancreatitis
- Neurological presentations: confusion, drowsiness, depression, psychosis, coma
- Renal presentations: renal stone, nephrocalcinosis, nephrogenic diabetes insipidus

ECG features of hypercalcaemia

- Short QT interval
- Flattened and widened T waves with ST elevation
- Prolonged PR interval
- Widened QRS complex
- Increased QRS voltage
- Notching of terminal portion of QRS complex from a prominent J wave
- AV block

Causes of hypocalcaemia

Endocrine

Hypoparathyroidism (PTH deficiency): parathyroid aplasia, autoimmune destruction (autoimmune polyglandular syndrome type 1), infiltration (haemochromatosis); total thyroidectomy; heavy metal deposition

Hypomagnesaemia

Pseudo-hypoparathyroidism (PTH resistance): chronic kidney disease; medications: calcitonin, bisphosphonates, mithramycin

Medullary carcinoma of thyroid (calcitonin secretion)

Reduced Intake or Absorption

- Malabsorption
- Severe vitamin D deficiency: Intestinal malabsorption; chronic kidney disease; liver disease; vitamin D dependent rickets type 1; nutritional deficiency

- Reduced absorptive area: small bowel bypass; short bowel
- Resistance to vitamin D

Increased Losses

- Osteoblastic metastases
- Acute necrotizing pancreatitis
- Rhabdomyolysis
- Citrate toxicity casuing calcium chelation: large volumes of fresh frozen plasma during massive blood transfusion
- Chronic kidney disease
- Diuretic therapy: frusemide; bumetanide
- Hyperphosphataemia

Presentations of hypocalcaemia (symptoms depend on the magnitude and rate of decrease in serum calcium)

- Neuromuscular: circumoral and digital paraesthesiae; generalized irritability; muscle cramps; tetany; latent tetany; carpopedal spasms; seizures; laryngospasm; neuromuscular irritability characterized by positive Chvostek and Trousseau signs
- Cardiovascular: hypotension; bradycardia; arrhythmia; atrio-ventricular block; heart failure
- Psychiatric: anxiety, confusion, psychosis
- Ocular: cataract, papilloedema

ECG features of hypocalcaemia

- Prolonged QT interval
- Flattening of ST segment
- T wave inversion
- AV block; ventricular fibrillation

Causes of hypophosphataemia

- Inadequate intake or absorption: malnutrition; chronic diarrhoea; Vitamin D deficiency or resistance; phosphate binding agents (antacids: magnesium and calcium salts); alcohol withdrawal
- Redistribution into cells: respiratory alkalosis; recovery phase of diabetic ketoacidosis; enteral or parenteral nutrition
- Increased renal excretion: primary hyperparathyroidism; osmotic diuresis; proximal renal tubular transport defects (Fanconi syndrome)

5 Dermatological Emergencies

Description of skin lesions

- Macule: flat circumscribed lesion <1 cm in diameter, not palpable and characterized by change in colour of skin; macules can be erythematous, hypopigmented, depigmented, hyperpigmented or any other colour (eg black-purple, yellow)
- Patch: flat circumscribed lesion >1 cm in diameter
- Papule: raised solid lesion <1 cm in diameter
- Nodule: raised solid lesion >1 cm in diameter; greatest mass below skin surface
- Plaque: a flat-topped nodule >1 cm in diameter
- Vesicle: clear fluid-filled lesion <1 cm in diameter
- Pustule: pus or exudate-filled lesion <1 cm in diameter
- Bulla: clear fluid-filled lesion >1 cm in diameter

Secondary changes in skin lesions

- Exudate: moist serum, blood or pus from an erosion, bulla or pustule
- Lichenification: grouped flat-topped papules associated with exaggerated skin markings, diffuse thickening and hyperpigmentation
- Excoriations: linear erosions caused by loss of epidermis and superficial dermis due to scratching
- Erosions: loss of superficial epidermis causing superficial depression
- Fissures: linear wedge shaped cracks in the epidermis extending down to the dermis and narrowing at the base
- Ulceration: full thickness loss of epidermis, some dermis and subcutaneous fat
- Scaling: dry flaky surface with normal or abnormal keratin from shed epidermal cells
- Crusting: dried exudates (serum, blood, pus, damaged epithelial cells)
- Scarring: atrophic (thinning or loss of epidermis and/or dermis); hypertrophic
- Maceration: appearance of surface softening due to constant moistness

Distribution of lesions

- Linear
- Grouped
- Circinate
- Annular
- Reticulate
- Serpiginous
- Geographical
- Segmental
- Zosteriform or dermatomal

A. Banerjee, *Emergency Clinical Diagnosis*, DOI 10.1007/978-3-319-50718-7_5

- Symmetrical
- Peripheral or central
- Limbs (extensor; flexural)

Skin rash assessment includes:

- Evaluation of general skin appearance: colour; texture; dryness; hydration; odour
- Site predilection: sun-exposed; acral; flexures; extensor surfaces
- If generalized, whether symmetrical (if so, whether central or peripheral) or not
- Shape of skin lesions: round, oval, annular, iris shaped, umbilicated
- Arrangement: isolated, grouped (linear, annular, serpiginous)
- Involvement of scalp, palms, soles, ears, sub-mammary and interdigital areas, hair-bearing areas (axillae, groins); perianal skin
- Involvement of skin appendages: hair; nails
- Mucosal involvement: oral cavity; lips; conjunctivae; nasal cavity

Causes of colouring in macules

- Red: hyperaemia; telangiectasia; petechiae; purpura; ecchymosis
- Blue: haematoma; dermal melanin; cyanosis
- Brown: dermal and epidermal melanin; haemosiderin
- Yellow: carotenoids; bile
- Grey-black: epidermal melanin; foreign bodies; heavy metals; tar
- White: depigmentation (loss of melanin)

Causes of fever and skin rash
Solid rash
Diffuse erythema

- Scarlet fever: sudden onset of sore throat, headache, high fever and chills, malaise, anorexia and nausea followed 1–2 days later by a generalised erythematous pinhead rash, initially on the neck, chest, axillae and abdomen, with sand-paper like texture (due to tiny papules) and sparing of the palms and soles; flushed cheeks with circumoral pallor and strawberry tongue (glossitis, with dilated papillae); pharyngeal exudate, punctate petechiae of the palate and uvula, cervical lymphadenopathy; streaks of petechiae along the axillary skin folds (Pastia lines)
- Drug eruption: morbilliform skin rash, eosinophilia, and systemic symptoms including high fever and organ involvement (DRESS refers to a drug reaction with eosinophilia and systemic symptoms, associated with a triad of fever, skin rash and internal organ involvement, including hepatitis, nephritis, pneumonitis, myocarditis, thyroiditis; there is a two to three-week period between initial exposure to the drug and onset of the reaction)
- Toxic shock syndrome
- Staphylococcal scalded skin syndrome (prodrome of fever, malaise and sore throat; skin tenderness and erythema, initially peri-orificial in the face, and in the neck, axillae and groins, with rapid progression over 24–48 h to diffuse erythroderma, accentuated in flexural areas; peri-oral erythema; large flaccid bullae may develop in the flexures and around orifices; diffuse desquamation leads to peri-oral, peri-nasal and peri-ocular crusting; resolution without scarring takes place within 2 weeks); early toxic epidermal necrolysis
- Erythroderma (red and scaly) secondary to drugs, eczema, psoriasis or T –cell lymphoma; may be idiopathic
- Scombrotoxicity

Petechial-purpuric rash
Palpable purpura

- Meningococcaemia (onset with prodrome of fever, headache and upper respiratory symptoms; a maculopapular rash may precede petechiae; the non-blanching petechial or purpuric rash may initially be found only in warm areas, such as groins and axillae; in patients with darker skin, the soles of the feet and palms of the hands

should be examined; the petechiae may have angular edges and a greyish interior; acrocyanosis of the ears, nose, lips, legs and genitalia; cold hands and feet; leg pain; confluent ecchmyoses with central necrosis can progress to gangrene)
- Gonococcaemia: haemorrhagic papules and pustules that develop a crust and become necrotic
- Henoch Schonlein purpura
- Staphylococcal endocarditis

Not palpable

- Idiopathic thrombocytopenic purpura
- Overwheming pneumococcal sepsis (in asplenic individuals)
- Disseminated intravascular coagulation (purpurafulminans)
- Leptospirosis
- Enteroviral infection
- Viral haemorrhagic fevers (Ebola, Marburg)
- Yellow fever; dengue fever
- Toxic shock syndrome
- Rat bite fevers: spirillum minus; streptobacillusmoniliformis
- Capnophagacanimorsus (DF-2) infection: in asplenic individuals, especially after dog bites
- Vitamin C deficiency (scurvy) (peri-follicular purpura; lower limb eccymoses; haemorrhagic gingivitis)
- Catastrophic anti-phospholipid antibody syndrome

Maculopapular rash

- Viral infections: rubella (mild prodrome; pink macular rash appearing on the face and spreading to the trunk and limbs,becoming confluent; red macules or petechiae on soft palate; post-auricular, posterior cervical and suboccipital lymphadenopathy); measles (prodromal 3 Cs of cough, coryza and conjunctivitis with photophobia; generalised erythematous maculopapular rash, starting on the backs of the ears and spreading to the head and neck and rest of the body, turning brown before disappearance; Koplik spots (1 mm white spots, resembling grains of sand, on an erythematous background, in the buccal mucosa in the lower premolar region)); enteroviruses; acute HIV infection; uncomplicated dengue; aminopenicillin therapy in the presence of Epstein-Barr virus
- Rickettsial infections
- Mycoplasma and chlamydial infections
- Bacterial/spirochaetal infections: secondary syphilis; leptospirosis; meningococcaemia
- Acute retroviral syndrome (HIV)

Nodular lesions

- Erythema nodosum
- Streptococcal infections
- Sarcoidosis
- Inflammatory bowel disease
- Disseminated fungal infection
- Disseminated tuberculosis/atypical mycobacteria
- Sweet's syndrome

Other

- Pseudomonas aeruginosa-echythmagangrenosum
- Lyme disease
- Typhoid

Fluid-filled
Vesiculo-bullous disorders
Diffuse

- Varicella (successive crops of erythematous macules, papules, clear vesicles placed eccentrically on an erythematous base-dew drop on rose petal appearance, pustules, followed by central umbilication, erosion and crusting evolving over 12–24 h; lesions are seen in different stages of evolution; usually no prodrome in children, or a prodrome of nausea, anorexia, myalgia and headache in adults; starts on trunk-centripetal distribution-and spreads to face and

limbs-centrifugal spread, sparing palms and soles; reinfection or a second clinical attack virtually unheard of)
- Toxic epidermal necrolysis
- Pemphigus vulgaris
- Erythema multiforme major (Stevens-Johnson syndrome: fever, sore throat, flaccid bullae, painful ulcers in the mouth, lips, anal and genital regions, and keratoconjunctivitis)
- Bullous pemphigoid
- Drug eruptions
- Disseminated herpes simplex (eczema herpeticum: in patients with atopic dermatitis and other widespread skin diseases, resulting from auto-inoculation usually from labial HSV or hetero-inoculation from an infected contact; rapidly spreading blistering eruption evolving into large erosions and ulcers, associated with fever)
- Bullous erythema multiforme
- Staphylococcal infections

Peripheral

- Zoster (unilateral painful eruption of grouped vesicles along a dermatome, with hyperaesthesia and occasionally regional lymph node enlargement)
- Hand-foot-and mouth disease
- Contact dermatitis

Pustular disorders

- Bacterial folliculitis
- Generalisedpustular psoriasis: small, sterile pruritic non-follicular pustules within large areas of erythema; oedema of the hands and feet (de novo or complicating atypical, acral or flexural disease)
- Acute generalized erythematous pustulosis

Risk factors for folliculitis
Staphylococcal

- Shaving, plucking or waxing hair
- Occlusion or maceration of skin
- Topical steroid therapy
- Atopic dermatitis
- Diabetes mellitus

Pseudomonal

- Inadequately chlorinated hot tubs, whirlpools and swimming pools

Lynch PJ, Edminster SC. Dermatology for the non-dermatologist: a problem-oriented system. Ann Emerg Med. 1984;13: 603–6

Red flags in skin rash

- Systemic symptoms
- Fever
- Altered mental state
- Co-morbidity: immunocompromised
- Large area of skin involvement
- Mucosal or ocular involvement

Causes of maculopapular rash
A maculopapular rash in the absence of fever or systemic illness does not constitute an urgent illness.Symptomatic treatment in the absence of a definitive diagnosis may be required.

Afebrile
- Central distribution: drug eruption; pityriasisrosea; viral infection
- Peripheral distribution: scabies; atopic dermatitis

Febrile
- Central distribution: viral exanthema (measles, rubella, rubeola, roseola- circular to elliptical rose-red macules or papules involving trunk, occasionally surrounded by a white halo, erythema infectiosum-slapped cheeks, with bright red erythema, infectious mononucleosis, enteroviral, adenoviral and arboviral infections); drug reaction; Kawasaki disease
- Peripheral distribution: Stevens-Johnson syndrome; erythema multiforme; early meningococcaemia; early toxic shock syndrome; secondary syphilis; Lyme disease

Causes of STAR complex (sore throat, arthropathy, and skin rash)

- Rubella
- Parvovirus B19 (slapped cheek syndrome; viral prodrome, slapped cheeks, peri-oral pallor, sparing of palms and soles)
- Hepatitis B
- Adenovirus
- Echovirus
- Coxsackie
- Epstein-Barr virus

Causes of purpura
Loss of dermal vascular connective tissue

- Senile purpura
- Steroid therapy
- Vitamin C deficiency
- Hereditary connective tissue diseases: Ehlers-Danlos syndrome; Marfan syndrome

Vascular
Vessel wall damage

- Mechanical: trauma, suction to skin, stasis, factitious
- Anoxic-microvascular obstruction: consumption coagulopathies: DIC, TTP, haemolyticuraemic syndrome; purpurafulminans; fat embolism; myeloproliferative disease

Inflammatory vasculitis (Palpable purpura)
Vasculitis/arteritis

- Hypersensitivity vasculitis: Henoch-Schonleinpurpura (tetrad of purpura, abdominal pain, renal disease and arthritis or arthralgia); collagen vascular disease
- Leukocytoclasticvasculitis
- Infective vasculitis: meningoccal, streptococcal, gonococcal
- Dysproteinemias

Rickettsial infections
Non-vasculitic (pseudo-purpura)

- Angiokeratoma
- Cherryangioma
- Pyogenic granuloma
- Kaposi's sarcoma

Intravascular (haematological)

- Thrombocytopenia
- Functional platelet disorders
- Coagulopathies

Causes of generalised itching

- Dry skin (xerosis)
- Atopic dermatitis (itchy, dry erythematous scaly patches with vesicles and exudation; flexural dermatitis with lichenification, egantecubital and popliteal fossae; involvement of eyelids; cheilitis; white dermographism; recurrent conjunctivitis, keratoconus, anterior and/or posterior subcapsular cataracts; personal/family history of atopic disease; increased susceptibility to viral infections; enhanced sensivity to irritation by detergents, wool and certain chemicals)
- Contact dermatitis
- Drugs: statins, ACE inhibitors, opiates, barbiturates, recreational drugs, antidepressants, oral retinoids
- Urticaria
- Conjugated hyperbilirubinemia (cholestasis)
- Scabies: linear burrows, erythematous papules, vesicles, excoriations, crusts and pustules which are symmetrical in distribution and typically involve the inter-digital web spaces, flexor aspects of the wrists, axillae and the waist, showing a predilection for warm moist areas. Thick scaly plaques characterize Norwegian or crusted scabies.
- Chronic kidney disease
- Biliary obstruction
- Papularurticaria
- Animal mites
- Flea bites
- Lice infestations (Pediculosis)
- Iron deficiency anaemia
- Polycythaemia

Evaluation of generalized itching

- Itch characteristics, onset, timing, duration, location
- Relieving factors
- Associated symptoms: skin rash, fever, weight loss
- Drug history
- Diet (iron deficiency)
- Alcohol misuse (liver disease)
- Emotional stress; mental health history

Factors that aggravate atopic dermatitis

- Diet: food allergens (egg, wheat, soy, peanuts)
- Drying of the skin
- Irritants: soaping, detergents
- Inhalants: pets, pollen
- Sweating
- Fabrics: synthetic; wool
- Contact sensitivity
- Stress; anxiety
- Hormonal: premenstrual flares
- Secondary bacterial infection
- Secondary herpes simplex viral infection

Causes of localised itching

- Allergic contact dermatitis (pruritic, erythematous papules or papul0-vesicles, progressing to vesicles, with oozing and crusting; accentuated by heat, sweating and friction)
- Lichen simplex
- Picker's nodule: localised prurigo nodularis
- Neuropathic itch
- Trigeminal trophic syndrome

Causes of urticaria (increased permeability of capillaries and small venules in the superficial dermis, raising the epidermis and causing itchy wheals-elevated, oedematous and non-pitting circular or annular plaques-which are evanescent and migratory and do not last more than 24 h. There is often central clearing as the lesions spread, leaving an arcuate or gyrate formation)

Chronic idiopathic (>6 weeks)
Acute (<6 weeks) (IgE-mediated)
Exogenous causes

- Physical: dermographism (trauma of scratching); acquagenic; cold; solar; heat; delayed pressure; vibration; cholinergic
- Contact
- Pharmacological: salicylates (aspirin, spearmint and wintergreen flavours, as in toothpaste); opiates; NSAIDs; penicillin; ACE inhibitors; food additives (dyes, preservatives, taste enhancers); herbal medication; vaccine; contrast media
- Food: seafood, strawberries
- Insect bites: popular urticari

Endogenous causes

- Infection: viral (hepatitis; infectious mononucleosis, HIV seroconversion), bacterial, mycoplasmal
- Intestinal parasites
- Connective tissue disorders
- Lymphoma
- Mastocytosis
- Urticarial vasculitis
- Inherited:
- Hereditary angioneurotic oedema (C1 esterase deficiency) (autosomal dominant) (episodic attacks of non-pitting and non-pruritic angioedema involving the hands, arms, leg, feet, face, trunk or genitalia, due to subcutaneous oedema; recurrent laryngeal oedema due to submucosal oedema of the upper airway; and recurrent acute abdominal pain with nausea and vomiting and diarrhoea, due to submucosaloedema of the gastrointestinal tract; positive family history of angioedema)

Pathogenetic mechanisms in urticaria
Immunological
IgE-dependent

- Specific antigen sensitivity
- Physical: dermographism, cold, exercise (cholinergic), heat, sun exposure (solar), water (acquagenic), pressure
- Contact: eg stinging nettles, animal saliva, moth or butterfly scales

Complement-mediated

- Serum sickness
- Reaction to blood products
- Hereditary angioneuroticoedema
- SLE

Non-immunological
Direct mast-cell releasing agents:

- Opiates: morphine, codeine
- Radiocontrast media

Agents that alter arachidonic acid metabolism:

- Aspirin
- NSAIDs
- Azo dyes
- Benzoate preservatives
- ACE inhibitors

Idiopathic

Cellulitis
Differential diagnosis of cellulitis (causes of **pseudocellulitis**)
Bilateral cellulitis is very rare in the absence of trauma

Superficial thrombophlebitis
Lymphangitis
Necrotising fasciitis (systemic toxicity; pain out of proportion to physical findings; redness, tense oedema, crepitus, vesicles and bullae, necrosis, anaesthesia of skin; septic shock)
Insect bite
Erysipelas (painful, indurated, tense erythematous plaque with raised and sharply demarcated borders; often facial, either unilateral or in a butterfly distribution)
Allergic contact dermatitis
Drug reactions: fixed drug reaction; vaccine/injection site; toxic erythema of cancer chemotherapy (Gemcitabine causing erysipeloid reaction, often in areas of pre-existing lymphoedema)
Acute gout/pseudogout
Acute osteomyelitis
Ruptured Baker cyst
Panniculitis, including lipodermatosclerosis (redness, induration and hyperpigmentation associated with chronic venous insufficiency; often bilateral)
Neutrophilic dermatoses: Sweet's syndrome; periodic fever syndromes

Risk factors for development of cellulitis

Skin break: bite, burn, laceration
Leg ulceration
Interdigital skin maceration or fungal infection
Lymphoedema
Chronic venous insufficiency
Atopic dermatitis
Tineapedis
Pre-existing skin lesions: furuncle
Retained foreign body
Injection drug use
Prior surgery

Risk factors for rapid progression or delayed treatment response (NICE)

- Obesity
- Co-morbidity: diabetes mellitus; chronic kidney disease; chronic liver disease
- Immunosuppression
- Alcohol misuse
- Peripheral arterial disease
- Chronic venous insufficiency
- Peripheral neuropathy

Blistering diseases
Causes of blisters and vesicles (circumscribed, elevated swellings that contain free fluid)
Sub-corneal (very thin roof): superficial blisters below the stratum corneum

- Pustular psoriasis: white pustules or pus-filled blisters surrounded by erythematous skin
- Miliaria: blocked eccrine sweat ducts
- Subcornealpustulardermatosis: large pus-filled blisters, usually arranged in a

complete or partial ring shape. Individual blisters may contain a pus level.
- Staphylococcal scalded skin syndrome: extensive blistering with loss of sheets of skin.
- Bullous impetigo: fragile flaccid blisters on an erythematous base, rupturing with production of a golden-yellow crust.

Intra-corneal (intra-epidermal) (thin roof)
(Deeper intra-epidermal blisters)

- Friction blisters: necrosis of epidermal keratinocytes due to pressure or friction on a localized area of skin, healing within 2–3 days if further friction is avoided
- Insect bites: arranged in groups usually; surrounding inflammation
- Acute eczema
- Herpes simplex: grouped blisters on an erythematous base, which rupture and often crust
- Herpes zoster
- Hand-foot-and-mouth disease: vesicles on hands, feet, buttocks and in the mouth, especially on the palate (stomatitis)
- Pemphigus vulgaris: painful oral ulcerations precede onset of large flaccid bullae, which are painful, non-itchy and become generalised; positive Nikolsky sign-extension of the bulla on application of lateral pressure to the periphery of an active lesion
- Varicella

Sub-epidermal (tense roof, often intact)

- Bullous pemphigoid: large tense fluid-filled blisters on an erythematous base or normal skin, sites of predilection being on the lower abdomen, inner thighs and flexor aspects of forearms; mild to moderate pruritus; Nikolsky sign negative
- Dermatitis herpetiformis: intensely itchy papulo-vesicular rash, usually distributed symmetrically on extensor surfaces (back of neck, elbows, knees, buttocks and, scalp hairline; mucosal involvement is uncommon; grouped excoriations are characteristic
- Erythema multiforme minor: target or iris lesions (comprising three concentric areas: circular macules or plaques with dusky purple or erythematous central area of epidermal keratinocyte necrosis with bulla and/or crust, a pale oedematous concentric rim, and a purplish or erythematous halo, that enlarge peripherally); vesicles progressing to bullae; predilection for sun-exposed skin; may exhibit Koebner phenomenon; no mucosal involvement
- Erythema multiforme major (Stevens-Johnson syndrome)
- Toxic epidermal necrolysis: prodrome of fever and skin tenderness; rapid onset of blistering with epidermal detachment; positive Nikolsky sign
- Linear IgA disease: vesicles and bullae, arranged in rings (annular lesions), on skin and mucous membranes
- Cold and thermal injury: burns; frostbite
- Dystrophic epidermolysisbullosa
- Oedema blisters: severe dependent oedema of the leg
- Pemphigoid ('herpes') gestationis

Aetiology of blistering

Mechanical and physical causes (mechanobullous diseases)

- Friction blister
- Burns
- Pressure
- Epidermolysisbullosa simplex: generalised; superficial; epidermolysis bullosa dystrophica (AR; AD); epidermolysisbullosaletalis: fatal; non-fatal
- Porphyria cutanea tarda (vesicles on hands and on any area of exposure to ultra-violet light)
- Recurrent bullous eruption of hands and feet (Weber-Cockayne disease)

Infective

- Bacterial: staphylococcus; streptococcus
- Viral: varicella zoster; herpes simplex; herpes zoster
- Bites and infestations: spiders; insects; scabies

Inflammatory

- Eczema
- Pompholyx (dyshidrotic eczema): itchy vesicles, restricted to palms of hands and soles of feet, that may coalesce to form bullae
- Drugs

Immunobullous diseases: due to auto-antibodies directed at differing components of the desmosome complex; skin biopsy and direct immunofluorescence are diagnostic

- Pemphigus vulgaris: flaccid blisters and erosions involving the skin and mucous membranes (oral, nasal, pharyngeal, genital)
- Bullous pemphigoid
- Cicatricialpemphigoid
- Dermatitis herpetiformis
- Linear IgA disease
- Pemphigoidgestationis

Metabolic

- Porphyria
- Pseudo-porphyria
- Amyloidosis

Features of Stevens-Johnson syndrome

Acute prodromal flu-like symptoms, high fever, sore throat, conjunctivitis
Skin: morbilliform to diffuse or macular erythema, atypical target lesions (red macule with or without central vesicle), epidermal detachment and erosions
Mucosal involvement (involving two or more mucosal sites): oropharynx, genital, nasal, conjunctiva, anus
Gastrointestinal tract: bleeding, diarrhea

Causes of erythema multiforme

- Drugs: non-steroidal anti-inflammatory agents; antimicrobials (sulphonamides, penicillins); psychotropic drugs; anti-epileptic drugs
- Infections: viral (herpes simplex; varicella zoster; cytomegalovirus; parvovirus B19; HIV); bacterial (mycoplasma; salmonella; tuberculosis); fungal (histoplasmosis)
- Inflammatory bowel disease: Crohn's disease; ulcerative colitis

Causes of vesiculopustular eruptions
Viral infections:

- Herpes simplex: clusters of small tense vesicles on an erythematous base, which may coalesce, before rupturing to form ulcers, with a thin yellowish crust of dried exudate
- Varicella: successive crops over 12–24 h of itchy macules, papules, vesicles and pustules, followed by umbilication and crust formation, often with a prodrome of nausea, anorexia, myalgia and headache in adults. Vesicles with clear fluid surrounded by a narrow erythematous halo may produce a "dew drops on rose petals" appearance.
- Herpes zoster
- Hand, foot and mouth disease: a mild febrile illness with sore throat, painful oral ulceration, and an erythematous rash involving the palms of the hands, soles of the feet, and occasionally knees, elbows, buttocks and/or genitals; mostly affects children aged 10 years and under
- Eczema herpeticum: acute development of multiple, grouped 2–3 mm umbilicated vesicles, progressing to punched out erosions and haemorrhagic crusting, often in areas of active dermatitis, and associated with high fever and worsening pruritus

Bacterial infections:

- Impetigo
- Staphylococcal scalded skin syndrome: erythema on face (peri-nostril and peri-ocular), neck, axillae, groins and perineum becoming generalized within 48 h; skin tenderness; flaccid bullae with positive Nikolsky sign-the moist reddened base after rupture gives a scalded appearance
- Staphylococcal folliculitis

Immuno-bullous dermatoses:
- Intraepidermal disorders
  - Pemphigus vulgaris
  - Pemphigus foliaceous
- Sub-epidermal disorders
  - Chronic bullous dermatosis of childhood
  - Dermatitis herpetiformis

Mechano-bullous disorders:
- Friction blisters
- Epidermolysisbullosa

Acute dermatitides
Toxic epidermal necrolysis
- Fever, malaise
- Diffuse erythema and skin tenderness
- Loss of sheets of epidermis; flaccid bullae
- Positive Nikolsky sign: separation of epidermis with gentle shearing pressure

Erythroderma (exfoliative dermatitis)
Diffuse erythema and scaling affecting 90% or more of body surface area, which can be primary or secondary (generalization of prior localized skin disease).

Causes

- Adverse drug reaction: penicillin; sulphonamides, antiepileptic drugs
- Exacerbation of pre-existing dermatitis: atopic; seborrhoeic; contact; stasis
- Psoriasis
- Pityriasisrubrapilaris (reddish follicular papules and/or plaques with thick, dry scales)
- Immunobullous disease: pemphigus; bullous pemphigoid
- HIV infection
- Graft versus host disease
- Haematological malignancies: lymphoma; leukaemia;
- Cutaneous T cell lymphoma (Sezary syndrome-triad of erythroderma, generalized lymphadenopathy and neoplastic T cells in the skin, lymph nodes and blood) (atypical lymphocytes with cerebriform nuclei constitute more than 20% of circulating peripheral blood mononuclear cells)

Associations

- Oedema (eczema; drugs)
- Serous exudate (eczema)
- Scaling (eczema, psoriasis)
- Hair loss
- Keratoderma of palms and soles
- Nail shedding or dystrophy
- Ectropion
- Hypo- or hyper-pigmentation
- Localised or generalized lymphadenopathy

Complications

- Secondary infection
- Electrolyte imbalance
- Hypotension
- Heat loss: hypothermia
- High output congestive heart failure
- Failure of thermoregulation
- Acute kidney injury
- Hypoalbuminaemia

Causes of erythema nodosum

- Idiopathic
- Bacterial infections: streptococcus; primary tuberculosis; mycoplasma pneumoniae; campylobacter
- Viral infections: Epstein-Barr virus
- Autoimmune: inflammatory bowel disease (ulcerative colitis; Crohn's disease); sarcoidosis
- Pregnancy
- Medications: sulphonamides, penicillin, oral contraceptive, salicylates
- Cancer: non-Hodgkin lymphoma; carcinoid

Causes of nodular skin lesions

- Neoplasm: basal cell carcinoma; squamous cell carcinoma; lymphoma; malignant melanoma; Kaposi's sarcoma
- Vasculitis: erythema nodosum
- Metabolic: xanthoma; gouty tophus
- Infection: mycobacteria; fungal; bacterial (leprosy)
- Chronic inflammation: sarcoidosis; rheumatoid nodules

- Sweet's syndrome (acute febrile neutrophilicdermatosis); fever, neutrophilia, tender erythematous skin lesions (papules, nodules and plaques)

Pigmented lesions
The ABCDE Symptoms rule suggestive of malignant melanoma

- Asymmetrical shape
- Border irregularity
- Colour irregularity
- Diameter >6 mm
- Evolution of lesion (eg change in size and/ or shape)
- Symptoms: bleeding or itching

Risk factors for malignant melanoma

- Excessive ultraviolet exposure
- Skin type 1 (always burns, never tans)
- History of multiple moles or atypical moles (dysplastic naevus syndrome)
- Family history of or previous personal history of melanoma
- Xerodermapigmentosum
- Large congenital naevus

Mnemonic for causes of painful skin tumours
BENGAL:

- Blue rubber bleb naevus
- Eccrinetumours
- Neural tumours: traumatic neuroma; neurofibroma
- Glomustumour: usually blue
- Angiolipoma
- Leiomyoma

Burn wound assessment

- Superficial (epidermal): red, dry, painful, blanches on pressure, capillary refill time <2 s; due to flash, mild scald, or sunburn
- Partial thickness: superficial dermal: pale pink, painful, blistering, slow capillary refill after blanching; deep dermal: dry or moist; mottled, pink and white, painful or with reduced pain sensation, blisters may be present, no blanching on pressure; due to scald (hot liquid contact)
- Full thickness: dry and white, brown or black; leathery or waxy, painless, no blisters, insensate; due to flame, prolonged contact, chemical, electrical or lightning injury

Types of cutaneous drug eruptions

- Exanthem: macular or maculopapupar rash
- Urticaria
- Photoallergic contact dermatitis
- Phototoxic reactions
- Bullous eruptions (Stevens-Johnson syndrome; drug-induced pemphigus)
- Vasculitis
- Fixed drug eruption
- Exfoliative dermatitis
- Acneiform eruption

Red flags with cutaneous drug eruptions
Skin

- Confluent erythema
- Facial oedema
- Skin pain
- Palpable purpura
- Blisters
- Epidermal detachment
- Positive Nikolsky's sign (shearing of epidermal layer on rubbing blister, perilesional skin or adjacent normal skin)
- Skin necrosis

Mucosae

- Mucous membrane erosions
- Tongue swelling

Systemic

- High fever > 40°
- Lymph node enlargement
- Arthralgia; arthritis
- Hepatic/renal dysfunction
  Hypotension

Causes of angioedema (painless swelling of face, eyelids, lips and tongue)

- Kinin-related: hereditary angioedema (C1-INH deficiency); acquired angioedema (accelerated consumption of C1-INH); lymphoproliferative disorders; autoimmune disorders; ACE inhibitors
- Mast cell-mediated
  - Food allergies: additives, egg, nut, shellfish, milk, wheat, soy
  - Drug allergies:aspirin, NSAIDs, oral contraceptive, narcotics
  - Insect stings
  - Physically induced: cold; heat; vibration; exercise; trauma; stress; ultraviolet light
  - Cytokine-asssociated angioedema syndrome (Gleich)
    - Hypereosinophilic syndrome
    - Idiopathic recurrent angioedema
    - Thyroid autoimmune disease

Features to suggest hereditary angioneurotic oedema (C1 esterase inhibitor deficiency)

- Recurrent angioedema, lasting more than 24 h (non-pruritic, non-pitting, non-erythematous and non-responsive to anti-histamines)
- Absence of urticaria
- Unexplained recurrent colicky abdominal pain
- Recurrent laryngeal oedema
- Positive family history

Presentations of anaphylaxis

A multi-system syndrome related to exposure to foreign protein (antigen) and presenting with life threatening airway, and/or breathing and/or circulation problems, associated with skin and/or mucosal changes

Anaphylaxis should be suspected with sudden onset and rapid progression of symptoms, usually within 15 min of exposure, including shock and respiratory symptoms (dyspnoea, wheeze, and stridor)

Upper airway problems (related to pharyngeal and laryngeal oedema)

- Swelling of tongue and throat, including uvula
- Hoarseness of voice
- Stridor
- Rhinorrhoea (nasal discharge)

Breathing problems (lower airway)

Dyspnoea
Wheezing
Chest tightness
Confusion
Cyanosis
Respiratory arrest

Circulation problems

- Cardiovascular collapse
- Shock: hypotension and tachycardia
- Cardiac arrest

Skin and/or mucosa changes

- Urticaria
- Angioedema
- Flushing

Gastrointestinal symptoms

- Severe cramping abdominal pain related to intestinal and uterine colic
- Diarrhoea
- Nausea and vomiting

Biphasic reactions involved a delayed reaction 4–10 h after the initial presentation

Triggers for anaphylaxis

IgE-mediated

Antibiotics: beta-lactam antibiotics (penicillins)
  Venoms: bee, wasp (insect stings)
  Natural rubber latex (gloves; tourniquets; blood pressure cuffs)

Food: shellfish; peanut; soybean; tree nut (cashew, walnut, Brazil nut); egg; milk; wheat; nitrates or nitrites
Food additives: spices, colourants, vegetable gums
Vaccines
Seminal fluid

Non-IgE-mediated (anaphylactoid reactions): these are clinically indistinguishable from anaphylactic reactions but do not involve previous antigen exposure

Iodinated radiopaque contrast media
Opiates, aspirin, NSAIDs
Blood transfusion
Immunoglobulin
Physical factors: exercise; cold; heat; sunlight/ultraviolet radiation

Risk factors for latex anaphylaxis

- Genetic predisposition (atopic individuals)
- Previous exposure to latex: chronic bladder care requiring intermittent catheterization or chronic indwelling catheter (spina bifida, meningomyelocele; cloacal abnormalities-bladder exstrophy)
- Health care workers exposed to latex
- Multiple surgical procedures

Factors influencing severity of anaphylactic reaction

- Initial severe symptoms
- History of severe, protracted or recurrent anaphylaxis
- Co-morbidities: asthma, congestive heart failure, renal disease
- Beta-adrenergic blocker therapy

Differential diagnosis of anaphylaxis

- Acute urticaria
- Dyspnoea: asthma; pulmonary embolism
- Syncope; vasovagal attack
- Stridor: laryngospasm; epiglottitis; foreign body
- Flushing: red man syndrome (vancomycin); scombrotoxic fish poisoning: histamine-like compound in improperly refrigerated fish such as tuna, mackerel, sardines, anchovies, mahi-mahi, and blue fish causing facial flushing and sweating, dizziness, nausea, headache, vomiting, and a generalised skin rash 30 min after ingestion; usually resolves within 24 h; carcinoid syndrome; systemic mastocytosis: episodes of flushing, urticaria, bronchospasm and hypotension; monosodium glutamate ingestion (Chinese restaurant syndrome): headache, chest pain, flushing, bronchospasm, and burning or numbness in theupper trunk, face and neck within 3060 min of eating food with a high concentration of monosodium glutamate
- Panic attack

Clinical settings for toxic shock syndrome (TSS)

Menstrual TSS

- Tampon-associated (especially highly absorbent brands)
- Not tampon-associated

Non-menstrual TSS

- TSS related to the female genitourinary tract
  Associated with barrier contraception use (diaphragm, contraceptive sponges)
  Occurring in the puerperium
  Following non-obstetric gynaecological surgery
  Associated with septic abortion
- TSS related to skin or soft tissue infections
  Primary staphylococcal infections (folliculitis, cellulitis, carbuncle, muscle abscesses)
  Staphylococcal super-infections of pre-existing lesions (burns, insect bites, varicella/zoster infections, surgical wounds)

- TSS related to respiratory tract infections:
  Upper respiratory tract focus (sinusitis, pharyngitis, laryngotracheitis, odontogenic infection)
  Lower respiratory tract focus (staphylococcal pneumonia)
- TSS related to skeletal infections:
  Osteomyelitis
  Septic arthritis

Diagnostic criteria for toxic shock syndrome
Major criteria

- Fever: temperature 38.7 C or >
- Rash: diffuse, macular erythroderma
- Mucosal membranes: hyperaemia, oropharyngeal or conjunctival
- Desquamation: 1–2 weeks after onset of illness (typically palms and soles)
- Hypotension: systolic blood pressure <=5th percentile by age (children under 16 years of age) or systolic blood pressure <= 90 mm Hg (adults), or orthostatic hypotension

Minor criteria: Multi-system dysfunction- at least three

- Chest: tachypnoea (>40/min); tachycardia (>160/min)
- Gut: vomiting and/or diarrhoea at onset of illness
- Renal function: diminished urine output or raised plasma creatinine>= twice the upper limit of normal, or pyuria (>= 5 leukocytes per high-power field) in the absence of urinary tract infection
- Hepatic: serum bilirubin or liver enzymes (AST/ALT) elevated >= twice the upper limit of normal
- CNS: confusion or irritability 9
- Haematologic:
  <100 × 10/l platelets
  9
  >10.0 × 10/l neutrophils

Causes of skin rash in the groin

- Tineacruris
- Contact dermatitis
- Scabies
- Pubic lice
- Sexually transmitted infection
- Psoriasis

Causes of diaper area (nappy) rash

- Poor hygiene practices
- Type of nappy: disposable/reusable cotton
- Exposure to irritants: moisture; chemicals (soap, detergent, alcohol-based baby wipes)
- Trauma: friction from nappies; over-vigorous cleaning
- Recent antbiotic therapy
- Infection: *Candida albicans* (sharply marginated redness; satellite papules and pustules; skin creasei involvement); bacterial (marked redness; exudates; erosions with crusting;vesicular and pustular lesions)
- Seborrhoeic dermatitis
- Atopic dermatitis

6 Ocular Emergencies

Causes of acute red eye

Uniocular

Painless

Normal vision:

Subconjunctival haemorrhage
Episcleritis
Pterygium
Pingueculum
Conjunctivitis

Painful

Normal vision:

Corneal stain:

Negative

- Anterior uveitis (iridocyclitis and iritis) (irregular pupil from posterior synechiae, circumcorneal congestion, anterior chamber flare and cells; keratic precipitates on posterior surface of cornea)
- Scleritis (redness of the sclera, localized or generalized; diffuse tenderness)
- Herpes zoster ophthalmicus (early)

Positive

- Corneal abrasion
- Herpes simplex keratitis
- Marginal ulcer

Vision reduced:

Corneal fluorescein stain negative

- Severe uveitis
- Acute angle closure glaucoma (circumcorneal congestion; non-reactive, semi-dilated vertically elliptical pupil; corneal oedema or haziness; shallow anterior chamber; severe pain; vomiting; haloes around lights; predisposing factors include a shallow anterior chamber, hypermetropia, and lens abnormalities such as cataracts)
- Secondary glaucoma

Corneal fluorescein stain positive

- Herpes simplex keratitis (punctate keratitis; small bullous epithelial lesions; dendritic ulcer-branching linear lesion; geographical ulcer)
- Bacterial keratitis
- Herpes zoster ophthalmicus: clear vesicles on inflamed and hyperaesthetic forehead, upper eyelid or on tip of nose (Hutchinson sign), in distribution of ophthalmic division of trigeminal nerve; punctate or dendritic lesions of cornea; follicular or papillary conjunctivitis; episcleritis
- Corneal burn

A. Banerjee, *Emergency Clinical Diagnosis*, DOI 10.1007/978-3-319-50718-7_6

- Acanthamoeba keratitis (contact lens wearer; disproportionate pain; superficial punctuate keratitis; ring infiltrates from coalescing paracentral infiltrates; radial keratoneuritis due to infiltrates along corneal nerves)

Binocular:
No pain/good vision:

- Bacterial conjunctivitis: purulent discharge
- Viral conjunctivitis
- Allergic conjunctivitis

Pain/vision good or poor:

- Viral keratoconjunctivitis
- Chlamydial keratoconjunctivitis
- Arc eye (photokeratitis or ultraviolet keratitis) (pain, lacrimation, foreign body sensation, photophobia, miosis; punctate conjunctival erosions; exposure to welder's arc, sun lamp in tanning salon or bright snow-covered environment)

Patterns of red eye
Normal/near normal vision

Painful/discomfort

Diffuse superficial redness of bulbar and palpebral conjunctiva, maximal in the fornices: conjunctivitis
Diffuse deep redness: anterior scleritis
Circum-limbal (corneo-scleral junction) redness: keratitis; anterior uveitis; corneal foreign body
Sectoral redness: episcleritis

Painless

- Subconjunctival haemorrhage: deep crimson red and confluent

Reduced vision

Normal intraocular pressure

- Abnormal cornosclera: corneal abrasion; keratitis
- Abnormal uvea: anterior uveitis; endophthalmitis

Raised intraocular pressure

- Acute glaucoma

Hypertensive uveitis

Red flags for red eye

- Moderate to severe ocular pain
- Photophobia
- Marked redness of one eye
- Loss of visual acuity
- Associated bowel or joint symptoms

Checklist for foreign body sensation in the eye

- Visual acuity
- Pupil size, shape and reactions
- Upper and lower fornices of the conjunctiva, including eversion of the upper lid
- Fluorescein staining of the cornea; linear vertical corneal abrasions suggest a subtarsal foreign body
- Anterior chamber: intraocular foreign body; hyphaema

Clues to cause of conjunctivitis

- Bacterial: mucopurulent or purulent discharge
- Gonococcal: profuse purulent discharge; severe chemosis and eyelid swelling
- Viral: watery, mucous discharge; lacrimation; foreign body sensation; pinpoint subconjunctival haemorrhages; preauricular lymphadenopathy
- Epidemic keratoconjunctivitis: chemosis; corneal infiltrates
- Herpes simplex: vesicles on eyelid margin or peri-ocular skin; dendritic ulcer
- Herpes zoster: rash or vesicles in distribution of naso-ciliary branch of ophthalmic division of trigeminal nerve; dendritic ulcer
- Allergic: seasonal; itching, lacrimation; personal or family history of atopy

Risk factors for bacterial keratitis

Local ocular factors

- Corneal: abrasion, foreign bodies, exposure, bullous keratopathy
- Abnormal tear function: dry eye; dacryocystitis
- Abnormal lid function: blepharitis; entropion; ectropion; cicatricialpemphigoid; lagopthalmos; trichiasis
- Cosmetic: contact lens wear; cosmetic eye makeup
- Drugs and treatments: topical corticosteroids; cyanoacrylate adhesive; ocular surgery

Systemic factors: immunosuppressive therapy; diabetes mellitus; coma; alcoholism; burns; Stevens-Johnson syndrome; AIDS

Causes of hyphaema

- Ocular trauma: blunt; penetrating
- Intra-ocular tumours: ocular melanoma; retinoblastoma; metastatic tumours
- Coagulopathy: von Willebrand disease; thrombocytopenia; haemophilia; leukaemia
- Neovascularisation of the iris: proliferative diabetic retinopathy; carotid stenosis
- Post-surgical: cataract extraction; trabeculectomy; pars plana vitrectomy

Causes of periorbital redness and swelling

Orbital inflammation

No proptosis

Infections

- Pre-septal cellulitis (secondary to lid trauma –e.g. insect or animal bite, minor trauma-e.g. eyelid abrasion; lid skin infections-stye, dacryocystitis, herpes simplex; conjunctivitis; associated with upper respiratory tract infections and sinusitis; normal visual acuity and pupillary reflexes)
- Dacryocystitis (tense painful erythematous swelling below the medial canthal ligament)
- Dacryoadenitis (painful erythematous swelling of the lateral upper eyelid, with or without ptosis)
- Blepharitis (erythema and thickening of eyelid margins; crusting and scales, with eyelash loss; eyelashes may stick together)
- Conjunctivitis
- Endophthalmitis

Non-infectious causes

- Allergic reaction

Proptosis

- Orbital infections: orbital cellulitis (lid oedema; pain with eye movements; conjunctival hyperaemia and chemosis; ophthalmoplegia; optic nerve involvement with reduced visual acuity; fever; loss of sensation related to the ophthalmic and maxillary divisions of the trigeminal nerve; may involve spread of infection from paranasal sinuses, especially the ethmoid or frontal sinuses); cavernous sinus thrombosis
- Endocrine: thyroid eye disease
- Inflammatory: systemic inflammatory disorders: Wegener's granulomatosis, sarcoidosis; orbital pseudotumour
- Neoplasm: lymphoma; lymphoproliferative disorders; rhabdomyosarcoma; choroidal malignant melanoma with extra-ocular spread; metastatic carcinoma
- Carotid-cavernous fistula (proptosis; conjunctival chemosis; exposure keratopathy; poorly reactive dilated mid-position pupil; retinal vein congestion; raised intraocular pressure)
- Retrobulbar haemorrhage/abscess

Risk factors for mucormycosis

- Diabetic ketoacidosis
- Haematological malignancy

- Bone marrow and solid organ transplant recipients
- Steroid therapy
- Intravenous drug use
- Burns

Causes of diplopia (double vision)

Monocular

Extra-ocular: optical lens or contact lens problem

Ocular

Strabismus

Lid: chalazion

Cornea: infection, trauma, distortion (keratoconus)

Iris: pharmacological mydriasis

Lens: cataract; subluxation

Retina: detachment, central retinal vein occlusion

Uncorrected refractive error (resolves with pinhole testing)

Binocular

- Cranial nerve palsies (infranuclear): III, IV, VI
- Myopathies: thyroid eye disease; myasthenia gravis
- Trauma: orbital blow-out fracture
- Orbital lesions: cellulitis; neoplasm
- Supranuclear lesions: internuclear ophthalmoplegia (horizontal diplopia with weakness of adduction of ipsilateral eye and nystagmus of the contralateral abducting eye); brainstem ischaemia (pons or midbrain lesions)

Checklist for diplopia

- Resting position of the eyes
- Eyelid function: ptosis
- Visual acuity in each eye separately and then both together
- Pupil size and reactivity
- Ocular motility; disconjugate eye movements; nystagmus
- Other cranial nerves
- Cerebellar function
- Fatigability of eye movements (myasthenia gravis)

Causes of acute visual loss

Uniocularvisual loss

Central:

Retinal:

- Age related macular degeneration (either dry, with drusen and pigmentary changes in the macula, or wet, with choroidal neovascularisation)
- Venous and arterial occlusions: central retinal vein/branch retinal vein occlusion (retinal haemorrhages in all four quadrants, dilated tortuous retinal branch veins, multiple cotton wool spots, macular and optic disc oedema, neovascularisation of the iris, retina or optic disc); central retinal artery/branch retinal artery occlusion(attenuated retinal arteries; retinal opacification, whitening and oedema-ground-glass retina; cherry red spot in macula due to cilio-retinal sparing; amaurosis fugax; relative afferent pupillary defect)
- Central serous retinopathy

Optic nerve (central scotoma; afferent pupillary defect)

- Optic neuritis: inflammatory neuropathy (idiopathic; multiple sclerosis; viral infection-varicella-zoster; post-viral; granulomatous inflammation-sarcoidosis, tuberculosis; HIV; drugs: ethambutol, tamoxifen)
- Demyelinating neuropathy: retrobulbar neuritis
- Compressive neuropathy
- Ischaemic optic neuropathy
- Traumatic optic neuritis

Media opacity

- Vitreous haemorrhage (reduced or absent red reflex; limited or no visualization of the optic fundus)
- Choroiditis

Peripheral:

Retinal:

- Retinal detachment (recent history of increased numbers of visual floaters and/or flashing lights; dark shadow or black spot in field of vision)
- CMV retinitis
- Retinal migraine

Optic nerve:

- Ischaemic optic neuropathy

Binocular visual loss:

Central:

Retinal:

- CMV retinitis
- Acute posterior multi-focal placoid pigment epitheliopathy
- Hypertensive retinopathy

Optic nerve:

- Infiltration
- Papilloedema

Cortical:

- Occipital lobe infarction: acute basilar artery occlusive disease; posterior circulation hypoperfusion (watershed infarction); superior sagittal sinus thrombosis
- Functional

Peripheral:

Retinal

- Retinal detachment (subacute onset of painless progressive visual field loss, often preceded by the acute onset of floaters and flashes, which are white in colour and may be associated with the phenomenon of a curtain descending over the vision; high myopia is a predisposing factor; the retina is indistinct and cloudy, being difficult to focus on during examination)

Optic nerve:

- Drusen

Cortical:

- Homonymous hemianopia
- Bitemporal hemianopia

Causes of sudden/recent loss of vision
Painless

(1) Few seconds duration
- Unilateral: giant cell arteritis; papilloedema; impending central retinal vein occlusion; ocular ischaemic syndrome
- Bilateral: papilloedema

(2) Few minutes duration
- Unilateral: amaurosisfugax; giant cell arteritis
- Bilateral: vertebro-basilar insufficiency

(3) Up to 1 h in duration
- Migraine

(4) Persistent
- Abnormal cornea: hydrops-acute corneal oedema
- Abnormal vitreous: vitreous haemorrhage
- Abnormal fundus: central retinal artery occlusion, central retinal vein occlusion, rhegmatogenous retinal detachment, exudative retinal detachment, intermediate uveitis, posterior uveitis
- Abnormal disc: anterior ischaemic optic neuropathy
- Abnormal macula: choroidal neovascular membrane; central serous retinopathy (typically in males aged 20 to 45 years; shallow serous macular neurosensory detachment, often surrounded by a halo light reflex; presents with acute visual loss and metamorphopsia)
- Normal fundus: cortical blindness; functional

Painful

- Abnormal cornea: acute angle closure glaucoma; bullous keratopathy; keratitis
- Abnormal uvea: anterior uveitis
- Abnormal disc: optic neuritis
- Normal fundus: retrobulbar neuritis

Checklist for assessment of the eye for visual loss

- Visual acuity
- Pupillary examination

- Visual fields
- Pen torch or slit lamp assessment of anterior segment
- Dilated funduscopy assessment of posterior segment

Testing for a relative afferent pupillary defect (swinging light test)

- Normal: both pupils constrict equally regardless of which eye is stimulated by light (intact direct and consensual pupillary light reactions)
- Abnormal: less pupil constriction, and apparent dilatation, in the eye with retinal or pre-chiasmal optic nerve disease, when the bright light is swung to the affected eye from the unaffected eye. The pupil of the abnormal eye dilates when illuminated and the contralateral pupil constricts when illuminated.

Causes of relative afferent pupillary defect (Marcus Gunn pupil)

- Optic nerve disorders: unilateral optic neuropathy (optic neuritis; ischaemic optic neuropathy; traumatic optic neuropathy; optic nerve tumour; orbital disease-thyroid-related orbitopathy; radiation optic neuropathy)
- Retinal disorders: ischaemic retinal disease (central retinal vein or artery occlusion; retinal detachment; ischaemic ocular disease (ophthalmic or internal carotid artery occlusion)); macular degeneration; retinal infection (CMV, herpes)

Types of visual field defects

Bitemporal hemianopia: pituitary adenoma; craniopharyngioma; parasellar meningioma; parasellar internal carotid artery aneurysm; glioma of optic chiasm

Binasal hemianopia

Homonymous hemianopia: incongruous: optic tract lesion; congruous: optic radiation lesion; occipital cortex (macular sparing)

Quadrantic homonymous hemianopia: inferior: parietal lobe (superior fibres of optic radiation); superior: temporal lobe (Meyer's loop)

Central scotoma: age-related macular degeneration; optic nerve disease

Causes of watering eye

Excessive lacrimation: overproduction of tears by lacrimal gland; normal lacrimal drainage system:

- Environmental: dust, smoke, wind
- Corneal irritation: abrasion, ulcer, foreign body, trichiasis
- Conjunctival irritation: conjunctivitis, foreign body, allergy
- Lid margin disease: blepharitis
- Lacrimal gland stimulation: dacryoadenitis; lacrimal gland tumour
- Aberrant regeneration post-Bell's palsy (crocodile tears, with lacrimation during eating, due to aberrant regeneration of salivary fibres towards the superficial greater petrosal nerve subserving lacrimation)

Epiphora: reduced outflow due to defective drainage of tears

- Pump failure: facial paralysis; lid retraction; lid laxity
- Punctal malposition: ectropion
- Punctal stenosis
- Canalicular obstruction: trauma with laceration; chronic infection with stenosis-trachoma
- Nasolacrimal duct obstruction: congenital; acquired (trauma; neoplasm) (associated with recurrent conjunctivitis, dacryocystitis, lacrimal sac mucocele or abscess)

Causes of ocular pain in the white (uninflamed) eye

- Ocular: optic neuropathy (demyelination; giant cell arteritis); dry eye
- Neurological: cluster headache; migraine; trigeminal neuralgia
- Vascular: haemorrhage (subarachnoid; subdural; extradural; intracerebral); carotid artery disease (dissection; aneurysm)
- Orbital: paranasal sinusitis; tumour invasion (e.g. nasopharyngeal)

Causes of painful ophthalmoplegia syndromes

Orbit

- Inflammatory pseudotumour (abrupt onset of pain, diplopia, visual loss, proptosis, chemosis, epibulbar injection and restricted ocular movements)
- Contiguous paranasal sinusitis
- Mucormycosis
- Metastatic tumour
- Lymphoma

Superior orbital fissure- anterior cavernous sinus

- Non-specific granulomatous inflammation (Tolosa-Hunt syndrome)
- Metastatic tumour
- Nasopharyngeal carcinoma
- Lymphoma
- Herpes zoster
- Carotid-cavernous fistula
- Cavernous sinus thrombosis

Parasellar area

- Pituitary adenoma
- Pituitary apoplexy (acute extrasellar extension), with classic triad of acute onset of severe headache, ophthalmoplegia and repeated vomiting
- Subarachnoid haemorrhage
- Intracavernous aneurysm
- Metastatic tumour
- Nasopharyngeal carcinoma
- Sphenoid sinus mucocele
- Chordoma
- Meningioma
- Apical petrositis (Gradenigo's syndrome)

Posterior cranial fossa

- Posterior cerebral artery aneurysm
- Basilar artery aneurysm

Miscellaneous

- Diabetic ophthalmoplegia
- Migraine
- Cranial arteritis

Features of cavernous sinus lesion

- Unilateral or isolated III, IV and VI nerve palsies
- Painful ophthalmoplegia
- Proptosis (pulsatile: carotid-cavernous fistula)
- Conjunctival congestion
- Optic disc oedema/pallor
- Anaesthesia in the territory of ophthalmic division of trigeminal nerve

Causes of pulsating globe

- Associated with orbital bruit: carotid-cavernous fistula; dural fistula; arteriovenous malformation
- Not associated with orbital bruit: orbital roof removal or trauma; neurofibromatosis; metastatic orbital tumours

Causes of IIIrd nerve palsy (diplopia; ptosis; mydriasis; eye abducted by lateral rectus; paresis of adduction and of upward and downward gaze; intorsion of the eye on attempted downgaze by superior oblique; pupil sparing is seen with ischaemic lesions)

- Nuclear lesions: dorsal midbrain: vascular (infarction), demyelination, tumour
- Fascicular lesions: ventral midbrain(Benedikt and Weber syndromes); interpeduncular (subarachnoid cistern) (giant aneurysms of anterior portion of posterior communicating artery; basal meninges-meningeal infection, neoplastic infiltration and inflammation; herniation of parahippocampalgyrus (uncal herniation) with raised intracranial pressure); cavernous sinus(cavernous sinus syndromes; sellar masses-pituitary adenoma; infection: sphenoid sinusitis, fungal infections- mucormycosis); superior orbital fissure (orbital cellulitis; pseudotumour; thyroid eye disease; tumours-optic nerve glioma/meningioma; Tolosa-Hunt syndrome)
- Infections and inflammations of IIIrd nerve: diabetes mellitus; demyelination

Causes of VIth nerve palsy (bilateral horizontal diplopia; convergent strabismus)

- Nuclear lesions in dorsal pons (Millard-Gubler syndrome; Foville's syndrome)
- Quadrigeminal plate: pineal tumour; meningioma; metastases
- Subarachnoid space: expanding supratentorial mass lesions causing stretch at the petroclinoid ligament, within Dorello's canal, by relative downward movement of the brain stem (false localizing sign of raised intracranial pressure); haemorrhage; meningeal or parameningeal infections, inflammation or infiltration
- Apex of petrous temporal bone: meningioma; cholesteatoma; plasmacytoma; spread of infection (mastoiditis; complicated otitis media)
- Tumours of the clivus: nasopharygeal carcinoma; chordoma
- Cavernous sinus
- Superior orbital fissure: tumour, pseudotumour, thyroid eye disease, orbital cellulitis
- Distended 3rd ventricle

Causes of anisocoria

- Physiological (20% of individuals)
- **Unilateral miosis**
  Horner's syndrome (partial ptosis, miosis, anhidrosis, apparent enophthalmos)
  Acute iridocyclitis: redness; cloudy anterior chamber
- **Unilateral mydriasis**
  Third nerve paralysis: posterior communicating aneurysm; temporal lobe (uncal) herniation
  Mydriatic use
  Traumatic mydriasis with iridoplegia
  Mechanical iris dysfunction: cataract extraction
  Adie (tonic) pupil: slow convergence reaction

Causes of Horner's syndrome

- First order neuron (central)
  Hypothalamus
  Brain stem: infarction (lateral medullary syndrome; dorsi-lateral pontine infarction); demyelination (multiple sclerosis); syringobulbia; bulbar poliomyelitis; encephalitis
  Cervico-thoracic spinal cord: trauma; syringomyelia; amyotrophic lateral sclerosis; glioma
- Second order neuron (pre-ganglionic)
  Lower brachial plexus: C7/T1 root avulsion
  Lower trunk of brachial plexus lesion: apex of lung lesion (Pancoast tumour)
  Neck: cervical rib; neurofibroma
- Third order neuron (post-ganglionic)
  Superior cervical ganglion: trauma; iatrogenic; jugular venous ectasia
  Internal carotid artery: dissection
  Cavernous sinus lesions
  Superior orbital fissure lesions

Causes of bilateral mydriasis

- Rostro-caudal deterioration: supra-tentorial masses
- Hypoxic-ischaemic encephalopathy
- Drugs: anticholinergics, tricyclic antidepressants, cocaine, adrenaline
- Post-ictal
- Bilateral optic nerve damage
- Parinaud's syndrome
- Emotional state
- Thyrotoxicosis

Causes of bilateral miosis

- Drugs: opiates; cholinergics; monoamine oxidase inhibitors
- Pontine lesions: massive haemorrhage

Causes of optic disc swelling

- Papilloedema (raised intracranial pressure) (swollen, blurred and elevated disk margins; engorged and pulseless veins; increased vascularity of disk margins)
- Inflammatory optic neuropathy: optic neuritis (central scotoma; loss of colour vision;

relative afferent pupillary defect); retrobulbar neuritis
- Ischaemic optic neuropathy: anterior ischaemic optic neuropathy; central retinal vein occlusion
- Optic nerve tumours: meningioma; glioma; metastases
- Compressive optic neuropathy: Graves' disease; sphenoidal ridge meningioma
- Ocular venous drainage obstruction: space occupying lesion in orbit; carotico-cavernous fistula; cavernous sinus thrombosis
- Pseudo-papilloedema: optic nerve drusen; hyperopia; myelinated nerve fibre layer

Causes of papilloedema (recurrent transient visual obscurations; enlarged blind spot; normal visual acuity)

Intracranial space occupying lesion
Increased CSF production: choroid plexus papilloma
Reduced CSF absorption: meningitis; subarachnoid haemorrhage
Cranial venous outflow obstruction: dural venous sinus thrombosis
Benign idiopathic intracranial hypertension
Endocrine: adrenocortical insufficiency; Cushing disease; hypothyroidism; hypoparathyroidism
Medication: tetracyclines (doxycycline); oral contraceptive; Vitamin A; isoretinoin
Obesity (BMI >30)

Effects of blunt trauma to the eye

- Eyelids: contusion, laceration (complicated: lid margin, medial canthal with or without lower lacrimal canaliculus involvement)
- Subconjunctival haemorrhage
- Cornea: abrasion, laceration (iris prolapse with tear-drop shaped pupil)
- Traumatic mydriasis
- Anterior chamber haemorrhage; hyphaema
- Iridodialysis
- Lens: concussional cataract (acute lens opacity); subluxation/dislocation (fluctuating vision; monocular diplopia; iridodonesis)
- Vitreous haemorrhage
- Retina: haemorrhage, oedema, detachment, commotio retinae
- Traumatic optic neuropathy (reduced central vision, afferent pupillary defect, poor colour vision)
- Orbital blowout fracture (diplopia on vertical gaze; orbital emphysema; infraorbital numbness)
- Orbital compartment syndrome (retrobulbar haemorrhage): proptosis; tense eyelids that are difficult to prise apart; diffuse subconjunctival haemorrhage; visual loss; raised intraocular pressure; relative afferent papillary defect

Orbital compression syndrome

- Raised intraocular pressure causing impaired perfusion of the optic nerve and globe
- Causes include post-traumatic retrobulbar haemorrhage, orbital emphysema (tension pneumo-orbit) related to orbital fracture, orbital cellulitis, rapidly growing orbital neoplasms or ruptured ophthalmic artery aneurysm, and iatrogenic (following eyelid and orbital surgery or retrobulbar anaesthetic injection)
- Presents with acute pain, proptosis, rapid visual loss, ophthalmoplegia, relative afferent pupillary defect, loss of pupillary light reflex
- Urgent orbital decompression using lateral canthotomy and inferior (with or without superior) cantholysis is needed

Penetrating trauma to the eye
Signs suggesting ruptured globe (protect eye with a plastic shield on making the diagnosis)

- Penetrating eyelid injury
- Loss of vision
- Corneal or scleral laceration
- Haemorrhagicchemosis
- Shallow anterior chamber
- Blood in anterior chamber (hyphaema)
- Iris prolapse
- Vitreous prolapse or haemorrhage
- Irregular pupil
- Low intraocular pressure

Risk factors for intraocular foreign body

- High velocity injury: hammering, chiselling, drilling metal
- Glass injuries
- Fireworks
- Shotgun wounds
- Darts

Potential complications of penetrating eyelid injury
Even a small and innocuous appearing eyelid laceration may be complicated by injury to the globe or with intracranial penetration. Visualisation of orbital fat in the laceration indicates penetration of the orbital septum. Eyelid injury may coexist with any of the following:

- Injury to the lid margin
- Injury to the medial canthal ligament, associated with displacement or distortion of the rounded appearance of the medial canthal angle
- Injury to lacrimal apparatus (canaliculi, common duct, lacrimal sac), seen with lacerations medial or nasal to the upper or lower eyelid punctum
- Injury to levator palpebrae complex, leading to ptosis
- Injury to the globe
- Injury to orbit
- Injury to paranasal sinuses
- Injury to cranium (the cranium may be entered via the orbital roof (superior orbital plate of the frontal bone), superior orbital fissure, or optic canal, the usual causative objects being pencils or pens, knives or chopsticks)

Eye injury checklist

- Mechanism of injury
- Pre-existing ocular disease
- Use of eye/face protection, e.g. safety glasses
- Contact lens usage
- Presenting complaints: pain, photophobia, tearing, change in vision
- Visual acuity
- Pupil size, reactivity; relative afferent pupillary defect
- Visual fields
- Extraocular movements, looking for evidence of entrapment
- Eyelids: swelling, laceration, ptosis; with lid lacerations be aware of occult penetrating intracranial injury caused by penetration of the orbital roof, superior orbital fissure or optic canal, and associated with intracranial injury and brain abscess
- Orbital rim: deformity, crepitus
- Conjunctiva: subconjunctival haemorrhage; chemosis; foreign body
- Cornea: abrasion, opacity, foreign body, contact lens
- Anterior chamber: blood, abnormal depth
- Iris: reactivity
- Lens: cataract, dislocation
- Vitreous: opacity
- Retina: haemorrhage, detachment

Sequence of visual acuity assessment

- Reading Snellen chart
- Finger counting
- Detecting hand motion
- Light perception

ENT and Maxillofacial Emergencies

7

Approach to the patient with vertigo

Vertigo is an illusory sensation of motion, that can be rotatory, linear, or vertical.

Spontaneous

- Single prolonged episode: vestibular neuronitis (associated hearing loss: labyrinthitis); labyrinthine concussion; lateral medullary or cerebellar infarction
- Recurrent episodes: Meniere disease (severe vertigo with tinnitus and progressive hearing loss); perilymph fistula; vestibular migraine (recurrent attacks of vertigo or dizziness lasting minutes to hours; associated with headache or other migrainous symptoms; postural imbalance; personal history of migraine); posterior circulation ischaemia

Positional

- Peripheral: benign paroxysmal positional vertigo
- Central

Causes of peripheral (labyrinthine) vertigo

- Trauma: head injury, barotrauma, perilymph fistula (vertigo triggered by straining); tympanic membrane rupture; round window rupture; labyrinthine concussion
- Iatrogenic: middle and inner ear surgery
- Infection: acute viral labyrinthitis (acute onset of sustained peripheral vertigo, nausea and vomiting, recent upper respiratory tract infection in 50%, symptoms predominantly with head movement, hearing loss, postural imbalance with falls toward affected side), herpes zoster, syphilis, suppurative labyrinthitis after suppurative otitis media; mastoiditis; vestibular neuronitis
- Metabolic: Meniere's disease (tetrad of recurrent attacks of vertigo lasting more than 20 min, fluctuating sensorineural hearing loss, tinnitus and subjective sensation of aural fullness; vestibular drop attacks may rarely occur), cochlear otosclerosis
- Ototoxic drugs: aminoglycosides (vestibular nerve); quinine, salicylates (vestibular)
- Degenerative: benign paroxysmal positional vertigo (repeated short-lived episodes of vertigo (<60 s), induced by positional change such as rolling over in bed, lying back in bed or sitting up from a supine position, and associated with transient rotatory nystagmus; caused by canalithiasis with free floating otoconia within the endolymph of the membranous labyrinth; particle repositioning manoeuvres such as the Epley manoeuvre can lead to symptom resolution)

A. Banerjee, *Emergency Clinical Diagnosis*, DOI 10.1007/978-3-319-50718-7_7

- Tumour: acoustic neuroma
- Drugs: quinine, salicylates
- Otitis media
- Motion sickness

Causes of central vertigo (brainstem, cerebellar or temporal lobe lesions)

- Cerebrovascular disease: vertebrobasilar insufficiency; cerebellar or brainstem stroke; cerebellar haemorrhage; vertebral artery dissection; subclavian steal syndrome; basilar artery migraine
- Cerebellar degeneration
- Multiple sclerosis
- Alcohol intoxication
- Posterior cranial fossa tumours of the brain stem or cerebellum
- Craniovertebral junction disorders: Arnold-Chiari malformations
- Trauma: basal skull fractures; vertebral artery injury
- Syringobulbia
- Temporal lobe epilepsy

Features suggesting central vertigo

- Gradual onset
- New onset headache
- Associated brainstem symptoms: dysarthria, dysphagia, diplopia
- Central neurological signs: gait ataxia; down-beat, vertical or changing-direction nystagmus
- Cranial nerve deficts

Features suggesting peripheral vertigo

- Acute onset
- Severe intensity of symptoms, especially with head movement to one side
- Positional symptoms
- Hearing loss, usually unilateral
- Tinnitus
- Otalgia
- Frequently severe autonomic symptoms
- Unidirectional, horizontal or rotatory jerk nystagmus on lateral gaze opposite side of lesion
- Visual fixation inhibits nystagmus
- Head movement increases symptoms
- Absence of cranial nerve palsies

Examination for balance includes consideration of

- Stance and gait tests
- Romberg sign
- Dix-Hallpike manoeuvre
- Oculomotor examination
- Vestibulo-ocular reflex
- Visual-vestibular interaction
- Dizziness-provoking manoeuvres

Dix-Hallpike manoeuvre (rapid movement from sitting to head hanging position)

- The patient sits upright, facing forwards with eyes open, and with legs extended
- Rotate head 45° to one side
- Lie down backwards rapidly with head extended 20°, hanging over the end of the table
- Hold in this position for 30 s
- The development of torsional nystagmus, with a latency of 5–10 s and with the fast phase directed towards the affected ear (closest to the ground) indicates benign paroxysmal positional vertigo. Nystagmus fades if the head is held in the provoking position
- Sit upright and then repeat with the head rotated 45° towards the other side
- The manoeuvre is contraindicated in the presence of cervical spine instability, prolpased intervertebral disc with radiculopathy, cervical myelopathy, previous cervical spine surgery, or vascular dissection syndromes

Localisation of vestibular lesions

- Inner ear: otalgia; tinnitus; aural fullness; hearing loss

- VIII nerve (internal auditory meatus): poor speech discrimination; facial weakness
- Cerebello-pontine angle: facial weakness; facial sensory loss; dysarthria; incoordination
- Brainstem: hemiparesis; hemi-sensory loss; dysphagia; dysarthria
- Cerebellum: incoordination; dysarthria
- Cortex: olfactory or gustatory hallucinations; vertiginous seizures

Differential diagnosis of dizziness

Near syncope or presyncope (sensation of impending faint or loss of consciousness): postural hypotension; cardiogenic hypotension (cardiac arrhythmia, valvular heart disease); vasovagal attack; carotid sinus hypersensitivity

Dysequilibrium (sensation of impaired balance and gait): multiple sensory deficits (peripheral neuropathy; visual impairment); cerebellar lesions

Vertigo (sensation of rotation of patient or environment, related to a mismatch of the vestibular, visual and somatosensory symptoms)

Light headedness: hyperventilation; hypoglycaemia; panic attack

Characteristics of cardiovascular dizziness

- Dizziness is described as light-headedness
- Associated with syncope, pallor, the need to sit/lie down
- Symptoms occur with prolonged standing

Causes of imbalance or vertigo on looking up

- Benign paroxysmal positional vertigo
- Posterior circulation ischaemia caused by cervical osteophytes leading to vertebral artery compression
- Chiari type 1 syndrome
- Parkinsonism
- Polyneuropathy

Types of nystagmus

Spontaneous, involuntary periodic and rhythmical oscillations of the eyes in which a slow phase alternates with a fast phase in the opposite direction.

Repetitive rapid (saccadic) eye movements, often alternating with a slow drift in the opposite direction; named for the direction of the fast component

Spontaneous

- Pendular (opposing movements of equal speed and amplitude): vertical; horizontal; see saw
- Horizontal
- Torsional (rotary)
- Downbeat (vertical jerk nystagmus with downward fast phase): cranio-cervical junction disorder (Chiari malformation); bilateral lesions of cerebellar flocculus or medial longitudinal fascicle
- Upbeat (vertical jerk nystagmus with upward fast phase): pontine lesions, along ventral tegmental tract; anterior cerebellar vermis (vestibulocerebellum)
- Periodic alternating: horizontal jerk nystagmus in which direction of fast phase changes spontaneously and cyclically with an intervening neutral period
- See saw: vertical-torsional oscillation of both eyes in which one eye rises and intorts and the other falls and extorts; rostral midbrain including midbrain-thalamic junction
- Dissociated (horizontal nystagmus that is greater in the abducting than inthe adducting eye)
- Medial longitudinal fasciculus lesion (inter-nuclear ophthalmoplegia)

Gaze-evoked (identified with patient fixating with both eyes)

- Gaze-evoked nystagmus: horizontal; vertical
- Optokinetic
- Endpoint: extreme lateral gaze

Clinical categorization of nystagmus
- Monocular
- Binocular asymmetrical or dissociative
- Binocular symmetrical:
  - Dysconjugate: seesaw; horizontal
  - Conjugate: pendular; jerk (fast corrective component)

Check list for evaluation of nystagmus

- Anomalous head posture
- Visual acuity: uniocular; binocular
- Laterality
- Latent/manifest
- Type; direction (horizontal, vertical, rotatory); frequency (fast; slow); amplitude (large, small); plane
- Conjugate (same in both eyes)/ dysconjugate
- Dissociation
- Occurrence in primary position (at rest) or gaze evoked

Causes of facial paralysis
Supranuclear (sparing of frontalis because of bilateral innervation)

- Stroke
- Tumour
- Multiple sclerosis

Infranuclear (unilateral facial weakness, including inability to wrinkle forehead, brow ptosis with inability to raise eyebrow, drooping of the angle of the mouth, asymmetrical smile, upper eyelid retraction, incomplete eyelid closure with risk of exposure keratopathy, lower eyelid atony leading to ectropion, inability to purse lips and to show teeth; aberrant regeneration may lead to gustatory epiphora and facial synkinesiae)

- Geniculate ganglion: Bell's palsy (herpes simplex type 1); Ramsay Hunt syndrome (herpes zoster of geniculate ganglion)-otalgia, vesicles in the external auditory canal, pinna or anterior 2/3rds of the tongue
- Middle ear: cholesteatoma; otitis media
- Parotid salivary gland: infection; tumour
- Lyme disease
- Granulomatous disorders: sarcoidosis
- GuillainBarre syndrome
- Temporal bone: fracture; tumour

The types of presentation of facial paralysis include

- Unilateral lower motor neuron: Bell's palsy
- Bilateral lower motor neuron: myasthenia gravis
- Unilateral upper motor neuron: hemispheric stroke
- Bilateral upper motor neuron: brainstem stroke (pseudobulbar palsy)

Causes of upper airway obstruction

- Trauma: laryngeal stenosis, acute laryngeal injury, airway burn, haemorrhage; retropharyngeal haematoma (associated with Capp's triad of tracheal or oesophagel compression, anterior displacement of the trachea, and subcutaneous bruising over the neck and anterior chest)
- Foreign bodies: teeth; dentures; fish bones
- Infection: retropharyngeal abscess (sore throat, fever, neck stiffness, dysphagia, odynophagia, stridor); peritonsillar abscess, Ludwig's angina (fever, trismus, lower facial and neck cellulitis, stridor, induration of floor of mouth; may complicate dental infection or tongue piercing), epiglottitis (high fever, sore throat, dysphagia, adoption of a position of leaning forward with mouth open, muffled voice, drooling of saliva), laryngitis, viral laryngotracheobronchitis (croup) (barking cough, hoarse voice, intermittent inspiratory stridor, retractions-often worse at night, variable respiratory distress; usually a benign, self-limited disease), diphtheria,bacterial tracheitis
- Vocal cord paralysis

- Tumours: benign and malignant laryngeal tumours; laryngeal papillomatosis
- Iatrogenic: post-intubation or post-tracheostomy sub-glottic stenosis

Features of inhalational burn injury

- Entrapment
- Fire in enclosed space
- Loss of consciousness at scene
- Carbonacous sputum
- Soot around mouth
- Singed nasal hairs
- Facial burns
- Pharyngeal oedema
- Stridor

Stridor

Stridor is a high-pitched, harsh noise, secondary to turbulent flow through a partially obstructed upper airway.

Stertor is a coarse inspiratory noise through a narrowed nose/pharynx.

Causes of stridor

Acute, febrile

- Viral croup (laryngotracheobronchitis)
- Bacterial tracheitis (high fever; no response to treatment for croup)
- Supraglottitis, including epiglottitis
- Retropharyngeal abscess
- Peritonsillar abscess
- Uvulitis
- Diphtheria
- Ludwig's angina

Acute, afebrile

- Foreign body inhalation/aspiration (sudden onset)
- Caustic/thermal injury
- Toxic gas inhalation
- Spasmodic croup
- Angioneuroticoedema
- Anaphylaxis
- Neck trauma: laryngeal fracture

Gradual onset; chronic

- Laryngotracheomalacia
- Vascular anomalies: double aortic arch; vascular sling
- Adeno-tonsillar hypertrophy
- Laryngeal web; diverticula; cyst; haemangioma
- Vocal cord paralysis: bilateral recurrent laryngeal nerve palsy
- Gastro-oesophageal reflux
- Laryngeal/pharyngeal tumours: papilloma
- Bilateral vocal cord paralysis
- Tracheal carcinoma
- Paratracheal compression by lymph nodes
- Crico-arytenoid rheumatoid arthritis
- Post tracheostomy intubation granulomata
- Psychogenic

Westley croup score

- Stridor: none (0); at rest on auscultation (1); at rest without auscultation (2)
- Chest wall retractions: none (0); mild (1); moderate (2); severe (3)
- Air entry: normal (0); decreased (1); severely decreased (2)
- Cyanosis: none (0); with agitation/activity (4); at rest (5)
- Consciousness level: normal (0); altered (5)

Possible score: 0–17

Croup severity: mild (<4); moderate (4–6); severe (>6)

Predictors of difficult airway

History: history of previous difficult intubation; upper airway inflammatory swelling, tumour, trauma; history of snoring/obstructive sleep apnoea.

Examination:

High body mass index

Stridor at rest

- Neck: short, thick (circumference >45 cm); limited flexion/extension: <90° to 165° respectively (immobile); neck extension undesirable: unstable cervical spine fracture; severe cervical stenosis; vertebral artery insufficiency; Chiari malformation

Mouth:
- Limited mouth opening: inter-incisal gap <4 cm in adult (TM joint disease; maxillary-mandibular fixation; severe facial burns)
- Temporomandibular joint range <4 cm (two finger breadths):trismus
- Protruding or receding mandible
- Inability to sublux the jaw (forward protrusion of the lower incisors beyond the upper incisors)
- Protruding maxillary incisors
- Long, high arched palate
- Macroglossia; large base of tongue (obscuring view of uvula and tonsillar pillars)
- Loose, damaged teeth
- Lack of dentitition (edentulous)
- Dental prostheses

Thyromental distance (thyroid cartilage notch to lower border of mentum) <6.5 cm with full head extension

Sternomental distance (upper border of manubrium sterni to tip of chin, with mouth closed and head fully extended) <12.5 cm

Airway masses: tongue, tonsils and larynx tumours; large goitre; mediastinal masses.

Tracheal deviation

Recognisable syndromes with airway abnormalities: Klippel-Feil syndrome; Treacher-Collins syndrome; Pierre-Robin syndrome

Causes of hoarseness of voice

- Laryngitis: viral; fungal (oral steroid inhaler use); senile atrophic
- Muscle tension dysphonia with or without vocal cord nodules: voice overuse or misuse (elevated loudness and pitch)
- Laryngeal papillomatosis
- Vocal cord paralysis
- Laryngeal cancer
- Spasmodic dysphonia

Presentations of tracheostomy emergencies

Acute respiratory distress (due to tube obstruction or dislodgement)

ABCD approach
- Airway: secretions; inability to pass suction catheter
- Breathing: work of breathing; bilateral breath sounds with equal chest rise; SpO_2; $ETCO_2$
- Circulation: heart rate, systolic blood pressure

Mnemonic
- D: dislodgement
- O: obstruction
- P: patient (pneumothorax, pulmonary embolism, pulmonary oedema)
- E: equipment failure

Haemorrhage: tracheo-innominate artery fistula

Causes of sore throat

- Infection

  Viral pharyngitis: herpes, influenza, enterovirus, rhinovirus, adenovirus; Epstein-Barr virus (infectious mononucleosis-palatal petechiae and lymphadenopathy)

Bacterial pharyngitis: Group A beta haemolytic streptococci (fever, tonsillo-pharyngeal exudate, soft palatal petechiae, red and swollen uvula, tender anterior deep cervical lymphadenopathy, scarlatininform rash, absence of cough), haemophilusinfluenzae, staphylococcus, streptococcus pneumonia; diphtheria (white membrane on both tonsils, uvula and soft palate; lymphadenopathy with oedema (bullneck); tracheitis and bronchitis);gonococcal; peritonsillar abscess (quinsy) (fever, sore throat, dysphagia, odynophagia, otalgia, muffled "hot potato" voice, drooling of saliva, halitosis, unilateral tonsillar swelling with medial shift of uvula away from the affected side, mucopurulenttonsillar exudates); retropharyngeal abscess; parapharyngeal abscess; epiglottitis

- Irritants: cigarette smoking or exposure to cigarette smoke; pollutants
- Neoplasm

- Blood dyscrasia
- Pathogens from the genital tract

It is important to recognize and treat Group A streptococcal pharyngitis because of the risk of suppurative (otitis media, sinusitis, peritonsillar and retropharyngeal abscesses) and non-suppurative (acute glomerulonephritis, acute rheumatic fever) complications.

Red flag symptoms with sore throat

Unilateral
Prolonged in smokers or heavy drinkers
Drooling of saliva
Muffled voice
Stridor
Immunosuppressed patient

Features of Lemierre syndrome (post-anginal sepsis)

- Septic thrombophlebitis of internal jugular vein, beginning in the tonsillar vein
- Septic pulmonary emboli and septic emboli to the abdominal viscera, muscles and joints

Causes of vesicular, bullous or ulcerative lesions of the oral mucosa
Infections

- Viral: primary acute herpetic gingivostomatitis; recurrent intraoral herpes; herpangina (Coxsackie A); hand, foot and mouth disease (Coxsackie A16); primary HIV infection
- Bacterial: acute necrotizing ulcerative gingivitis (Vincent's angina); primary syphilis; gonorrhoea
- Fungal: cervico-facial actinomycosis; candidiasis

Dermatological conditions

- Mucous membrane pemphigoid
- Erythema multiforme major (Stevens-Johnson syndrome)
- Pemphigus vulgaris
- Lichen planus

Other

- Acute myeloid leukaemia
- Lymphoma
- Recurrent aphthous ulcer
- Traumatic ulcer: dentures; foreign body
- Squamous cell carcinoma

Causes of epistaxis
Local (anterior), always septal:

- Trauma: nose picking, nasal and other facial fracture, foreign body
- Iatrogenic: nasal surgery, nasogastric tube
- Infection: infective rhinitis
- Vascular: Little's area (anterior)-95%, antero-inferior nasal septum; posterior degeneration (elderly)
- Neoplasm: benign (juvenile nasopharyngeal angiofibroma presents with epistaxis and nasal obstruction, typically in adolescent males); malignant
- Drugs: cocaine
- Allergy: allergic rhinitis
- Congenital: intranasal meningiomas

Systemic:

- Inherited: hereditary haemorrhagic telangiectasia; von Willebrand disease
- Bleeding disorders: thrombocytopenia; coagulopathies; platelet dysfunction
- Drugs: oral anticoagulants
- Neoplastic: leukaemia
- Granulomatous disease: sarcoidosis, Wegener's granulomatosis
- Post-traumatic internal carotid artery pseudoaneurysm
- Hypertension

Features of anterior epistaxis

- Bleeding from one nostril
- Self-limited
- Controlled by pressure (septal compression)

Features of posterior epistaxis (always lateral)

- Profuse bleeding
- Bleeding from both nostrils
- Bleeding site not identified on nasal speculum examination
- Bleeding not controlled with adequate bilateral anterior nasal packing

Causes of ear discharge (otorrhoea)

Purulent

External auditory canal

- Otitis externa
- Foreign body

Middle ear:

- Acute suppurative otitis media with tympanic membrane perforation
- Chronic suppurative otitis media +/− cholesteatoma
- Infected grommets (tympanostomy tubes)
- Mastoiditis

Clear (CSF)

- Temporal bone fracture
- Perilymphatic fistula

Causes of tinnitus

a. Subjective tinnitus

   Outer Ear:impacted wax; foreign body; neoplasm

   Middle ear and mastoid: trauma: fracture of the temporal bone; infection: acute suppurative otitis media; otosclerosis; cholesteatoma; barotrauma

   Cochlea: age-related (presbyacusis); infection, eg purulent meningitis; noise induced damage; ototoxic drugs, eg aminoglycosides; Meniere's disease

   8th nerve: cerebellopontine angle lesions:- acoustic neuroma; basal meningitis:- tuberculosis, sarcoidosis, malignant infiltration

   Brainstem: demyelination: multiple sclerosis; neoplasm; infarction

   Cerebral hemispheres: bilateral temporal lobe lesions, eg infarction, neoplasia

b. Objective tinnitus
   - Vascular, non-pulsatile: venous hum (sigmoid sinus; jugular vein); dehiscent jugular bulb; high-flow states (anaemia, thyrotoxicosis, pregnancy)
   - Pulsatile: vascular tumours of the temporal bone: glomus tympanicum tumour; paraganglioma; endolymph sac tumour; elevated intracranial pressure; carotid-cavernous fistula; carotid artery aneurysm
   - Non-vascular: myoclonus of stapedius, tensor tympani and levatorpalatini muscles; patulous Eustachian tube

Causes of earache (otalgia)

Pinna

- Perichondritis: trauma (burns; ear piercing); inflammatory (relapsing polychondritis); cellulitis

External auditory canal

- Otitis externa (pain on palpation of the tragus or on application of traction to the pinna; erythema and oedema of the external auditory canal, with granulation tissue at the junction of the cartilaginous and osseous portions of the canal; discharge; conductive hearing loss; tinnitus; cellulitis of the face; lymphadenopathy) (otitis externa can be caused by ear canal trauma, contact dermatitis, secondary infection from otitis media via tympanostomy tubes, or ear drainage from perforated tympanic membrane)
- Necrotising or malignant otitis externa (more likely in elderly, diabetic or immunocompromised patients) (severe otalgia and headache, fever, purulent discharge, granulation tissue in posterior and inferior ear canal, cervical lymphadenopathy, trismus, facial nerve paralysis)

- Furunculosis (infected hair follicle)
- Herpes zoster oticus (Ramsay Hunt syndrome)
- Foreign body

Middle or inner ear, temporal bone

- Acute suppurative otitis media (bulging red thickened and immobile tympanic membrane; triad of otalgia, fever and conductive hearing loss)
- Complicated chronic suppurative otitis media; cholesteatoma
- Bullous myringitis (severe ear pain and aural fullness; bullae on lateral surface of tympanic membrane)
- Acute otitic barotrauma: flying
- Neoplasm of ear
- Mastoiditis

Referred pain (non-otological causes)

- Pharynx: tonsillo-pharyngitis; post tonsillectomy; pharyngitis; peritonsillar abscess; neoplasm
- Temporomandibular joint: dysfunction; arthritis
- Dental: abscess; caries-lower molar teeth; impacted molar; erupting tooth; periodontal infection
- Oral: aphthous ulcers
- Paranasal sinuses: maxillary sinusitis
- Osteoarthritis of cervical spine; cervical spondylosis
- Malignancy of tonsil, pharynx, larynx, upper oesophagus
- Parotid: parotitis

Risk factors for otitis externa

- Moist ear canal: swimming; ear syringing
- Generalised skin conditions: seborrhoeic dermatitis; eczema
- Ear canal obstruction: impacted wax; canal stenosis or exostosis; foreign body; sebaceous cyst
- Ear canal trauma: cotton buds; finger nails; ear plugs

Causes of dental pain

- Pulpitis related to dental caries
- Dentoalveolar abscess (peri-apical)
- Periodontal abscess
- Pericoronitis
- Osteomyelitis of the jaw

Causes of painful mouth

Idiopathic:

Recurrent aphthous ulcers: painful round ulcers with red margins

Infections:

Candidiasis
Dental sepsis
Herpes simplex gingivostomatitis: multiple grouped lesions
Herpangina
Hand-foot and mouth disease: painless round erosions with red margins
Vincent's angina (acute necrotising ulcerative gingivitis) (painful bleeding gums, ulceration of inter-dental papillae with necrotic slough, halitosis, metallic taste in the mouth; associated with poor dental hygiene and immunosuppression)
Infectious mononucleosis

Trauma due to:

Teeth
Dentures

Carcinoma
Associated with systemic disorder:

- Drug allergy
- Deficiency of vitamin B12/folate
- Acute leukaemia
- Leukopenia
- Inflammatory bowel disease
- Reiter's syndrome
- Behcet's disease

Associated with skin disorder:

- Lichen planus
- Erythema multiforme
- Pemphigoid
- Pemphigus vulgaris

Causes of recurrent oro-genital ulceration

- Behcet's disease
- Reiter's syndrome
- Inflammatory bowel disease
- Cyclical neutropenia
- Bullous skin disorders
- Fixed drug reactions
- Erythema multiforme
- Sweet' s syndrome

Causes of acute facial swelling with inflammation

- Bacterial infections: cellulitis; erysipelas
- Viral infections: herpes zoster
- Paranasal sinusitis
- Odontogenic infections: dental abscess
- Parotid salivary gland infection
- Orbital infection
- Lymphadenitis
- Lupus erythematosus

Causes of facial pain

- **Local**:
  Teeth: impacted wisdom teeth; dental abscess
  Paranasal sinusitis
  Temporomandibular joint disorder
  Vascular: giant cell arteritis
  Nasopharynx: tumour (Trotter's triad of facial or ear pain, conductive deafness and palatal paralysis)
  Salivary gland disorder: infection; inflammation due to duct obstruction; tumour; granuloma
  Eye: glaucoma; uveitis; optic neuritis

- **Lesions between cavernous sinus and pons**:
  Root: cerebellopontine angle tumour
  Basal meninges: granuloma; tumour
  Ganglion: herpes zoster; middle fossa fracture

- **Central**:
  Thalamic infarct
  Brainstem glioma
  Posterior inferior cerebellar artery thrombosis
  Syringomyelia/syringobulbia
  Tabesdorsalis

- **Facial neuralgias**:
  Trigeminal neuralgia (paroxysms of brief lightning-like spasms which are either spontaneous or precipitated by cutaneous or auditory stimuli; trigger points may reproduce pain; no objective sensory or motor deficit)
  Post-herpetic neuralgia (herpes zoster)
  Migrainous neuralgia (cluster headache)
  Atypical facial pain

Facial injuries checklist

- Airway
  Blood in airway: oropharyngeal/nasal bleeding
  Airway oedema
  Tongue base retro-displacement with symphyseal or bilateral angle of mandible fracture
  Maxillary and mandibular fractures causing distortion of airway
  Displaced tooth fragments
- Cervical spine
- Upper third of face:
  Contusion, laceration, depression of forehead
  Crepitus; subcutaneous emphysema
  Disruption of supraorbital rims
  CSF in wound, CSF rhinorrhoea
  Forehead numbness
- Middle third of face:
  Peri-orbital swelling/crepitus
  Occlusion
  Visual acuity
  Eye movements; diplopia
  Ocular injury: subconjunctival haemorrhage
  Malposition of the globe
  Nasal deformity (comparison with pre-injury photos, eg driver's licence); crepitus; septalhaematoma; epistaxis; CSF rhinorrhoea

Cheek deformity
Numbness in infraorbital nerve distribution: lateral side of nose, upper lip and maxillary gingiva on affected side
Trismus

- Lower third of face:
  Occlusion
  Step deformity
  Open bite deformity
  Trismus
  Intra-oral laceration
  Sublingual haematoma
  Numbness in inferior alveolar nerve distribution: half of lower lip, chin, teeth and gingiva
  In the presence of a chin laceration or abrasion following a fall, bilateral condylar neck fractures are possible, associated with anterior open bite
  Unilateral condylar neck fractures are associated with deviation of the chin, an open bite on the uninvolved side, temporomandibular joint tenderness, and laceration of the external auditory canal with or without haemotympanum

Signs of facial injury on plain x-ray
Direct signs

- Linear radiolucent shadows
- Cortical defect
- Double density caused by overlapping bone fragments

Indirect signs

- Paranasal sinus opacification by fluid
- Air in soft tissues: orbital emphysema
- Soft tissue swelling

Features of naso-ethmoidal fracture

- Nasal deformity with widening of root of nose
- Bilateral periorbital ecchymosis
- Telecanthus: widening of inter-canthal distance between medial canthi (normal:30–31 mm)
- CSF rhinorrhoea
- Epiphora
- Epistaxis
- Anosmia

Features of orbital floor blow-out fracture

- Periorbital swelling
- Vertical gaze diplopia, with limited upward gaze
- Infraorbital nerve territory numbness
- Epistaxis
- On xray: orbital emphysema; fluid level within ipsilateral maxillary antrum; hanging drop appearance caused by prolapsed orbital contents
- Occasionally, the fracture may involve the medial orbital wall, with periorbital swelling, subcutaneous emphysema, lateral gaze diplopia due to medial rectus entrapment, and epistaxis/CSF rhinorhoea

Features of zygomatic arch fracture

Flattening of the lateral cheek, which is rapidly obscured by swelling
Trismus, due to impingement of the zygomatic arch fragment on the coronoid process of the mandible)
The zygomatic arch has an elephant's trunk appearance on x-ray

Features of zygomaticomaxillary complex fractures

- Involve the zygomatic arch, inferior oribital rim and lateral wall of the
- maxillary antrum
- Subconjunctival and periorbitalhaemorrhage
- Ipsilateral epistaxis
- Bruising in the buccal sulcus
- Trismus
- Infraorbital numbness

Features of Le Fort fracture

- Le Fort I fracture: mild swelling of the upper lip; mobile maxillary alveolar segment; ecchymoses in the labial or buccal vestibule; floating palate, displaced posteriorly; cracked pot sound on percussion of the maxillary teeth
- Le Fort II (pyramidal) fracture: marked swelling of the middle 1/3 of the face; bilateral periorbital bruising and subconjunctivalhaemorrhage; lengthened face with a dish-face deformity; epistaxis/CSF rhinorrhoea; diplopia; step deformities at the infraorbital rims and fronto-nasal junction; depressed nose; infraorbital numbness; mid-facial mobility; anterior open bite
- Le Fort III fracture: massive facial swelling (panda face); bilateral periorbital bruising and subconjunctival haemorrhage; epistaxis/CSF rhinorrhoea; dished in or concave face with depressed nose; limited ocular movement, diplopia; dystopia (hooding of eyes); mastoid processs ecchymosis (Battle's sign); anterior open bite

Causes of trismus (inability to open the mouth)
Intra-articular

- Tempormandibular arthritis; ankylosis; displacement of anterior disc

Extra-articular

- Masticatory space infection
  Odontogenic: pulpitis; periodontal infection; pericoronitis (impacted third mandibular molar)
  Non-odontogenic: peritonsillar abscess; parotid abscess; malignant otitis externa; retropharyngeal abscess; Ludwig's angina
- Massseter muscle spasm: tetanus
- Drugs: phenothiazines; metoclopramide
- Post-dental treatment: extraction of mandibular molar; mandibular block

Features of temporo-mandibular joint pain

- Pre-auricular pain
- Painful click/crepitus with mouth opening
- Limited mouth opening
- Deviated or painful jaw movements

Features of temporo-mandibular dislocation

- The head of the condyle is displaced from the glenoid fossa in the squamous temporal bone
- Anterior dislocation is usual, with the condyle displaced anterior to the articular eminence of the temporal bone; posterior dislocation involves displacement of the condyle posteriorly towards the mastoid
- Severe pre-auricular pain
- Visible and palpable pre-auricular depression
- Asymmetrical deviation of the chin, if unilateral, or protrusion of the chin, if bilateral
- Inability to occlude teeth

Features of penetrating neck trauma
Signs of laryngeal/cervical tracheal injury

- Dyspnoea
- Altered voice; hoarseness
- Haemoptysis
- Stridor
- Tracheal deviation
- Air bubbling through wound
- Subcutaneous emphysema

Signs of pharyngeal/oesophageal injury

- Dysphagia
- Drooling of saliva
- Blood in saliva
- Sucking neck wound
- Bleeding from mouth or in naso-gastric tube aspirate

Signs of carotid artery injury

- Active external pulsatile bleeding
- Expanding haematoma
- Refractory hypovolaemic shock
- Audible bruit
- Neurological signs

Gynaecological Emergencies 8

Secondary dysmenorrhea is associated with underlying pelvic pathology and can lead to ED attendance.

Causes of secondary dysmenorrhoea
Lower genital tract:
Painful cryptomenorrhoea:

- Imperforate hymen
- Transverse vaginal septum
- Congenital absence of cervix

Acquired cervical stenosis
Uterus:

- Congenital uterine abnormalities: non-communicating horn
- Adenomyosis
- Pedunculatedsubmucous fibroid
- Endometrial polp
- Intrauterine adhesions
- Intrauterine device use

Pelvis:

- Endometriosis (may be associated with dysmenorrhoea, dyschezia, chronic pelvic pain, infertility, haematuria, and rectal bleeding)
- Chronic pelvic inflammatory disease
- Pelvic adhesions

Key historical features in secondary dysmenorrhoea

- Typically, the onset is after several years of painless periods
- The pain may not respond to non-steroidal anti-inflammatory agents or oral contraception
- Gynaecological symptoms: dyspareunia; abnormal vaginal discharge; menorrhagia; inter-menstrual or post-coital bleeding
- Gastrointestinal symptoms: rectal pain and bleeding (endometriosis)

Causes of abnormal vaginal bleeding
Abnormal menstrual bleeding:

- Excessive
- Reduced
- Inappropriate (by age)

Non-menstrual bleeding:

- Post-coital
- Intermenstrual
- Postmenopausal

Categories of excessive vaginal bleeding

- Menorrhagia: excessive menses (>80 ml monthly menstrual loss, ie >90th centile

A. Banerjee, *Emergency Clinical Diagnosis*, DOI 10.1007/978-3-319-50718-7_8

for menstrual blood loss) but normal cycle (>7 days with one or more days of excessive loss)
- Short cycle (<21/7) but normal menses (polymenorrhoea)
- Short cycle + excess bleeding (polymenorrhagia)
- Excessive menses at long intervals
- Metrorrhagia: irregular intervals with excessive menses

Causes of abnormal genital tract bleeding in the reproductive age group
Pregnancy –related
Early pregnancy

- Implantation bleeding
- Pregnancy failure: miscarriage (haemodynamic status; state of internal os; products of conception)
- Ectopic pregnancy
- Gestational trophoblastic disease (molar pregnancy)

Later pregnancy (antepartum haemorrhage-from 24 weeks of pregnancy)

- Placenta praevia: painless bleeding; soft, non-tender uterus; high presenting part or malpresentation
- Placental abruption: severe abdominal or back pain; uterine contractions may be present; uterine tenderness
- Vasa praevia
- Uterine inversion
- Retained placenta
- Endometritis

Non-pregnancy-related

Dysfunctional uterine bleeding: anovulatory bleeding; corpus luteum dysfunction. Structural abnormalities

- Genital tract neoplasia: cervix; endometrium; vulva; vagina; Fallopian tube
- Polyps: cervix; endometrium

Infection:

- Endometritis
- Atrophic endometritis (post-menopausal)
- Cervicitis

Endocrine dysfunction:

- Hypothalamus/pituitary
- Adrenal
- Thyroid

Foreign bodies
Iatrogenic:

- Intrauterine devices
- Hormonal treatment

Blood dyscrasias:

- Platelet disorders:idiopathic thrombocytopenic purpura
- Clotting factor abnormalities: von Willebrand disease

Symptoms accompanying menorrhagia that indicate significant pathology

- Malignancy: persistent inter-menstrual or post-coital bleeding; unexplained vulval lump or vulval bleeding due to ulceration
- Other structural disease: pelvic pain; pressure symptoms

Causes of premenarcheal genital tract bleeding

- Trauma
- Lower genital tract neoplasm: cervix; vagina
- Foreign body
- Exogenous oestrogen
- Sporadic gonadotrophin surge
- Precocious puberty or pseudopuberty
- Gastrointestinal bleeding
- Urinary tract bleeding

Causes of menorrhagia

- Dysfunctional uterine bleeding (60%)
- Other gynaecological causes (35%)
  Uterine/ovarian tumours
  Endometrial hyperplasis
  Endometriosis
  Pelvic inflammatory disease
  Intrauterine contraceptive device
- Endocrine and haematological causes (<5%)
  Thyroid disease: hypothyroidism; hyperthyroidism
  Platelet problems: thrombocytopenia
  Clotting abnormalities: haemophilia; von Willebrand disease; anticoagulation
  Polycystic ovaries syndrome
  Excesssive exogenous oestrogen use
  Hyperprolactinemia

Causes of postmenopausal bleeding

- Neoplastic: cervical carcinoma; endometrial carcinoma; uterine sarcoma; cancer of the vagina/vulva/fallopian tube; oestrogen-secreting ovarian tumour; secondary deposits; endocervical polyps; endometrial polyps
- Atrophy: oestrogen-deficient atrophic vaginitis; urethral caruncle
- Infection: vaginitis; endometritis
- Iatrogenic: bleeding on hormone replacement therapy; bleeding on tamoxifen; ring pessary
- Miscellaneous:trauma during sexual intercourse (associated with atrophy)
- Spurious: haematuria; rectal bleeding

Causes of acute pelvic pain
Genital tract:

- Pregnancy related: miscarriage (threatened, incomplete); ectopic pregnancy; incarceration of uterus
- Ovarian: cyst (follicular; corpus luteum) accident- rupture/torsion(sudden onset colicky pain radiating from groin to flank-reverse renal colic); mittelschmerz (ovulation pain); bleeding corpus luteum; ovarian hyperstimulation syndrome (complicates assisted reproduction therapy, especially exogenous gonadotrophin therapy during the luteal phase, and may be associated with ascites, oliguria or anuria, and pleural effusion;this results from increased capillary permeability causing fluid shifts from the intravascular space to third space compartments)
- Fallopian tubes: torsion
- Uterine: degeneration of fibroid, tumour, pyometra; torsion of pendunculated fibroid
- Acute infection: pelvic inflammatory disease (triad of pelvic pain, cervical motion and adnexal tenderness and fever)-upper genital tract infection involving endometrium (endometritis), Fallopian tubes (salpingitis); tubo-ovarian abscess (pelvic mass on bimanual examination) and pelvic peritoneum (peritonitis)
- Endometriosis

Non-genital:

- Gastrointestinal: acute appendicitis, Meckel's diverticulum, inflammatory bowel disease, bowel perforation, bowel obstruction, strangulated hernia
- Metabolic: porphyria, sickle cell crisis
- Urinary tract: acute infection, calculus
- Vascular: aortic aneurysm
- Abdominal wall: rectus sheath haematoma; herpes zoster

Risk factors for ovarian torsion

- History of ovarian cysts
- Pregnancy
- Ovarian hyperstimulation syndrome
- History of pelvic inflammatory disease
- Tubal ligation

Features suggestive of ovarian cancer

- Persistent and progressive pelvic and/or abdominal pain

- Increasing abdominal girth; bloating
- Anorexia; fatigue; weight loss
- Altered bowel habit
- Back pain
- Pelvic or abdominal mass
- Ascites

Risk factors for ovarian cancer

- Advanced age
- Nulliparity
- Endometriosis
- Hormone replacement therapy
- Positive family history of ovarian cancer
- Previous benign ovarian cyst
- Pelvic radiotherapy for cervical cancer

Causes of pelvic pain related to menstrual cycle

- Severe dysmenorrhoea
- Cervical pain due to blood clots
- Prolapsed intraluminal fibroid polyp
- Ruptured corpus luteum cyst
- Ovarian hyperstimulation syndrome
- Mittelschmerz (mid-cycle pain)

Causes of vulval pain

- Infections:infected Bartholin cyst (unilateral lower labial pain and swelling); infected sebaceous cyst; acute herpes simplex vulvovaginitis; infected eczema
- Trauma: accidental; sexual; surgical; gynaecological
- Dermatological causes: erosive lichen planus; epidermolysisbullosa; lichen planus; Behcet disease

Causes of acute abdomen in pregnancy
Pregnancy-related pain
1st trimester

- Pregnancy loss: inevitable or incomplete miscarriage
- Ectopic pregnancy
- Ovarian cyst accidents: haemorrhage into or rupture of corpus luteum or follicular cyst
- Incarceration of a retroverted uterus

2nd trimester

- Late miscarriage
- Uterine fibroids: red degeneration

3rd trimester

- Placental abruption
- Uterine rupture
- Fulminant pre-eclampsia with subcapsular hepatic haemorrhage

Incidental (non-pregnancy-related)

- Acute appendicitis
- Acute cholecystitis; biliary colic
- Intestinal obstruction
- Renal: acute pyelonephritis; renal calculi
- Malignancy

Causes of sudden cardiovascular collapse in pregnancy

- Amniotic fluid embolism
- Pulmonary thrombo-embolism
- Venous air embolism
- Occult haemorrhage: placental abruption; hepatic rupture (fulminating pre-eclampsia; HELLP)
- Intracerebralhaemorrhage
- Drug toxicity, including local anaesthetics
- Sepsis
- Myocardial infarction

Ectopic pregnancy
Risk factors

- Previous history of ectopic pregnancy, spontaneous miscarriage or induced abortion
- Fallopian tube damage
  - Pelvic inflammatory disease, especially Chlamydial

Previous surgery on Fallopian tubes, including tubal surgery
Previous pelvic surgery (eg Caesarean section, ovarian cystectomy) or abdominal surgery (appendicectomy; bowel surgery) leading to pelvic adhesions
- Infertility
  Documented tubal disease
  Endometriosis
  In vitro fertilisation (assisted reproductive technology)
- Contraception failure
  Intrauterine contraceptive device in situ
  Progestogen-only oral contraceptive
- Maternal age >35 years

Typical presentation of ectopic pregnancy

- Amenorrhoea or abnormal menses, followed by slight vaginal bleeding
- Unilateral pelvic pain
- Pain radiating to the shoulder tip

Atypical presentations of ectopic pregnancy

- Diarrhoea and vomiting
- Dizziness, presyncope or syncope
- Right upper quadrant pain

Signs of ectopic pregnancy

- Tenderness: abdominal, pelvic; adnexal; cervical motion; rebound
- Postural hypotension
- Shock

Causes of vaginal discharge

Physiological (cervical mucus, vaginal transudate, bacteria, squamous epithelial cells) (leucorrhoea)

- Cyclical alteration in cervical mucus: ovulation
- Pregnancy

Pathological:

Sexually Transmitted infections of lower (vaginitis and cervicitis) and upper genital tract

- Chlamydia trachomatis
  Neisseria gonorrhoeae
  Trichomonasvaginalis
  Herpes simplex virus

Non-sexually transmitted genital tract infections

- Vulvovaginal candidiasis
- Bacterial vaginosis (3 out of 4: homogeneous milky or creamy vaginal discharge; fishy or amine odour; pH of secretions >4.5; and true clue cells on microscopic examination)

Non-infective

- Foreign body: retained tampon, condom
- Cervical polyps and ectopy
- Genital tract malignancy
- Fistulae
- Allergic reactions
- Vaginitis from vaginal sprays and soaps
- Extragenital causes

Associated symptoms with vaginal discharge

- Itching
- Superficial dyspareunia
- Vulval/vaginal pain
- Dysuria
- Abnormal vaginal bleeding (heavy, intermenstrual, post-coital)
- Deep dyspareunia
- Pelvic pain
- Fever

Risk factors for pelvic inflammatory disease

- Young age at first intercourse
- Multiple sexual partners
- Low socio-economic status
- Failure to use barrier methods of contraception
- Vaginal douching

Causes of genital ulceration

Sexually transmitted infections

- Genital herpes: primary/recurrent herpes simplex: grouped vesicles which rupture to form superficial shallow polycyclic and painful erosions with an erythematous base; with primary infections, lymphadenopathy and systemic symptoms may coexist
- Primary syphilis: single painless papule evolving to a chancre, an ulcer with regular indurated edges; mild, firm, non-tender and non-fluctuant inguinal lymphadenopathy
- Chancroid: multiple painful serpiginous friable ulcers, with contact bleeding; purulent exudates; tender, unilateral suppurative inguinal lymphadenopathy with erythema and oedema of the overlying skin
- Lymphogranulomavenereum: small shallow painless genital papule or ulcer, without induration; unilateral tender inguinal/femoral lymphadenopathy
- Granuloma inguinale: single or multiple painless beefy red (highly vascular) papules or ulcers, with contact bleeding; no lymphadenopathy; may have subcutaneous granulomas

Sexual trauma

- Malignancy: squamous cell carcinoma, basal cell carcinoma, vulvar intra-epithelial neoplasia, extra-mammary Paget's disease

Bullous dermatoses

- Contact dermatitis; erythema multiforme; toxic epidermal necrolysis; pemphigus; cicatricial pemphigoid

Non-bullous dermatoses

- Aphthous ulcers
- Lichen planus; erosive lichen planus
- Behcet's syndrome: triad of recurrent oral aphthous ulcers, recurrent painful genital ulcers, and uveitis; also skin lesions and multi-system involvement may be present
- Pyoderma gangrenosum: recurrent painful ulcers with undermined and violaceous or bluish borders, and mucopurulent or haemorrhagic exudate
- Fixed drug eruption
- Lupus erythematosus
- Crohn's disease
- Vasculitis

Causes of pruritus vulvae

- Vaginitis/infection: vulvo-vaginal candidiasis; Trichomonasvaginalis; bacterial vaginosis; herpes simplex infection; scabies; pediculosis pubis; human papillomavirus; molluscum contagiosum
- Vulvar dermatitis: contact dermatitis; lichen simplex; lichen planus; hidradenitis suppurativa; psoriasis; seborrhoeic dermatitis
- Other: vulvar intra-epithelial neoplasia; mechanical trauma

9 Neurological and Psychiatric Emergencies

Stroke

Stroke is a clinical diagnosis, associated with an acute presentation of ongoing focal neurological deficit that cannot be explained by hypoglycaemia or other stroke mimics and which is related to a vascular cause.

Causes of acute stroke

- Ischaemic stroke (85%)
  Thrombotic
    Large artery atherosclerosis: extracranial (carotid, vertebral, aortic arch); intracranial
    Small artery(lacunar): intracranial
    Sinovenous

  Embolic
    Cardiogenic: Cardio-embolism is the commonest cause of ischaemicstroke amongst the elderly.
    Paradoxical (peripheral source with inter-atrial defect-patent foramen ovale): cryptogenic stroke

  Haemodynamic
    Hypotensive(e.g., watershed-type infarcts-at frontal-parietal border, gyrus angularis, putamen and insula)
    Mechanical obstruction
    Vascular dissection
    Haematological
      Polycythaemia
      Thrombocytosis
      Hyperviscosity syndromes
      Hypercoagulable states

- Haemorrhagic stroke (15%)
  Intracerebral haemorrhage
    hypertension
    trauma
    bleeding disorders: leukaemia; thrombocytopenia
    bleeding from an arterio-venous malformation
    berry (saccular) aneurysm rupture
    rupture of mycotic aneurysm
    anticoagulant therapy
    haemorrhagic metastases
    bleeding into a primary brain neoplasm
    haemorrhagic infarction
    amyloid angiopathy
    recreational drug ingestion, e.g. cocaine, amphetamine-like compounds
    haemorrhagic leukoencephalopathy
  Subarachnoid haemorrhage
    Aneurysmal rupture
    Arteriovenous malformation

A. Banerjee, *Emergency Clinical Diagnosis*, DOI 10.1007/978-3-319-50718-7_9

Clinical findings suggesting cardio-embolic stroke

- Abrupt onset of symptoms
- Previous infarctions in various arterial sites (anterior and posterior circulation), especially if separated by time
- Other signs of systemic thromboembolism: splenic or renal infarcts; peripheral limb ischaemia

Causes of acute stroke in childhood

- Vascular
  Vasculitis: systemic lupus erythematosus, Kawasaki's disease, haemolytic uremic syndrome
  Trauma: Neck trauma with vertebral artery injury; intra-oral trauma with carotid artery injury
  Malformations: arteriovenous malformations, aneurysms, moya moya
  Arterial dissection (spontaneous or traumatic)
  Tumours
- Infections: meningitis; encephalitis; cerebral abscess; mycotic aneurysms (septic emboli)
- ENT infections: mastoiditis, otitis media, tonsillar or retropharyngeal abscesses, sinusitis leading to venous sinus thrombosis
- Haematological:sickle cell disease; vitamin K deficiency; coagulopathies, e.g. haemophilia; thrombophilias: deficiency of protein C, protein S, antithrombin III; polycythaemia; acute myeloid leukaemia
- Embolic: cardio-embolic: chronic cyanotic congenital heart disease (right to left shunts), paradoxical emboli (patent foramen ovale); valvular heart disease, including endocarditis; atrial tumours; arrhythmias; cardiomyopathy
  Fat emboli
- Drugs: cocaine; amphetamines; oral contraceptive pill; ergot toxicity
- Metabolic: homocystinuria; Fabry's disease; mitochondrial encephalopathies (MELAS syndrome); organic acidurias; hyperlipidaemias
- Neurocutaneous syndromes: neurofibromatosis; tuberous sclerosis; Sturge-Weber syndrome

Anatomical classification of stroke
Anterior circulation

- Large vessels: internal carotid artery and its main branches-MCA and ACA; complete MCA occlusion; occlusion of lenticulo-striate branches of MCA; posterior MCA occlusion; anterior MCA occlusion; ACA occlusion
- Small vessels: branches from the MCA and ACA

Posterior circulation

- Large vessels: vertebral arteries, which join to form the basilar artery and its main branches, the posterior cerebral arteries: basilar artery occlusion (massive brain stem infarction; locked-in syndrome; Anton's syndrome)
- Small vessels: branches from all these vessels; e.g. lateral medullary syndrome (posterior inferior cerebellar artery); penetrating branches of basilar artery: pontine lacunar infarction syndrome; circumferential branches of basilar artery: midbrain infarction

Lacunar (small, deep micro-infarcts): occlusion of deep perforating arteries, which arise from both the anterior and posterior circulation, and supply the white matter of the cerebral hemispheres and brainstem.

Subclavian steal syndrome

Border zone infarcts

Lacunar infarcts: small, deep cerebral infarcts in arterial territories of lenticulostriate and thalamoperforating arteries, paramedial branches of the basilar artery and branches of the anterior choroidal artery.

- Pure motor hemiparesis (internal capsule, pons, cerebral peduncle): contralateral hemiparesis; isolated limb paresis

- Pure hemi-anaesthesia, involving face, arm and leg (sensory stroke) ; dysaesthetic symptoms have also been reported in the thalamic pain syndrome of Dejerine-Roussy (thalamus)
- Ataxic hemiparesis (ipsilateral motor hemiparesis with cerebellar ataxia) (pons, internal capsule)
- Dysarthria/clumsy hand syndrome (pons, internal capsule): dysarthria, dysphagia, contralateral facial and tongue weakness, contralateral arm and hand weakness
- Sensorimotor stroke (thalamus): contralateral hemiparesis, hemisensory loss

Definitions:

- Maximum deficit from a single vascular event
- No visual field deficit
- No new disturbance of higher cerebral function
- No signs of brainstem disturbance

FAST recognition of anterior circulation stroke

- Face: does one side of the face droop? ; ask the person to smile
- Arms: is one arm weak or numb? ; ask the person to raise both arms;does one arm drift downwards?
- Speech: is speech slurred? ask the person to repeat a simple sentence; is the sentence repeated correctly?
- Time: if the person shows any of these symptoms, call 999 or 911

ROSIER scale for emergency stroke recognition

- Loss of consciousness or syncope: −1
- Seizure activity: −1
- New acute onset (or on awakening from sleep)
  Asymmetrical facial weakness: 1
  Arm weakness: 1
  Leg weakness: 1
  Speech disturbance: 1
  Visual field defect 1

Range: −2 to + 5

Features of anterior cerebral artery lesions
Hemispheric

- Either: contralateral hemiparesis, lower limb > upper limb, face; contralateral grasp reflex with paratonic rigidity (gegenhalten)
- Both: urinary incontinence; akinetic mutism; paraplegia; anarthria; apraxia of gait; corpus callosum infarction causing interhemispheric disconnection syndromes (split brain syndrome)-anterior (akinetic mutism), posterior (alexia without agraphia) or complete (visual disconnection); frontal release signs (glabellar, snout, sucking, rooting, grasping and palmomental reflexes)

Medial lenticulostriates

- Either: facial weakness
- Left: dysarthria ± motor aphasia

Features of middle cerebral artery lesions
Hemispheric

- Either: contralateral hemiparesis, face + upper limb > lower limb weakness; contralateral hemi-sensory loss; contralateral homonymous hemianopia
- Left (dominant):motor aphasia (anterior); receptive aphasia (posterior); global aphasia (total MCA)
- Right (non-dominant): visuo-spatial dysfunction; hemi-spatial neglect, anosognosia, constructional apraxia

Lateral lenticulostriates

- Either: variable lacunar syndromes

Features of posterior cerebral artery lesions
Hemispheric

- Either: contralateral hemianopia: homonymous hemianopia; homonymous hemianopia with central or macular sparing (due to overlap of posterior and middle cerebral arteries at the occipital pole); superior quadrantic homonymous hemianopia (lingual gyrus); inferior quadrantic homonymous hemianopia; visual neglect
- Both: cortical blindness –visual agnosia (preserved optokinetic nystagmus); memory deficits
- Dominant: alexia without agraphia; Gerstmann syndrome (acalculia, agraphia, finger agnosia, right-left disorientation)
- Non-dominant: prosopagnosia (difficulty in recognizing familiar faces)

Thalamo-perforators

- Either: hypersomnolence; sensory disturbances (hemisensory loss)

Possible levels of lesion causing hemiparesis

- Cortex: cortical dysfunction
- Corona radiata
- Internal capsule
- Brain stem
  Midbrain: ipsilateral III nerve palsy (Weber)
  Pons: ipsilateral VI ± VII palsy (Millard-Gubler)
  Medulla: descending spinal tract and nucleus of V nerve

Features of posterior circulation stroke

The 5Ds are dizziness, diplopia, dysarthria, dysphagia and dystaxia (disequilibrium), in varying combinations, with usually at least two being present simultaneously.

Crossed syndromes of ipsilateral cranial nerve palsy (facial involvement) and contralateral motor and/or sensory tract dysfunction (long tract signs) are highly characteristic of posterior circulation stroke, being indicative of brainstem ischaemia.

Medulla Oblongata

- Lateral medullary syndrome (Wallenberg): ipsilateral nystagmus, Horner syndrome (descending sympathetic tract), loss of pain and temperature sensation in the face (spinal trigeminal nucleus), limb ataxia (inferior cerebellar peduncle), dysarthria, dysphagia, dysphonia (nucleus ambiguuus with vocal cord and palatal paralysis); contralateral loss of pain and temperature sensation in the trunk and limbs (spinothalamic tract) (crossed sensory loss); vertigo
- Medial medullary syndrome (Dejerine): ipsilateral tongue weakness with slurring of speech (XII nerve palsy); contralateral hemiplegia
- Hemi-medullary syndrome (lateral and medial medullary infarction) (Babinski-Nageotte) (Babinski-Nageotte); ipsilateral limb ataxia, facial sensory loss, Horner syndrome; contralateral hemiplegia, hemi-sensory loss; vomiting, vertigo, nystagmus

Pons

- Lateral pontine syndrome (Marie-Foix): contralateral hemiplegia and hemi-sensory loss (loss of pain and temperature); ipsilateral ataxia, VII and VIII nerve palsy
- Inferior medial pontine syndrome (Foville): contralateral hemiplegia and weakness of lower half of face, loss of proprioception and vibration; ipsilateral ataxia (middle cerebellar peduncle) and VI nerve palsy
- Locked-in syndrome (bilateral vertebral artery occlusion): quadriparesis (bilateral pyramidal tract lesions in the pons); loss of speech; alertness, with preserved awareness and cognition; normal sensation; bilateral facial and oropharyngeal palsy; preservation of blinking, eyelid elevation and upward gaze (III nerve intact), allowing for communication
- Ventral pontine syndromes
  Millard-Gubler syndrome: contralateral hemiplegia; ipsilateral VI and UMN VII nerve palsy

Raymond syndrome: contralateral hemiplegia; ipsilateral VI nerve palsy.

Midbrain

- Weber syndrome: ipsilateral III nerve palsy; contralateral hemiplegia
- Benedikt syndrome: ipsilateral III nerve palsy; contralateral hemi-ataxia and chorea
- Claude syndrome: ipsilateral III nerve palsy; contralateral upper and lower limb ataxia and tremor
- Parinaud syndrome (superior colliculus of dorsal midbrain): bilateral vertical upward gaze palsy; convergence-retraction nystagmus; lid retraction

Rostral brainstem

- Top of the basilar syndrome (Anton): hypersomnolence; delirium; memory loss; confusion; mutism; visual hallucinations; eyelid retraction; unawareness or denial of blindness; vertical upward and downward gaze paralysis; skew deviation of eyes

Features of cerebellar infarction

- Early symptoms: headache, dizziness, nausea, vomiting, loss of balance
- Signs: truncal and appendicular ataxia; nystagmus; dysarthria
- Later signs:
  Brain stem compression: VI nerve paresis; complete loss of lateral gaze (compression of VI nucleus and lateral gaze centre); peripheral facial paresis (compression of facial colliculus)
  Acute hydrocephalus

Presentations of carotid artery dissection

- Headache
- Neck and facial pain
- Amaurosis fugax
- Partial ptosis with miosis (Horner's syndrome); acute Horner syndrome with face or neck pain is due to internal carotid artery dissection until proven otherwise
- Neck swelling
- Pulsatile tinnitus
- Hypogeusia
- Focal weakness

Presentations of vertebral artery dissection

Severe occipital headache and posterior neck pain

Lateral medullary syndrome: ipsilateral facial pain and numbness (dysaesthesiae), dysarthria or hoarseness (IX, X), contralateral loss of pain and temperatures sensation in trunk and limbs; ipsilateral loss of taste (nucleus tractus solitarius), hiccups, vertigo, nausea and vomiting, diplopia or oscillopsia, dysphagia (IX, X), disequilibrium, unilateral hearing loss

Medial medullary syndrome: contralateral weakness or paralysis (pyramidal tract); contralateral numbness (medial lemniscus)

Brainstem/cerebellum: limb/truncal ataxia; nystagmus; impaired fine touch and proprioception; contralateral impaired pain and temperature sensation in limbs (spinothalamic tract)

Causes of stroke in pregnancy and puerperium

Cardiac disease

- Paradoxical embolism
- Peri-partum cardiomyopathy

Thrombophilias

- Protein C or S deficiency
- Factor V Leiden mutation

Haematological disorders

- Thrombotic thrombocytopenic purpura
- Disseminated intravascular coagulation

Vascular causes

- Arterial dissection
- Cerebral venous thrombosis

Other causes

- Eclampsia
- Metastatic choriocarcinoma

Stroke mimics
Stroke is a clinical diagnosis. It is important to consider the possibility of stroke mimics, for which the treatment is different. Stroke mimics are more likely to present with positive symptoms (e.g. motor, visual or somato-sensory), while stroke is associated with negative symptoms.

Toxic/metabolic (metabolic encephalopathies):

- Hypoglycaemia: focal neurological signs, often involving the brainstem
- Hyperglycaemia with hyperosmolar state
- Hyponatraemia
- Hepatic encephalopathy

CNS disease

- Space occupying lesion:brain tumours (primary or metastatic)-often associated with haemorrhage into tumour, rapid onset of oedema, or obstructive hydrocephalus, compression of the intracerebral microcirculation resulting in ischaemia, post-ictal weakness associated with a seizure; chronic subdural haematoma; arteriovenous malformation; cerebral abscess
- Seizure: Post-ictal state after unwitnessed or unrecognised stroke (Todd's paralysis-usually hemiparesis; hemi-sensory deficit); partial seizures
- Syncope
- Cerebral vasculitis
- Infection: meningitis; encephalitis; cerebral abscess: rapidly progressive localized intracerebral mass lesion; non-specific signs and symptoms of raised intracranial pressure; focal neurological deficit
- Migraine: complicated migraine (hemiplegic migraine); migraine with aura; aura without headache
- Acute demyelinating disorders: multiple sclerosis (initial diagnosis or acute exacerbation)
- Functional hemiparesis: conversion disorder
- Old stroke with intercurrent illness
- Transient global amnesia
- Reversible cerebral vasoconstriction syndrome; posterior reversible encephalopathy syndrome
- Acute peripheral polyneuropathy (Guillain-Barre syndrome; Miller-Fisher variant)

Stroke mimics should be considered in the presence of:

- Reduced level of consciousness
- Gradual onset of symptoms
- Fever
- Absence of focal signs
- Fluctuating signs

Stroke chameleons represent atypical manifestations of stroke, which may lead to non-recognition:

- Acute dyskinesias, such as hemiballismus
- Acute confusional states (non-dominant anterior circulation strokes involving the temporo-parietal region)
- Abnormal sensations or loss of sensation (parietal cortical and thalamic strokes)
- Cortical blindness, with normal pupillary light reactions and normal optic disks on funduscopy

Transient ischaemic attack mimics (causes of transient neurological symptoms)

These are important to consider and recognize where possible, given that up to 60% of patients attending TIA clinics turn out not to have a transient ischaemic attack

Seizure with or without Todd's paralysis
Migraine aura; complicated migraine; Bickerstaff migraine (bilateral visual disturbance-visual

field deficits, scintillating scotomata), dysarthria, perioral numbness, loss of consciousness
Hypoglycaemia
Space occupying lesions
Acute vestibular syndrome (labyrinthine disorders)
Syncope
Transient global amnesia: temporary loss of anterograde memory loss
Amyloid spells (cerebral amyloid angiopathy): stereotyped transient positive (aura-like spreading paraesthesiae, positive visual phenomena or limb jerking) and negative (TIA-like limb weakness, numbness, dysphasia or visual loss) symptoms
Paroxysmal symptoms due to demyelination: multiple sclerosis
Subclavian steal

Causes of transient ischaemic attack

- Large artery atherosclerosis: carotid stenosis, vertebro-basilar disease, aortic atherosclerosis
- Cardio-aortic embolism: atrial fibrillation, left ventricle thrombus, valvular disease
- Small artery occlusion: intracranial small vessel disease from hypertension, increased age
- Cryptogenic

Features which do not support the diagnosis of transient ischaemic attack (TIA mimics)

- Alteration or transient loss of consciousness (syncope)
- Positive symptoms
- Generalised weakness
- Isolated dizziness/vertigo
- Confusion
- Urine incontinence
- Loss of balance
- Amnesia
- Falls
- Isolated diplopia
- Isolated dysphagia
- Drop attacks
- Sensory symptoms in part of one limb or in the face

Features of transient ischaemic attacks

Seventy-five percent last less than 1 h

Carotid artery territory

- Unilateral hemiparesis
- Unilateral hemi-sensory loss
- Unilateral visual disturbance: homonymous hemianopia; blindness (amaurosis fugax)
- Aphasia; dysphasia

Vertebral artery territory

- Bilateral motor/sensory loss
- Bilateral visual loss
- Ataxia
- Combinations of vertigo, diplopia, dysphagia, dysarthria

Risk stratification for TIA
ABCD2 score

- Age >60: 1
- Blood pressure >140/90 mm Hg: 1
- Clinical features
  Unilateral weakness 2
  Speech deficit 1
- Duration of symptoms
  10–59 min: 1
  >59 min: 2
- Diabetes mellitus: 1

Cardio-embolism
High risk sources

- Mechanical prosthetic valves
- Mitral stenosis with atrial fibrillation
- Atrial fibrillation (other than lone AF)
- Left atrial/atrial appendage thrombus
- Dilated cardiomyopathy
- Akinetic left ventricular segment
- Atrial myxoma
- Infective endocarditis

Medium risk sources

- Mitral valve prolapse
- Mitral annulus calcification

- Mitral stenosis without atrial fibrillation
- Left atrial turbulence
- Atrial septal aneurysm
- Patent foramen ovale
- Atrial flutter
- Lone atrial fibrillation
- Bio-prosthetic cardiac valve
- Non-bacterial thrombotic endocarditis
- Congestive heart failure
- Hypokinetic left ventricular segment
- Myocardial infarction (from 4 weeks to 6 months)

Coma evaluation

Coma refers to a Glasgow Coma Score of 8 or under. ABCDE evaluation comes first

General

Skin: rash; jaundice; track marks
Temperature: fever, hypothermia
Blood pressure
Odour on breath
Cardiovascular: arrhythmia
Abdomen: organomegaly

Neurological assessment

Meningeal signs
Funduscopy: papilloedema; subhyaloid haemorrhages; hypertensive retinopathy; diabetic retinopathy
Tympanic membranes
Brain stem function:
Pupillary reactions: size, symmetry, light reaction
Spontaneous eye movements
Oculocephalic (doll's eye) responses
Oculovestibular (caloric) responses
Corneal responses
Abnormal eye positions: dysconjugate gaze; skew deviation (vertical separation of ocular axes); tonic deviation
Gag responses
Respiratory pattern
Cheyne-Stokes breathing: alternating hyperventilation and apnoea
Central neurogenic hyperventilation: rapid, regular, deep
Apneustic: rapid, with sudden pauses of inspiration, lasting 2–3 s
Ataxic: irregular unpredictable and chaotic
Motor function in limbs
Spontaneous and stimulus-induced movements
Tone; clonus
Deep tendon reflexes; plantar responses

- Posturing: decorticate (bilateral upper limb flexion and lower limb extension); decerebrate (bilateral upper and lower limb extension)

Clinical categorisation of coma

- No focal or meningeal signs: toxic-metabolic encephalopathy (normal pupils (except with opiates); multi-focal myoclonus)
- Meningeal signs; no focal signs: subarachnoid haemorrhage; meningitis; meningoencephalitis
- Focal signs: intracranial haemorrhage, space occupying lesion (tumour; abscess; infarction)

Pupillary signs in coma

- Enlarged and reactive: sympathomimetic intoxication (amphetamines, cocaine)
- Fixed and dilated: anticholinergic intoxication
- Mid-position and unreactive: focal mid-brain dysfunction, related to enlarging supratentorial space-occupying lesion
- Constricted: opioid intoxication
- Unilateral dilated: ipsilateral IIIrd nerve compression caused by uncal herniation

Mnemonic for causes of coma

- A: alcohol; acidosis
- E: epilepsy; electrolyte; encephalopathy; endocrine
- I: insulin
- O: opium; oxygen (hypoxia)
- U: uraemia (metabolic)

- T: trauma; tumour; temperature
- I: infection (CNS or other)
- P: psychiatric; poisoning
- S: shock; space occupying lesion; stroke

Causes of coma

Supra-tentorial structural lesions:

Mass lesion with tentorial herniation; bilateral hemisphere damage; bilateral thalamic lesion (asymmetrical neurological deficits of movement, posturing reflexes, and gaze; dilated fixed pupil; partial or secondarily generalized seizures)

- Subarachnoid haemorrhage
- Extradural haematoma
- Subdural haematoma
- Tumour
- Intracranial haemorrhage
- Infarct
- Abscess
- Venous sinus thrombosis
- Head injury
- Infra-tentorial structural lesions

Brain stem compression (posterior cranial fossa lesion) or primary brain stem disease (basilar artery thrombosis) (early development of quadriparesis; cranial nerve palsies; loss of brain stem reflexes; apnoea)

- Infarct
- Haemorrhage
- Tumour
- Inflammatory lesion

Diffuse (bilateral hemispheric dysfunction) (preserved pupillary light reflexes; nystagmus; myoclonic jerks; tremor; bilateral asterixis; primary generalized seizures)

- Metabolic encephalopathy: hypoglycaemia; hyperglycaemia; hyponatraemia; hypernatraemia; hypercalcaemia; hypocalcaemia
- Hypoxia; hypercapnia
- Acidosis
- Hepatic encephalopathy
- Uraemia
- Adrenocortical failure
- Inborn errors of metabolism: organic acidurias and organic acidaemias,
- Urea cycle defects, mitochondrial and carnitine disorders, fatty acid
- Oxidation defects, leukodystrophies
- Toxic: ethanol; methanol
- Drug overdose: sedative-hypnotics (benzodiazepines); opiates; tricyclic antidepressants
- Epilepsy: non-convulsive status epilepticus (nystagmoid jerks of eyes, myoclonic limb movements, akathisia)
- Environmental: hypothermia; heat stroke; carbon monoxide
- Infections
- Meningitis
- Encephalitis

Features suggestive of metabolic encephalopathy

- Delirium
- Fluctuating level of consciousness
- Motor phenomena: tremor; asterixis; multifocal myoclonus
- Hallucinations
- Impaired remote memory
- Sparing of pupillary reactions
- Normal ocular movements

Differential diagnosis of coma (coma mimics)

- Akinetic mutism
- Locked-in syndrome: alert and awake; unable to communicate except through blinking and vertical eye movements; quadriplegia with all other voluntary movements abolished, including those depending on innervation by lower cranial nerves; due to destructive lesions of the basis pontis interrupting the corticospinal and corticobulbar pathways, with sparing of auditory tracts and ascending sensory tracts
- Persistent vegetative state: loss of cognitive function, retained automatically controlled visceral functions, papillary

reflexes, and reflex postural responses to noxious stimuli
- Generalised muscle paralysis due to neuromuscular blocking drugs or an acute neuromuscular disease
- Catatonia: rigidity, mutism, unresponsiveness to environmental stimuli, eyes open; optokinetic and vestibulo-ocular responses maintained; waxy flexibility, catalepsy, posturing and grimacing
- Abulia: severe apathy

Mimics of brain death (coma with absent brain stem reflexes and apnoea, after exclusion of reversible confounders)

- Severe metabolic disease with potentially reversible coma
- High spinal cord injury
- Peripheral nerve or muscle dysfunction or neuromuscular blockade accounting for unresponsiveness: Guillain Barre syndrome
- Organophosphate/baclofen toxicity
- Profound hypothermia

Features of psychogenic coma

Normal physical examination
Symmetrical reduced tone
Normal symmetrical reflexes
Flexor plantar responses
Nystagmus with ice water calorics

Causes of reduced level of consciousness in children

- Shock (hypovolaemic, distributive-anaphylactic, cardiogenic)
- Sepsis
- Metabolic diseases
- Intracranial infection
- Raised intracranial pressure
- Convulsions; post-ictal
- Intoxication (alcohol), poisoning
- Trauma (blood loss; traumatic pneumothorax; cardiac tamponade)
- Stroke
- Hypertensive encephalopathy
- Acute hydrocephalus

Glasgow Coma Score

Eye opening
4: Spontaneous eye opening
3: Eye opening to verbal command
2: Eye opening to pain
1: None
Best verbal response
5: Orientated
4: Confused conversation
3: Inappropriate words
2: Incomprehensible sounds (moaning, groaning)
1: None
Best motor response
6: Obeys commands
5: Localizes pain (movement localized to painful stimulus)
4: Withdraws from pain
3: Abnormal flexion to pain (decorticate posturing) (upper limb adduction; flexion of arms, wrists and fingers; extension and internal rotation of lower limbs, plantar flexion of ankles)
2: Extension to pain (decerebrate posturing) (upper limb adduction;extension of legs; plantar flexion of ankles)
1: None

Problems with use of the Glasgow Coma Score

- Inter-rater variability
- Confounding factors
  Eye opening: swelling of eyelids (ocular or facial trauma); IIIrd nerve palsy
  Best verbal response: dysphasia/aphasia; sedation; tracheal intubation/tracheostomy; dementia; alcohol or drug intoxication; tongue oedema; fractures of mandible/maxillae; language difficulty; psychiatric disease; mutism
  Best motor response: neuromuscular blockade; spinal cord/brachial plexus injury; splints/immobilization devices

Seizure characteristics

- Paroxysmal episodes
- Abrupt onset
- Self limited
- Stereotyped

- Lateral tongue bite is pathognomic; bites of the tip of the tongue can be associated with syncope
- Post-ictal confusion/sleep

Seizure presentations

- Generalised convulsive movements
- Transient loss of consciousness
- Transient focal motor or sensory attacks
- Facial muscle and eye movements
- Episodic phenomena during sleep
- Prolonged confusional state
- Automatisms
- Psychic experiences
- Aggressive or vocal outbursts

Features of generalized tonic-clonic seizures

- Vocalisation at the onset
- Tonic phase (10–30 s) with apnoea, cyanosis, hypersalivation, urine and faecal incontinence, mydriasis and upward eye deviation
- Clonic phase (30–60 s)
- Typically, last less than 1 min

Features of complex partial seizures

- Formed hallucinations: visual; auditory; gustatory; olfactory
- Dyscognitive experiences: depersonalization; dreamy states: déjà vu; jamais vu
- Affective states: fear, depression, elation
- Automatisms (ictal and post-ictal repetitive non-purposeful behaviour): lip smacking, chewing, repeating words or phrases
- Transient amnesia
- Typically, last less than 3 min

Features of absence seizures

- Brief discontinuation of activity
- Unresponsiveness, unawareness and subsequent lack of recall
- Associated features (with complex absence seizures) include clonic movements (blinking of eyelids, nystagmus, limb jerking), changes in tone (reduced or decreased), subtle automatisms (oral, vocal or gestural), and autonomic features (changes in skin colour, mydriasis, urine incontinence)

Features of occipital lobe seizures

- Visual symptoms: positive (light flashes, colours) or negative (scotomas, field defects) phenomena
- Complex visual phenomena, e.g. hallucinations (relatively uncommon)

Causes of symptomatic (provoked) seizures

- Acute metabolic disturbance: hypoglycaemia; hyperglycaemia; hyperosmolar state; hyponatraemia, hypocalcaemia, hypomagnesaemia
- Acute/subacute neurological disorders: CNS infection; mass lesion/vascular malformation; stroke (cerebral haemorrhage); subarachnoid haemorrhage; HIV encephalopathy; hypertensive encephalopathy
- Medication toxicity
- Alcohol or drug (heroin, cocaine, amphetamine, methadone) overdose or withdrawal
- Head injury
- Hyperthermia; febrile convulsion

Seizure mimics

- Convulsive syncope
- Migraine
- Sleep disorders
- Conversion disorder
- Paroxysmal cardiac arrhythmia
- Breath-holding spells

The **diagnosis of epilepsy** should only be made by a neurologist with training and expertise in epilepsy as misdiagnosis is common.

The International League Against Epilepsy (ILAE) task force for the diagnosis of epilepsy includes:

- At least two unprovoked (or reflex) seizures occurring more than 24 h apart, or

- One unprovoked (or reflex) seizure and capability of further seizures similar to the general recurrence risk after two unprovoked seizures (at least 60% over the next 10 years), or
- The diagnosis of an epilepsy syndrome

International Classification of Epileptic Seizures

Focal (or partial)

- Simple partial (no loss of consciousness)
- Complex partial (with impaired consciousness at the onset, or simple partial onset followed by impaired consciousness)
- Complex partial seizure evolving to generalized tonic-clonic seizure

Generalised (convulsive or non-convulsive with bilateral discharge involving sub-cortical structures): absence, myoclonic, clonic, tonic, tonic-clonic, atonic

Unclassified

Features of generalized genetic epilepsies

- Childhood or teenage onset; onset above the age of 25 years is unusual
- Triggered by sleep deprivation or alcohol
- Early morning tonic-clonic seizures or myoclonic jerks
- Short absence seizures

Features of simple febrile seizure

- Child aged 6 months to 5 years
- Generalised clonic or tonic-clonic seizure, lasting less than 15 min
- No neurological abnormality by examination or by developmental history
- No recurrence within the following 24 h
- Fever and seizure not caused by meningitis, encephalitis, or other brain illness

Features of complex febrile seizures

- Lasts longer than 15 min
- Focal seizure, with or without secondary generalisation
- Todd's paralysis may be present
- Repetitive seizures may occur

Features suggestive of CNS infection causing seizure

- Complex febrile seizure
- Prolonged post-ictal drowsiness, altered consciousness or neurological deficit, lasting longer than 1 h
- Incomplete immunization against Haemophilus influenzae b and Streptococcus pneumoniae
- Previous or current antibiotic treatment
- Physical signs of meningitis or encephalitis (especially in children aged 2 years and above): bulging fontanelle. Photophobia, neck stiffness, focal neurological signs

Causes of seizure clusters (three or more seizures within a 24-h period with a return to baseline between events) and **breakthrough seizures** (seizures that occur despite use of anti-epileptic drugs in a patient who has achieved seizure control)

- Sub-therapeutic drug levels: non-compliance to anti-epileptic drug treatment; drug interactions (new medication interfering with protein binding and metabolism of anti-epileptic drug)
- Infection; fever
- Severe stress
- Sleep deprivation
- Metabolic/hormonal changes
- Alcohol; substance abuse

Causes of intractable epilepsy

Non-epileptic event
Sub-optimal anti-epileptic drug therapy
Poor compliance to anti-epileptic drug therapy
Mis-classification of epilepsy syndrome
Lesional epilepsy
Progressive epilepsy of neurodegenerative disease
New structural CNS disorder

Status epilepticus-precipitating factors

- Abrupt withdrawal of anti-epileptic drugs
- Stroke
- Alcohol withdrawal or intoxication
- Toxicity: recreational drugs: cocaine; prescription drugs: theophylline; environmental exposure: carbon monoxide, lead, organophosphates
- Hypoxia
- Metabolic disorder: electrolytes; hypoglycaemia; uraemia
- Infections:meningo-encephalitis; granuloma
- Pregnancy related eclampsia
- Trauma: head injury; post-intracranial surgery
- Tumours: primary or metastatic brain tumour

Non-convulsive status epilepticus mimics

- Prolonged migraine aura
- Transient global amnesia
- Dissociative disorders
- Accidental overdose
- Meningoencephalitis

Seizure mimics

Convulsive syncope (associated with pallor, sweating, and post-ictal fatigue; there may be a fixed gaze, upward eye deviation, and neck rigidity; the motor phenomena may include focal or multi-focal myoclonic jerks, tonic spasm, focal seizures, or generalized tonic-clonic convulsions)
Complicated migraine
Transient ischaemic attack
Sleep disorders (parasomnias) (narcolepsy-tetrad of excessive daytime sleepiness, hypnagogic hallucinations, sleep paralysis, and cataplexy or sudden loss of lower limb tone)
Paroxysmal movement disorders: acute dystonic reaction
Breath-holding attacks
Cardiac events: arrhythmia; conduction defect
Non-epileptic attacks
Paroxysmal vertigo
Rage attack (episodic dyscontrol syndrome)

Characteristics of non-epileptic seizures

- Last longer than 5 min
- Gradual onset
- Eyes closed during seizure, and eyelid opening is resisted
- Tongue tip bite
- Fluctuating in severity
- Episodes of prolonged motionless collapse or pseudo-sleep
- Ictal and post-ictal crying, screaming and/or vocalization
- Discontinuous, irregular or asynchronous limb movements
- Pelvic thrusting
- Opisthotonus (arching of back)
- Side-to-side head movements
- Episodes can be affected by bystanders (intensified or alleviated)
- Does not occur during sleep
- Preserved awareness in the presence of bilateral motor involvement
- Inappropriate affect or lack of concern (la belle indifference)
- Emotional outbursts may be associated with attacks
- Absence of self injury
- Abrupt ending with rapid recovery
- Short post-ictal period, with recall for period of unresponsiveness
- Unusual triggers
- Recurrent attacks may occur in medical settings (e.g. clinics)
- Treatment resistance to multiple anti-epileptic drugs
- Very high frequency of seizures, including multiple daily attacks

Causes of acute onset of chorea

- Drugs: anti-epileptic drugs; oral contraceptive; L-Dopa, cocaine, amphetamines; neuroleptics
- Infections: HIV encephalopathy, toxoplasmosis, Sydenham's chorea, tuberculoma, cryptococcal granuloma

- Metabolic: hypoglycaemia, hyperglycaemia; hypothyroidism, hyperthyroidism; hypocalcaemia
- Structural basal ganglia and cerebellar lesions: mass lesions
- Vascular: ischaemic stroke; haemorrhagic stroke
- Inflammatory: multiple sclerosis, sarcoidosis
- Autoimmune: SLE; chorea gravidarum

Acute extrapyramidal syndromes

Causes: dopamine receptor blockers-antiemetics, calcium channel blockers, calcium channel antagonists, antipsychotics

Types of syndrome

- Acute dystonias: oculogyric crisis; opisthotonus; trismus; torticollis; laryngospasm with stridor
- Pseudo-Parkinsonism: bradykinesia; rigidity; tremor; postural instability
- Akathisia: pacing; inability to sit still; repetitive motor movements

Categories of spinal cord syndromes

Complete spinal cord lesion: loss of all motor and sensory function below the level of injury

Partial spinal cord lesions

Anterior cord syndrome (bilateral loss of motor function, pain and temperature sensation; preservation of light touch, vibration sense and proprioception)

Brown-Sequard syndrome of functional hemisection of the cord (ipsilateral loss of proprioception, light touch, vibration sense and motor function-with spastic weakness; contralateral loss of pain and temperature sensation)

Central cord syndrome (motor> sensory loss; upper > lower extremity loss and distal> proximal muscle weakness ("man-in-a-barrel syndrome"); bladder dysfunction, usually urinary retention; sacral sparing)

Posterior cord syndrome: loss of touch and temperature; preservation of proprioception, stereognosis, two-point discrimination and graphaesthesia below the lesion; preservation of motor function

Foramen magnum syndrome

Cauda equina compression: reduced bladder and bowel control; reduced perineal sensation (S2, S3)

Conus medullaris compression: areflexic bladder; loss of bowel control; loss of ankle jerks; bilateral extensor plantar responses; saddle anaesthesia (S2-S4)

Causes of central cord syndrome

Trauma (hyperextension); cervical spondylosis
Fracture dislocation
Compressive fracture
Syringomyelia; hydromyelia
Intramedullary spinal cord tumours

Features of spinal cord ischaemia

Anterior spinal artery syndrome

- Rapidly progressive flaccid paraplegia
- Loss of pain and temperature to a sensory level
- Preserved proprioception and vibration sense
- Urinary incontinence

Posterior spinal artery syndrome

- Loss of proprioception and vibration sense
- Loss of pain and temperature at involved segment of cord
- No motor deficit

Causes of acute paraparesis

Intramedullary lesion (dissociated anaesthesia; early bladder involvement; symmetrical involvement)

- Demyelination: MS; ADEM; subacute combined degeneration
- Ischaemia: infarction (trauma; global ischaemia-shock, cardiac arrest, aortic dissection; anterior spinal artery thrombosis; thromboembolism; aortic aneurysm repair; pregnancy; vasculitis); haemorrhages
- Myelitis: viral (immunocompetent: HSV2. VZV, EBV, poliomyelitis; immunocom-

promised: CMV, HTLV1-tropical spastic paraparesis); bacterial (*Listeria monocytogenes*); parasitic (toxoplasmosis, schistosomiasis); para-infectious
- Mass: astrocytoma; ependymoma; syingomyelia; haematomyelia; dermoid; haematoma

Extramedullary intradural lesion

- Neurofibroma
- Meningioma
- Arachnoiditis
- Metastases

Extradural lesions (root pain; spinal tenderness; early pyramidal involvement; asymmetrical involvement)

- Epidural abscess
- Pathological fracture (metastases- breast, lung, prostate)
- Traumatic fracture-dislocation
- Tuberculosis spinal
- Disc lesions: prolapse
- Haematoma: trauma; dural arterio-venous malformation; anticoagulant therapy

Causes of acute transverse myelopathy
Demyelinating:

- Multiple sclerosis
- Devic's demyelinating neuromyelitis optica
- Subacute myelo-optic neuropathy
- Guillain-Barre radiculomyelopathy
- Acute disseminated encephalomyelitis

Virus –related

- Post-infective, post-vaccination myelopathies
- Infections
- AIDS-related

Non-viral infections

- Spirochaetes: syphilis, Lyme disease
- Parasites: schistosomiasis, larva migrans

Autoimmune

- Collagen diseases
- Stings, bites

Drugs

- Heavy metals
- Orthocresyl phosphate
- Intrathecal drugs

Physical agents

- Burns
- Electric shock
- Irradiation

Toxic and deficiency states

- Neurolathyrism
- Nutritional: vitamin B12 deficiency

Causes of acute generalised weakness

- CNS causes:
  Brain stem: bilateral basal brain stem stroke; compression; basal demyelination (central pontine myelinolysis; demyelinating disease: multiple sclerosis, ADEM, neuromyelitis optica)
  Cervical spinal cord: trauma; compression; stroke (anterior spinal artery occlusion); demyelination
- Anterior horn cell (motor neuronopathies): motor neuron disease; poliomyelitis, West Nile virus
- Peripheral nerve (acute acquired polyradiculoneuropathy): Guillain-Barre syndrome; Miller-Fisher syndrome (oculo-bulbar symptoms; ataxia; areflexia); critical illness neuropathy; metabolic diseases-diabetes mellitus, acute porphyria; acute motor axonal neuropathy; tick paralysis; diphtheria; arsenic intoxication
- Neuromuscular junction transmission disorders: myasthenia gravis, Eaton-Lambert syndrome, botulism

- Muscle (myopathies): endocrine myopathy (hypothyroidism), polymyositis, acute rhabdomyolysis, critical illness myopathy
- Metabolic/endocrine disorders: familial hypokalemic paralysis; hypokalaemia; hypocalcaemia; hypophosphataemia; hyponatraemia; hypomagnesaemia; adreno-cortical insufficiency
- Connective tissue diseases and vasculitis; giant cell arteritis/polymyalgia rheumatic; systemic lupus erythematosus; polymyositis

Checklist for weakness

- Cortical signs: aphasia; agnosia; apraxia; neglect; visual field deficit
- Presence or absence of facial involvement
- Bulbar signs
- Distribution of weakness
- Presence of upper or lower motor neuron signs
- Bowel or bladder involvement
- Fluctuating pattern of weakness
- Fatigability of initially normal strength

Motor neuron signs

	Upper motor neuron	Lower motor neuron
Weakness	More diffuse	More focal
Atrophy	Mild, general	Severe, focal
Fasciculations	Not seen	May be present
Muscle tone	Increased	Reduced
Muscle stretch reflexes increased		Decreased
Clonus	May be present	Absent
Pathological reflexes may be present		Absent

Causes of acute flaccid weakness

- Spinal cord: spinal shock (early stage of acute cord disease); transverse myelitis (mixed upper and lower motor); spinal cord compression
- Anterior horn cell: poliomyelitis; other enterovirus infections; motor neuron disease (subacute)
- Peripheral nerve (polyradiculoneuropathy): acute inflammatory demyelinating polyneuropathy (Guillain-Barre syndrome: acute onset of ascending predominantly motor polyradiculoneuropathy; autonomic dysfunction); tick paralysis; diphtheria; heavy metal intoxication; toxins: n-toluene, glue sniffing; acute intermittent porphyria
- Neuromuscular junction: myasthenia gravis; drug-induced myasthenia; Eaton-Lambert syndrome; botulism; organophosphate poisoning
- Muscle: polymyositis; periodic paralysis; toxic myopathy; neuroleptic malignant syndrome; malignant hyperthermia; myoglobinuria/rhabdomyolysis
- Pseudoparesis (localised); skeletal disease; traumatic injury; osteomyelitis; septic arthritis

Localisation of neurological lesions

Upper motor neuron

- Increased tone of clasp-knife type(spasticity)
- Weakness most evident in anti-gravity muscles
- Increased(brisk) reflexes
- Clonus
- Extensor plantar responses

Lower motor neuron

- Fasciculation
- Reduced tone(flaccidity)
- Weakness
- Wasting
- Reduced or absent reflexes
- Flexor or absent plantar response

Primary muscle disorders

- Wasting
- No fasciculation

- Weakness
- Tone normal or reduced
- Reflexes normal or reduced

Neuromuscular junction lesions

- Prominent, variable and fatigable weakness
- Normal muscle bulk, tone and reflexes
- Ocular, bulbar and small muscles of the hand particularly affected
- No sensory deficit

Non-organic weakness

- Collapsing quality with sudden giving way
- Variable non-anatomical distribution
- Muscle bulk, tone, reflexes and plantar responses normal

MRC grading of muscle power

5: Normal power
4: Inability to maintain position against moderate resistance
3: Inability to maintain position against slight resistance or gravity
2: Active movement with gravity eliminated
1: Trace of contraction
0: No contraction

Descending paralysis acute diffuse weakness beginning in bulbar region and progressing to paralysis

Ds of botulism

- Dry mouth
- Diplopia
- Dilated pupils
- Droopy eyes (ptosis)
- Diminished gag reflex
- Dysphagia
- Dysarthria
- Dysphonia
- Difficulty lifting head
- Descending paralysis
- Diaphragmatic paralysis

Causes of ascending flaccid paralysis and acute ataxia

- Neuropathies: Guillain-Barre syndrome (symmetrical ascending paralysis, with distal small muscles first affected; affects both upper and lower limbs; commences in lower limbs, and trunk, bulbar, facial and respiratory muscles may be involved; rapid onset; preceding upper respiratory tract infection; ventilatory failure, autonomic failure; no or mild sensory deficit) and Miller-Fisher variant; diphtheritic polyneuropathy; porphyrias; meningoradiculopathies
- Neuromuscular junction disorders: botulism; myasthenia gravis
- Myopathies due to electrolyte imbalance: hypokalaemia; hypophosphataemia; hypomagnesaemia
- Heavy metal intoxication
- Spinal cord disease
- CNS disorders: rabies, acute paralytic poliomyelitis
- Tick paralysis: dermacentor variabilis

Causes of proximal muscle weakness with elevated creatine kinase

- Inflammatory: myositis
- Non-inflammatory myopathies: hypothyroidism; hypokalemia; alcohol; drugs: HMG CoA reductase inhibitors (statins), AZT

Causes of rapidly progressive weakness

- Myopathies: inflammatory; idiopathic (polymyositis, dermatomyositis, paroxysmal rhabdomyolysis); toxic: colchicine, cholesterol-lowering agents (CLAM); viral: influenza, Coxsackie B; parasitic: trichinosis; protozoal: toxoplasmosis; metabolic: glycogen and lipid disorders, especially carnitine palmitoyl transferase deficiency; endocrinopathies: hyperthyroidism, corticosteroid related; electrolyte

imbalance: hypokalaemia and hyperkalaemia, hypocalcaemia and hypercalcaemia, hypophosphataemia and hypermagnesaemia; periodic paralysis
- Neuromuscular junction: myasthenia gravis, congenital myasthenias, Lambert-Eaton syndrome, botulism, hypermagnesaemia
- Polyradiculoneuropathy: Guillain-Barre syndrome, porphyria, diphtheria, proximal diabetic neuropathy
- Anterior horn cell: poliomyelitis, West Nile virus, rabies, amyotrophic lateral sclerosis
- Radiculopathy: Cyomegalovirus polyradiculopathy

ABCD assessments in patients presenting with acute weakness

- Airway and breathing: tachypnea; shallow breathing; use of accessory muscles; paradoxical abdominal movement during the respiratory cycle; forced vital capacity <10–12 ml/kg
- Circulation: autonomic instability (sinus tachycardia; bradycardia)

Features suggesting functional weakness (a combination of absence of signs of organic disease alongside positive evidence of a functional disorder)

- Normal tone and reflexes
- La belle indifference
- Hoover's sign: hip extension is weak on direct testing, but is normal with flexion of the contralateral hip against resistance, when involuntary hip extension occurs.
- Collapsing weakness: limb collapses from a normal position with a light touch
- Co-contraction: the contraction of an antagonist muscle can be felt during testing of the agonist muscle

Potential acute presentations of multiple sclerosis with demyelination symptoms

- Optic neuritis, with unilateral eye pain and loss of central vision
- Brainstem lesions: acute onset diplopia, especially vertical; internuclear ophthalmoplegia
- Spinal cord lesions: Lhermitte's syndrome of electric sensations passing down the legs on neck flexion; limb weakness (useless hand, foot drop) bladder and bowel disturbance; acute respiratory muscle weakness with ventilatory failure
- Cerebellar lesions: ataxia
- Adventitious movements: tremor; reflex spasms

Causes of foot drop
Lower motor neurone lesion

Unilateral: radiculopathy (L5/S1 root); plexopathy; mononeuropathy (sciatic nerve; common peroneal nerve)
Bilateral: polyneuropathy; muscular dystrophy: scapuloperoneal type

Upper motor neurone lesion

Cerebral motor cortex: parasagittal lesion
Spinal cord lesion

Causes of ataxia
Acute

- Infections/post-infectious causes: acute cerebellar ataxia (post-infectious: varicella); cerebellar abscess
- Posterior cranial fossa mass lesions: haemangioblastoma, metastases, extra-axial meningioma, choroid plexus papilloma (adults); medulloblastoma, astrocytoma, ependymoma, brain stem glioma (children)
- Drug intoxications: ethanol; anti-epileptic drugs (phenytoin, carbamazepine); sedative-hypnotics (benzodiazepines)
- Vestibular: labyrinthitis; benign paroxysmal positional vertigo
- Demyelination: multiple sclerosis; ADEM
- Seizure/post-ictal state
- Post-concussion syndrome

- Cerebellar stroke/haemorrhage
- Vertebral artery dissection
- Causes of intermittent ataxia
- Conversion disorder

Intermittent

- Migraine
- Epilepsy
- Transient ischaemic attack

Signs of ataxia
Cerebellar ataxia

- Truncal ataxia, with wide-based gait
- Limb ataxia: dysmetria; intention tremor; dysdiadochokinesia; impaired finger-to-nose, finger-to-finger or heel-to-shin test
- Speech: dysmetria (staccato speech)
- Ocular signs: gaze-evoked nystagmus; skew deviation; dysconjugate saccades
- Negative Romberg sign

Sensory ataxia

- Reduced or absent deep tendon reflexes
- Positive Romberg sign

Vestibular ataxia

- Vertigo
- Past-pointing of limb movements

Causes of amnesia
Chronic/persistent

- Alzheimer's disease (often with evidence of mild dysfunction in other cognitive domains, e.g. perception, language, executive function); a temporal gradient is often evident in the amnesia of AD, with more distant events being more easily remembered than recent happenings, often characterised by relatives as a defect in short term memory with preserved long term memory. Verbal repetition (repetitive questioning) regarding day to day matters, reflecting the amnesia, is one of the most common symptoms
- Alcohol-related memory problems: Wernicke-Korsakoff syndrome; alcohol-related dementia
- Sequelae of herpes simplex encephalitis
- Limbic encephalitis (paraneoplastic or non-paraneoplastic)
- Hypoxic brain injury
- Bilateral paramedian thalamic infarction/posterior cerebral artery occlusion ("strategic infarct dementia")
- Third ventricle tumour, cyst; fornix damage
- Temporal lobectomy (bilateral; or unilateral with previous contralateral injury, usually birth asphyxia)
- Focal retrograde amnesia (rare)

Acute/transient

- Closed head injury
- Drugs
- Transient global amnesia
- Transient epileptic amnesia
- Migraine
- Profound hypoglycaemia
- Multiple sclerosis

Dystonic reactions
Types

Oculogyric crisis
Buccolingual crisis
Torticollic crisis
Tortipelvic crisis
Opisthotonos

Causes

Neuroleptic agents: phenothiazines, thioxanthenes, butyrophenones
Anti-emetic agents: dopamine agonists; metclopramide; trimetobenzamide
Others: tricyclic antidepressants; cocaine; serotonin reuptake inhibitors; monoamine oxidase inhibitors

Headache
The distinction between primary and secondary headache is crucial to guide definitive manage-

ment in the emergency department. Primary headache syndromes are defined by history, classical presentations, and the absence of an underlying cause. Secondary headache is more commonly seen in emergency settings, with an increasing requirement for the consideration of CT brain scanning. The International Headache Society classification system provides a system for recognition of clinical presentations of headache.

Improvement with treatment does not exclude a serious underlying cause for headache.

The following modes of onset of headache are usually seen:

Acute onset of severe headache

- Subarachnoid haemorrhage
- Intracerebral haemorrhage
- Temporal (giant cell) arteritis (unilateral headache, jaw/tongue claudication, age 50 or more at the onset of symptoms; temporal artery tenderness, or a reduction in the pulse; ESR of 50 mm/h or more; positive temporal artery biopsy, within 3 days of commencing high dose steroid therapy)
- Thunderclap headache (abrupt onset reaching maximum intensity within 5 min)
- Acute hydrocephalus
- Meningitis; encephalitis
- Acute hypertension (e.g. phaeochromocytoma); hypertensive encephalopathy
- Internal carotid artery dissection
- Intracranial venous thrombosis
- Idiopathic intracranial hypertension (headache associated with transient visual obscurations, photopsia, pulsatile intracranial noises, retrobulbar pain, diplopia and visual loss; raised intracranial pressure in the absence of ventricular dilatation, intracranial mass lesion or abnormalities in CSF)
- Reversible cerebral vasoconstriction syndrome
- Primary headache; benign exertional or coital headache; first episode of cluster headache or crash migraine; tension headache; paroxysmal hemicrania

Sub-acute onset, and often progressive, headache (suggests space-occupying lesion):

- Subdural haematoma
- Intracranial tumour
- Intracranial abscess
- Temporal arteritis
- Chronic meningitis

Chronic and non-progressive headache

- Chronic migraine with or without analgesic overuse
- Chronic tension headache (musculo-skeletal headache)
- Post-herpetic neuralgia
- Post-traumatic headache
- Analgesia-induced headache or rebound headache: ergotamine; opioids; opioid combinations; 5-HT1 agonists; caffeine; alcohol; vasodilators; nifedipine; indomethacin; sympathomimetic agents

Recurrent episodic headache

- Migraine
- Cluster headache
- Trigeminal neuralgia
- Paroxysmal hypertension
- Coital headache

Neurological evaluation in headache

- Cranial nerves: pupils; visual fields; eye movements; facial power and sensation; bulbar function (soft palate, tongue movement)
- Tone, power, reflexes and coordination of all four limbs
- Plantar responses
- Gait including heel-toe walking
- Funduscopy
- Signs of meningeal irritation

Features suggestive of raised intracranial pressure

- Early morning headache
- Vomiting
- Drowsiness
- Posture-related headache
- Headache with pulse-synchronous tinnitus

Features of cluster headache

Periodic
Intense unilateral headache and retro-orbital pain, lasting from 15 min to 3 h
Ipsilateral nasal congestion, rhinorrhoea, conjunctival injection, lacrimation, facial flushing, eyelid oedema, Horner's syndrome
Clusters of daily headaches lasting 4–8 weeks and separated by headache-free intervals

Features of tension headache

- Sensation of pressing or tightening, and non-pulsatile
- Frontal and occipital location
- Bilateral mild to moderate headache
- Not aggravated by physical activity
- No nausea and vomiting
- Associated with photophobia and/or phonophobia

Red flags for secondary headache (headache with structural or metabolic cause)

Sudden onset of severe headache
Time from onset to peak headache intensity within 1 min (thunderclap headache)
New onset of, or change in, character of headache after 50 years of age
Focal neurological signs or symptoms (including ataxia; cognitive dysfunction)
Headache with seizure
Headache secondary to head trauma
Headache precipitated by exertion, sexual activity (orgasm) or Valsalva manoeuvre
Associated with fever and skin rash
Coexisting neck stiffness
New onset headache in a patient with HIV infection or cancer
Jaw claudication
Prior neurosurgical procedure or CSF shunt
Pregnancy or post-partum

Causes of thunderclap headache (reaches peak intensity within 5 min of onset).

Secondary thunderclap headache

- Subarachnoid haemorrhage
- Sentinel headache
- Cervico-cephalic arterial dissection: internal carotid (unilateral headache, unilateral facial, orbital and neck pain; pulsatile tinnitus; ipsilateral partial Horner syndrome with miosis and partial ptosis, amaurosis fugax; contralateral MCA/ACA stroke); vertebral (unilateral occipital headache; posterior neck pain; lateral medullary ischaemia with features of posterior circulation syndromes: ataxia, vertigo, dysarthria, diplopia, and dysphagia)
- Cerebral venous sinus thrombosis
- Pituitary apoplexy (pre-existing pituitary adenoma): acute headache, ophthalmoplegia; reduced visual acuity; altered mental state; obstructive hydrocephalus (3rd ventricle obstruction or haemorrhage); acute adrenocortical insufficiency from secondary hypoadrenalism
- Hypertensive emergency
- Reversible cerebral vasoconstriction syndrome (recurrent sudden onset severe or thunderclap headache over 1–3 months; self-limited; low recurrence risk; diffuse and multifocal segmental arterial constriction on magnetic resonance angiography or CT angiography; CT or MRI may be normal)
- Phaeochromocytoma
- Colloid cyst of third ventricle
- Spontaneous intracranial hypotension (postural headache, worse in the upright posture and relieved or improved with recumbency; related to spontaneous CSF leak through a dural tear; associated with neck stiffness, tinnitus, hyperacusis, photophobia, interscapular and radicular upper limb pain, vertigo, visual field defects and cranial nerve palsies)
- Spontaneous retroclival haematoma

Primary thunderclap headache (normal brain imaging and CSF analysis).

Types of coital headache

- Dull: muscle tension

- Explosive: thunderclap
- Postural: CSF leak from dural root sleeve rupture

Risk factors for subarachnoid haemorrhage

- Hypertension
- Alcohol use
- Cocaine
- Linked genetic disorders: adult polycystic kidney disease; Ehlers-Danlos syndrome type IV; neurofibromatosis type 1
- First degree relatives with subarachnoid haemorrhage

Causes of subarachnoid haemorrhage

- Aneurysmal
- Non-aneurysmal: peri-mesencephalic; arterio-venous malformations; neoplasm; pituitary apoplexy; vasculitis; cerebral venous thrombosis; drugs: cocaine, amphetamines; haematological: coagulopathy, leukaemia

Presentations of subarachnoid haemorrhage

- Acute severe, worst ever, headache, with peak intensity at onset, associated with neck pain, photophobia, nausea and vomiting; transient loss of consciousness and seizures are common at the onset
- Acute neck or low back pain (nerve root irritation from pooling of arachnoid blood)
- Sentinel headache (warning leak)
- Acute confusion
- Cardiac arrhythmia, secondary to autonomic or electrolyte imbalance

Localising features with intracranial aneurysms

Anterior communicating artery

- Optic tract:homonymous hemianopia; altitudinal field defect
- Optic chiasm: bitemporal hemianopia
- Optic nerve: unilateral amblyopia

Internal carotid artery-posterior communicating artery aneurysm

- IIIrd nerve palsy

Middle cerebral artery aneurysm: hemiparesis; hemi-sensory loss; visual disturbance; aphasia; seizure.

World Federation of Neurological Surgeons grading scale for subarachnoid haemorrhage

Grade	GCS	Motor deficit
I	15	Absent
II	13 or 14	Absent
III	13 or 14	Present
IV	7–12	Absent or present
V	3–6	Absent or present

Risk factors for spontaneous intracerebral haemorrhage

- Small vessel disease of the brain: hypertensive vasculopathy; cerebral amyloid angiopathy (lobar intracerebral haemorrhage in the elderly)
- Coagulopathy: bleeding disorders, anticoagulants, thrombolytic agents
- Structural lesions: bleeding into brain tumour; intracranial vascular malformations (arteriovenous malformations, dural arteriovenous fistulae, cavernomas, saccular aneurysms); haemorrhagic transformation of ischaemic stroke; infections (mycotic aneurysms, aspergillosis, herpes simplex encephalitis); Moyamoya disease
- Dural venous sinus thrombosis (haemorrhagic venous infarction)
- Recreational drugs: cocaine, amphetamines

Risk factors for cerebral venous sinus thrombosis

- Pregnancy; puerperium
- Transient situations: dehydration, sepsis
- Malignancy
- Head injury

- Paranasal sinusitis
- Thrombophilia: protein S or protein C deficiency
- Medication: oral contraceptive pill; steroids
- Inflammatory bowel disease: ulcerative colitis
- Behcet syndrome

Features associated with cerebral venous sinus thrombosis

Recognition can be delayed as the clinical features are variable and non-specific and CT scan findings are often subtle.

- Headache, which can be new, atypical, progressive over days to weeks, or thunderclap
- Acute confusional state
- Reduced or altered level of consciousness; coma
- Seizures, often followed by post-ictal paresis
- Papilloedema
- Cranial nerve palsies
- Focal neurological deficit: hemiparesis, hemi-sensory disturbance
- Superior sagittal sinus thrombosis may be associated with paraparesis
- Cavernous sinus thrombosis presents with chemosis, proptosis and painful ophthalmoplegia
- Hyperdensity of a cortical or deep cerebral vein or of a dural venous sinus on CT scan
- Enhancement of dural lining of venous sinus with a filling defect within a cortical vein or dural sinus on contrast-enhanced CT scan
- Evidence of a hypecoagulable state

Features of reversible cerebral vasoconstriction syndrome

The syndrome is under-recognised and often misdiagnosed, as the clinical features are non-specific

- Recurrent sudden onset and severe headaches over 1–3 months, with or without seizure and focal headache, with resolution
- Resolution within 1–3 months, with a low incidence of recurrence
- Typically affects females aged 20–50 years
- Precipitants include pregnancy or the post-partum state, vasoactive drugs (recreational drugs such as cocaine, SSRI, triptans, ergot alkaloid derivatives), and catecholamine-secreting tumours
- Associated with multi-focal segmental constriction of cerebral arteries (string of beads appearance on cerebral angiography)
- Many patients have initially normal vascular imaging
- Complications include ischaemic stroke (can be a cause of cryptogenic stroke), non-aneurysmal subarachnoid haemorrhage (localized convexity SAH), intracerebral haemorrhage, cerebral oedema and posterior reversible leukoencephalopathy syndrome

Features of idiopathic intracranial hypertension

- Headache, often worse on lying down, which is refractory to treatment
- Visual disturbance: blurring of vision, diplopia (usually horizontal), transient visual obscurations, progressive loss of peripheral vision, sudden visual loss
- Typically affects obese young women
- Papilloedema, which can be bilateral or unilateral, and occasionally VIth nerve palsy
- Raised CSF pressure in the absence of an intracranial mass lesion or ventricular dilatation

Risk factors for idiopathic intracranial hypertension

CNS infection
Cerebral venous sinus thrombosis

Drugs: oral contraceptives, tetracyclines, anabolic steroids, Vitamin A, cis-retinoic acid, amiodarone, nirofurantoin, ciclosporin, psychotropic drugs
Endocrine: hypoparathyroidism; hypothyroidism; obesity
Guillain Barre syndrome
Pregnancy
Iron deficiency anaemia
Systemic lupus erythematosus

Migraine syndromes
Migraine with aura

- Classic (visual auras are monochromatic, angulated, bright and scintillating, starting centrally and spreading peripherally, and are associated with visual field defects)

Complicated:

- Hemiplegic migraine (recurrent transient hemiplegia or hemparesis associated with migraine headache)
- Ophthalmoplegic migraine (migraine-like attack followed by periorbital pain and external ophthalmoplegia)
- Migraine with brainstem aura (basilar artery migraine) (the aura includes two or more of: bilateral visual disturbances including diplopia, dysarthria, dizziness, vertigo, tinnitus or ataxia)
- Acute confusional state
- Alice-in-Wonderland syndrome (altered visual perception of sizes of body parts or sizes of external objects, especially at night, including micropsia, macropsia, pelopsia (sensation of proximity) or teleopsia (sensation of increased distance away))
- Status migrainous: a debilitating migraine attack associated with severe headache lasting more than 72 h, disregarding interruption due to sleep

Migraine without aura (common migraine)
Migraine variants

- Abdominal migraine (recurrent episodes of central abdominal pain in children aged 3–10 years)
- Benign paroxysmal vertigo of childhood
- Paroxysmal torticollis
- Ocular migraine (associated with visual loss)

Features suggesting migraine

- Recurrent headache
- Stereotyped premonitory symptoms
- Characteristic triggers
- Predictable timing around menstruation or ovulation
- Relieved with sleep
- Positive family history
- Childhood precursors: motion sickness, episodic vomiting, episodic vertigo

Causes of neck stiffness (meningism)

- Infection: meningitis; viral upper respiratory tract infection with cervical lymphadenitis; upper lobe pneumonia
- Acute torticollis (wry neck)
- Neck sprain
- Dystonic drug reaction
- Sandifer syndrome (gastro-oesophageal reflux)
- Tonsillar herniation

Risk factors for bacterial meningitis

- Age: infants
- Community clusters: college or university halls of residence, military barracks, day care facilities
- Travel to meningitis belt of sub-Saharan Africa; Hajj or Umrah pilgrims on annual pilgrimage to Mecca
- Para-meningeal infections: middle ear (otitis media); orbit (orbital cellulitis); paranasal sinuses; mastoiditis
- CSF shunts (ventriculoperitoneal shunts); dural defects; external ventricular drains
- Neural tube defects: dermal sinuses
- Head injuries: basal skull fractures with dural tears; penetrating cranial injuries
- Immunosuppression: glucocorticoids; cancer chemotherapy
- Alcoholism
- Diabetes mellitus

- Intravenous drug abuse
- Functional/anatomical asplenia: splenectomy; sickle cell disease
- HIV/AIDS
- Malignancy

Risk factors for neonatal meningitis

- Low birth weight (<2500 g)
- Premature rupture of membranes
- Premature delivery
- Traumatic delivery
- Maternal peri-partum infection
- Foetal hypoxia

Clinical features of acute meningitis

- Neonates: lethargy, irritability, poor feeding, high pitched cry, fever/hypothermia, bulging fontanelle (age <2 years)/acute increase in head circumference, apneoic episodes, seizures, jaundice, pallor, hypotonia, hypoglycaemia
- Infants and children: irritability, headache, nausea and vomiting, fever, altered mental state (confusion, delirium, drowsiness, coma) neck stiffness, bulging fontanelle, photophobia, meningeal signs, focal neurological deficit, convulsive status epilepticus
- Adults: classical triad of fever, headache and meningeal signs including neck stiffness (resistance to passive neck flexion), Kernig's sign (involuntary knee flexion with forced hip flexion; with hips and knees in flexion, passive knee extension is limited by hamstring spasm and/or pain), and Brudzinski's sign (passive neck flexion causes hip and knee flexion); nausea and vomiting, lethargy, irritability, confusion/delirium, photophobia, focal neurological deficit, coma

Indications for CT head scan prior to lumbar puncture with suspected meningitis

- Instability: signs of shock, purpuric skin rash (lesions >2 mm in diameter)
- Suspicion of space occupying lesion or raised intracranial pressure: new onset focal seizures; focal neurological signs, including cranial nerve palsies; papilloedema; altered, reduced or fluctuating level of consciousness; GCS 8 or under, or a drop of 3 or more; decerebrate or decorticate posturing; poorly responsive or fixed, dilated or unequal pupils; absent dolls eye movement; Cushing triad (hypertension, bradycardia, irregular respirations)
- Immunocompromised state: HIV, immunosuppressive therapy, solid organ or haematopoietic stem cell transplantation
- Local site for lumbar puncture: skin infection; anatomical abnormality
- Coagulation abnormalities

Atypical presentations of meningitis are commoner in

- Neonates, infants and the elderly
- Diabetes mellitus
- Immunosuppression: neutropenia; organ and tissue transplant recipients
- Ventriculo-peritoneal shunts
- Chronic kidney disease
- Chronic lung disease
- HIV/AIDS

Features associated with meningococcal septicaemia

- Fever
- Arthralgia; myalgia (leg pain)
- Septic shock
- Purpuric skin rash (lesions >2 mm diameter): a rash may be less visible in darker skin (check soles of feet, palms of hands and conjunctivae)
- Seizures
- Acute respiratory distress syndrome
- Multi-organ dysfunction

Causes of fever with altered level of consciousness

- Infections: encephalitis; meningitis; cerebral malaria; brain abscess; sepsis with DIC
- Heat over-production: neuroleptic malignant syndrome; malignant hyperthermia;

sympathomimetic toxicity (cocaine, amphetamines); convulsive status epilepticus; catatonia
- Impaired heat dissipation: heat stroke; anticholinergic toxicity
- Structural brain lesions: hypothalamic/brain stem lesion; subarachnoid and intraventricular haemorrhage

Risk factors for brain abscess (triad of headache, fever and focal neurological deficit)

- Direct extension from chronic middle ear (otitis media, mastoiditis), paranasal sinus (frontal, ethmoidal and sphenoidal sinusitis), dental, facial and scalp infections
- Trauma: skull fracture; penetrating orbital wounds (orbital roof, superior orbital fissure and optic canal)
- Extra-cranial spread from chronic pulmonary infection (lung abscess; bronchiectasis), endocarditis
- Congenital heart disease (cyanotic heart disease including Tetralogy of Fallot; right to left shunts; patent foramen ovale)
- Meningitis
- Immunosuppression: cancer chemotherapy
- CSF shunts
- Diabetes mellitus
- Recent neurosurgical procedure

Clinical features of acute encephalitis

- Fever
- Lethargy
- Photophobia
- Altered, reduced or fluctuating level of consciousness
- Neck pain/stiffness
- Cognitive dysfunction: acute memory disturbance
- Behavioural changes: personality change, disorientation, hallucinations, agitation, psychosis
- Focal neurological signs: dysphasia, hemiparesis, hemianopia
- Seizures
- Associated features: skin rash; upper respiratory tract infection
- SIADH

Clinical clues to the cause of acute viral encephalitis

- Skin rash: enterovirus; adenovirus; measles
- Conjunctivitis: adenovirus; enterovirus; measles
- Parotitis: mumps; enterovirus; HIV; Epstein-Barr virus
- Pharyngitis: adenovirus; enterovirus; Epstein-Barr virus
- Lymphadenopathy: Epstein-Barr virus; cytomegalovirus
- Pneumonia: measles; varicella; cytomegalovirus; adenovirus; influenza
- Enteritis: enterovirus
- Hepatitis: adenovirus; cytomegalovirus; varicella; Epstein-Barr virus
- Behavioural change; complex partial seizures: herpes simplex

Pneumocephalus (air or gas within the skull)

- Can be extra-axial (epidural, subdural or subarachnoid) or intra-axial (parenchymal, intraventricular, intravascular)

Causes

- Head and facial trauma: fractures of base of skull or paranasal sinuses; compound skull fracture with dural laceration
- Iatrogenic: intracranial or sinus surgery; external ventricular drain insertion; ventriculo-peritoneal or ventriculo-pleural shunting; nasogastric tube insertion
- Barotrauma: scuba diving, flying
- Otogenic
- Meningitis with anaerobic gas-forming organisms
- Neoplasm of paranasal sinuses or intracranial
- Congenital skull or tegmen tympani defects

Features of raised intracranial pressure

Symptoms

- Headache
- Nausea and vomiting
- Reduced visual acuity
- Diplopia

Signs

- Progressive decline in level of consciousness
- Reduced upward gaze
- Bilateral VIth nerve palsy
- Papilloedema
- Altered vital signs

Categories of hydrocephalus

Obstructive

- Aqueduct of Sylvius: lateral and 3rd ventricles dilated
- Foramen of Monro: lateral ventricles dilated
- Foramina of Luschka and Magendie: 4th ventricle blockage followed by 3rd and lateral ventricles
- Subarachnoid space around brain stem: post-infectious or post-subarachnoid haemorrhage

Non-obstructive

- Normal pressure hydrocephalus (triad of dementia, gait disturbance and urine incontinence; diffuse ventriculomegaly out of proportion to degree of sulcal prominence)

Causes of acute hydrocephalus

- Infection: bacterial meningitis; parasitic infections (neurocysticercosis, with intraventricular cysts); cerebellar encephalitis
- Intracranial haemorrhage: subarachnoid haemorrhage (obstruction at level of ventricular system, basal cisterns, or arachnoid villi); intracerebral haemorrhage, with or without intraventricular extension; cerebellar haemorrhage
- Mass lesions in ventricles or peri-ventricular spaces (foramen of Monro, pineal region, cerebral aqueduct of Sylvius; 4th ventricle): colloid cyst of 3rd ventricle
- Ischaemic stroke
- Head injury: cerebral swelling/haematoma; subarachnoid/intraventricular haemorrhage
- After intracranial operations

Potential presentations of CSF shunt complications

Shunt malfunction

- Persistent headache
- Vomiting
- Drowsiness; lethargy
- Neck pain and stiffness
- Failure of upward gaze
- Bulging fontanelles and diastasis of sutures in infants
- Reduced visual acuity
- Papilloedema

Shunt infection (local soft tissue infection, meningitis, peritonitis)

- Malaise
- Fever
- Headache
- Vomiting
- Neck pain and stiffness
- Redness around shunt
- Abdominal distension
- Recurrent lower shunt obstruction

Shunt overdrainage

- Extra-axial collection of fluid and/or blood
- Slit ventricle syndrome (intermittent severe headache, often relieved on lying down)

Evaluation of shunt malfunction

- CT scan (enlargement of ventricles or other signs of raised intracranial pressure; slit ventricles)

- Plain x-ray of entire shunt system (lateral skull, antero-posterior chest and antero-posterior abdomen) (disconnection, kinks, breaks, migration of shunt tubing)
- Blood tests: CRP; white cell count
- Abdominal ultrasound (abdominal complications of ventriculoperitoneal shunts such as pseudocysts)
- Shunt reservoir tap (CSF white cell count, culture, bacterial antigen detection)

Checklist for mild to moderate head injuries

- Mechanism of injury
- Witnessed loss of consciousness >5 min
- Anterograde amnesia >5 min or retrograde amnesia >30 min in relation to the event
- Vomiting
- Headache
- Seizure
- Glasgow Coma Score and serial changes
- Drug/alcohol intoxication
- Anticoagulant therapy; bleeding and clotting disorders
- Scalp wound or bruising
- Signs of basal skull fracture: CSF leak from nose or ear; panda eyes; Battle sign (mastoid region bruising); haemotympanum
- Focal neurological deficit
- In children, suspicion of non-accidental injury

Mechanisms of brain damage following head injury

Primary brain damage (at the time of impact)

- Cortical laceration
- Cortical contusion
- Intracerebral haematoma
- Diffuse axonal injury
- Subcortical grey matter injury

Secondary brain damage

Intracranial causes

- Extra-axial haematoma: extradural; subdural
- Subarachnoid haemorrhage; intraventricular haemorrhage
- Cerebral oedema
- Infection
- Hydrocephalus
- Leptomeningeal cyst (growing fracture): dural tear with progressive widening of skull defect or skull fracture
- Focal encephalomalacia: tissue loss with surrounding gliosis

Extracranial

- Hypovolaemic shock (blood loss, profound diuresis from mannitol)
- Hypoxia (airway obstruction)
- Hypercapnia
- Electrolyte abnormalities
- Hyperthermia (temperature > 38 °C)
- Coagulopathy
- Abnormal blood glucose

Confounding factors in head injury assessment

- Alcohol intoxication
- Drug overdose
- Epileptic seizure
- Cognitive impairment: dementia

Features indicating clinical deterioration after head injury

- Early: agitation; confusion; drowsiness; recurrent vomiting; severe headache
- Late: fall in Glasgow Coma Score by 2 points or more; dilated pupil;
- focal neurological deficit; seizure; Cushing response of hypertension, bradycardia and widening of the pulse pressure

Causes of delayed deterioration after head injury (including patients who talk and die)

Delayed intracranial haematoma: extradural haematoma; acute subdural haematoma

Delayed intracerebral haemorrhage related to contusions

Diffuse cerebral oedema
Seizures
Hydrocephalus
Tension pneumocephalus (intracranial air causing a mass effect)
Metabolic: hyponatraemia; hypoxia; hypoglycaemia; adrenocortical insufficiency; drug/alcohol withdrawal; hepatic encephalopathy
Vascular events: dural venous sinus thrombosis; carotid artery dissection; subarachnoid haemorrhage; cerebral embolism (including fat embolism)
Meningitis
Transtentorial or cerebellar herniation

Predisposing factors for chronic subdural haematoma

- Chronic alcoholism
- Coagulopathy
- Elderly
- Coagulopathy; anticoagulant therapy; thrombocytopenia
- Arachnoid cyst

Potential presentations of subdural haematoma

- Altered or fluctuating level of consci ousness
- Headache
- Dementia
- Seizure
- Hemiparesis
- Recurrent falls
- Transient neurological deficit mimicking transient ischaemic attack
- Parkinsonism
- Symptoms of raised intracranial pressure

Potential symptoms of concussion

- Disorientation
- Confusion
- Delayed verbal and motor responses
- Amnesia
- History of loss of consciousness
- Drowsiness
- Irritability
- Headache
- Nausea and vomiting
- Dizziness
- Slurring of speech
- Photophobia (light sensitivity); phonophobia (noise sensitivity)
- Sleep disturbance

Signs of temporal bone fracture

- Conductive hearing loss
- Haemotympanum
- CSF otorrhoea
- Peripheral nystagmus
- Facial nerve paresis or paralysis

Acute Psychiatric Disorder
Triage safety questions

Is the patient a danger to him or herself?
Is the patient at risk of leaving before assessment?
Is the patient a danger to others?
Is the area safe?

Predictors of organic disorder as cause of acute behavioural disturbance

First presentation of mental disorder
Sudden onset-over hours to days
Delirium
Level of consciousness fluctuating or decreased (clouding of consciousness)
Disorientation
Wavering attention
Hallucinations (especially visual, tactile or olfactory)
History of drug use
Recreational
Overdose
Prescribed or over-the-counter
Recent or new medical problems
Neurological signs or symptoms:nystagmus, ataxia
Abnormal pupil size, symmetry and reactivity
Movement disorders
Abnormal vital signs

Features indicative of psychiatric illness

- Gradual onset-weeks to months
- Continuous course
- No clouding of consciousness
- Auditory hallucinations
- Flat affect
- Past psychiatric history
- Normal physical examination

Checklist for mental state assessment

- General appearance and behaviour (clothing, grooming, hygiene, hair and nails, facial expression, eye contact and rapport)
- Motor activity: body posture, gait, gestures, dystonias, dyskinesias, psychomotor retardation
- Alertness (level of consciousness)
- Cognition: orientation (time, place, person); registration; recall; concentration and attention; general knowledge
- Mood (happiness, irritability, stability)
- Affect (range: flat, normal, expansive; stability: stable, labile; appropriateness: appropriate, inappropriate)
- Memory (immediate, short term, long term)
- Thought content (delusions, obsessions, suicidal ideation, depressive thoughts, anxiety) and form (thought block, thought withdrawal, thought insertion, thought broadcasting, derailment or flight of ideas)
- Hallucinations (visual, tactile, auditory, olfactory, gustatory, visceral)
- Attention and concentration
- Speech (speech rate, volume, tonality, content and quantity)
- Judgement

Acute behavioural disorder including violent behaviour

Causes

- Substance abuse: intoxication and withdrawal-alcohol, psychostimulant drugs (PCP, LSD, amphetamines), benzodiazepines
- CNS disorders: head injury (chronic subdural haematoma); stroke; tumour; encephalitis; meningitis
- Metabolic: hypoglycaemia, hyponatraemia, hypercalcaemia
- Hypoxaemia/hypercarbia
- Sepsis
- Organ failure: liver, kidneys
- Endocrine: thyroid storm; corticosteroids
- Neuroleptic malignant syndrome (rigidity, autonomic instability and delirium)
- Serotonin syndrome
- Mental health conditions: psychosis; affective disorders with psychotic symptoms (mania; depression); delusional disorders; personality disorders; anti-social behaviour; mental retardation
- Dementia

Markers for organic causes

Sudden onset, within minutes to hours
Age >40 years with no prior psychiatric history (first episode)
Recreational or prescribed drug use
Clouding of consciousness
Decreased level of consciousness; loss of consciousness
Fluctuating course
Global impairment of cognitive function
Confusion
New or worsening headache
Speech, movement or gait disorder in absence of alcohol or substance abuse
Disorientation
Psychomotor retardation
Visual, olfactory or tactile hallucinations
Disorganised delusions
Labile affect (emotional lability)
Abnormal vital signs
Focal neurological signs
Toxidrome features

Acute psychosis

An organic cause must always be considered initially in the presence of a de novo presentation with acute psychosis.

In an acute psychosis, there is a predominance of positive symptoms, including:

- Delusions (false, fixed, irrational and often unusual beliefs): paranoid (mostly persecutory); grandiose (imparting special powers or missions, including religious); somatic (of terminal illness); thought interference
- Hallucinations (sensory perception without an appropriate stimulus): typically auditory (third person hallucinations, involving hearing voices speaking about the patient, which may be derogatory, threatening, or commanding); third party commentary may involve the patient hearing someone describing their actions as they are being carried out; rarely visual, olfactory or tactile (which usually suggest an organic aetiology)
- Thought disorder, including tangential thinking, circumstantiality, loose associations, clang associations, perseveration, neologisms, echolalia, thought-blocking
- Behavioural disturbance, including bizarre behaviour, agitation and aggression
- Catatonia

Initial screening should include:

- Vital signs
- Capillary blood glucose
- Past medical history
- Symptoms and signs of acute intoxication or withdrawal
- Signs of trauma
- Collateral documentation: e.g. ambulance sheet
- Brief history of recent events

Additionally, there may be negative symptoms:

- Emotional withdrawal (flat affect)
- Poverty of speech (alogia)
- Loss of interest (anhedonia)
- Loss of motivation, initiative and drive (apathy)
- Reduction in physical activity
- Lack of attention to appearance or personal hygiene
- Indecisiveness (ambivalence)

The **first episode of psychosis** due to psychiatric illness is often a late presentation, initiated by others. Prodromal symptoms of psychosis (which is usually of gradual onset) include:

- Reduced concentration and attention
- Reduced drive and motivation; lack of energy; apathy
- Depressed mood
- Irritability
- Sleep disturbance
- Social withdrawal; changes in relationships with family and friends
- Reduced self care
- Suspiciousness; paranoid ideas
- Fleeting auditory hallucinations
- Unusual thinking, which can be more abstract or obtuse
- Deterioration in role function: non-attendance or deterioration in performance at workplace or at school

Life threatening causes of acute psychotic presentations include:

- Hypoglycaemia
- Wernicke's encephalopathy
- Withdrawal of alcohol or barbiturates
- Intracranial causes: tumour; stroke
- Infections: meningitis; encephalitis; AIDS; neurosyphilis
- Poisoning: heavy metal toxicity; carbon monoxide poisoning
- Recreational drugs: amphetamines, cocaine, phencyclidine
- Prescribed medication: steroids; quinolones; digoxin; benzodiazepines
- Seizures: post-ictal; complex partial seizures

Causes of violence

Functional (psychiatric disorder): schizophrenia; mania; agitated depression; anti-social behaviour; adjustment disorders; acute reaction to stress.

CNS: delirium; dementia; infection; seizure; stroke; head injury.

Metabolic: hypoglycaemia; hypoxia.

Drugs: alcohol, sedatives, cocaine, phencyclidine; anti-cholinergics, steroids, LSD.

Hypothermia; hyperthermia.

Assessment of risk of violence
History

- Male gender
- Previous history of violence and pattern of violence
- Substance dependence: alcohol or drug intoxication
- Forensic history: criminal record-imprisonment for violent offences; cruelty to animals, fire setting (pyromania)
- Carrying weapons (knifes, guns)
- Psychosis
- Organic mental disorders, global or with frontal lobe involvement
- In police custody

Mental state

- Persecutory delusions
- Delusions of passivity
- Delusions or hallucinations with violent content
- Delusions of control
- Threats and thoughts of violence
- Emotional state: psychomotor agitation, manic excitement
- Impulsivity
- Lack of empathy, anti-social or psychopathic traits

Signs of impending violence

- Loud, threatening, or profane speech
- Increased muscle tension, such as sitting on edge of, or gripping arms, of chair; clenched teeth and fists
- Hyperactivity, such as pacing
- Slamming doors; knocking over furniture; throwing objects
- Carrying weapons or other objects that may be used as weapons

Causes of aggression and out-of-control behaviour in children

- Disruptive behaviour disorders: attention deficit hyperactivity disorder, conduct disorder
- Mood disorders: irritability with depression and with mania
- Substance abuse: intoxication
- Developmental disabilities: mental retardation, autism
- Psychosis
- Head injury

Presentations of childhood psychosis

- Decline in social and cognitive functions: social withdrawal, worsening school performance, bizarre or eccentric thoughts and behaviours, self neglect, suspiciousness, anxiety, irritability, aggression
- Psychotic symptoms

Features of acute mania

- Inflated self esteem; grandiosity
- Pressured speech
- Flight of ideas; racing thoughts
- Hyperactivity; increased interest in multiple activities
- Increased sexual behaviour; provocative clothing
- Buying sprees
- Reduced sleep

Clinical depression can be recognised by:

- Continuous low mood or sadness
- Feelings of helplessness and hopelessness
- Loss of interest in daily activities, including social activities and sex (anhedonia)
- Loss of appetite

- Sleep changes: insomnia; early hour waking; over-sleeping (hypersomnia)
- Loss of energy; fatigue, exhaustion
- Feelings of worthlessness; excessive or inappropriate guilt; low self esteem
- Nihilistic thoughts
- Reckless behaviour: substance abuse; compulsive gambling; reckless driving
- Concentration problems:difficulty focusing and making decisions
- Somatic symptoms, which are unexplained and not responsive to conventional treatment: headache; chronic pain (back, abdominal, muscle)
- Thoughts of suicide
- Unexplained weight loss or gain

Deliberate self harm
Risk assessment

- Methods and frequency of current and past self-harm
- Current and past suicidal intent: lethality of method chosen; premeditation (advance planning-personal business finalized, e.g. preparation of will, arrangements for pets); suicide note; avoidance of discovery; final acts in anticipation
- Depressive symptoms: affective (pessimism; self-dislike; worthlessness); physical (loss of appetite; change in sleep patterns; loss of libido; loss of energy; agitation)
- Psychiatric illness

Risk factors for suicide

- Male gender
- Advancing age
- Lack of employment
- Alcohol and drug abuse
- Family/childhood: parental depression, substance abuse, suicide, and divorce; bullying
- Low social support (social isolation); living alone (separated; divorced; widowed)
- Significant life events: financial setback; disciplinary crises; marital crises
- Depression
- Psychiatric illness: mood disorders; schizophrenia; anxiety disorders; boderline personality disorder
- Chronic debilitating physical illness (especially with chronic pain); terminal illness
- History of sexual or physical abuse in childhood
- Family history of suicide

Features suggestive of factitious disorder

- Multiple hospital attendances and admissions
- Multiple aliases and hospital registration numbers
- Familiarity with medical jargon
- current or prior employment as a health care professional
- Few inter-personal relationships; no available next of kin
- Unexplained physical findings
- Failure to respond to standard treatments
- Multiple surgical scars
- History of substance abuse disorders

Features of delirium

- Acute and rapid onset
- Fluctuating clinical state with lucid intervals
- Impairment of/clouding of consciousness: reduced awareness of the environment and inability to maintain attention (perseveration in answer to a question; wandering off during a conversation)-shortened attention span. The alertness or arousal to the surrounding environment fluctuates between falsely increased alertness and a lowered awareness of the surroundings.
- Confusion worse at night with morning lucid interval; increased severity at evening or night time (sun-downing) when environmental stimulation is lowered.

- Global disturbance of cognition affecting multiple cognitive domains-memory, attention, concentration, orientation, language, visuo-spatial ability, or perception. Short-term, immediate, and working memory are commonly affected but long-term memories can also be disturbed.
- Disorganised thinking, e.g. rambling or incoherent speech, constructional apraxia (impaired ability to copy geometrical figures), dysnomia
- Psychomotor disturbance: agitation; reduced activity
- Disturbance of sleep-wake cycle: e.g. frequent daytime naps (daytime drowsiness), night-time agitation (insomnia at night); sleep fragmentation
- Emotional lability: anxiety, fear, depression, tearfulness, elation, fatuousness
- Perceptual abnormalities (illusions; hallucinations, especially visual, also tactile, auditory, olfactory)
- Paranoid ideas/delusions
- Reversible: usually resolves

Factors predisposing to delirium

- Age 65 years or over
- Cognitive impairment
- Severe illness (e.g. heart failure)
- Physical frailty
- Visual impairment
- Surgery, especially recent orthopaedic surgery

Factors precipitating delirium (transient disorder of cognition)
Metabolic:

- Acute kidney injury
- Liver failure
- Hypoglycemia; hyperglycemia
- Electrolyte imbalance: hyponatremia; hypernatremia; hypercalcemia; hypocalcemia

Peri-ictal:

Post-ictal
Complex partial and petit mal status

Trauma:

- Head injury: subdural haematoma

Infection:

- Cerebral infection: meningitis; encephalitis: HIV; syphilis
- Systemic infection: septicaemia, pneumonia, urinary tract infection
- Malaria

Respiratory and cardiac disease: heart failure, pulmonary embolism, myocardial infarction

Gastrointestinal: faecal impaction

Genitourinary: urine retention; bladder catheter

Neoplastic:

- Carcinomatosis
- Intracranial neoplasm: primary/metastatic

Nutritional:

- Vitamin deficiency: B12, thiamine (Wernicke encephalopathy), nicotinic acid
- Severe malnutrition

Withdrawal states:

- Alcohol
- Benzodiazepines; barbiturates; hypnotics

Toxic:

- Alcohol intoxication
- Polypharmacy
- Drug-induced: L-dopa and dopamine agonists, anticholinergics, opioids, benzodiazepines, glucocorticoids

- Neuroleptic malignant syndrome
- Heavy metals (lead)
- Solvents and pesticides

Endocrine:

- Hyperthyroidism (thyroid storm: disproportionate fever; sinus tachycardia or supraventricular arrhythmia; gastrointestinal symptoms-vomiting, diarrhea; and CNS symptoms-agitation, confusion, delirium or coma)
- Hypothyroidism
- Cushing's disease
- Addison's disease: acute adrenocortical failure
- Hyperparathyroidism

Raised intracranial pressure
Sensory deprivation

Subtypes of delirium
Hyperactive

- Agitation
- Restlessness
- Attempts to remove catheters and tubes
- Hitting; biting
- Emotional lability

Hypoactive

- Flat affect
- Withdrawal
- Apathy
- Lethargy; reduced responsiveness

Mixed

- Concurrent or sequential appearance of hyper- and hypo-active delirium

10 Toxicological Emergencies

ABCD assessment in poisoning

- Airway: signs of obstruction (caustic ingestion; ACE inhibitors); loss of protective airway reflexes (CNS depression; seizures); increased secretions (organophosphates); risk of aspiration; predicted rapid progression to respiratory failure (paralysis-botulinum toxin; pneumonitis-hydrocarbons, inhalants)
- Breathing: non-cardiogenic pulmonary oedema/acute lung injury
- Circulation
- Disability: GCS; mental state; pupil size and reaction; hypoglycaemia (ethanol, oral hypoglycaemic agents, beta-blockers, salicylates)
- Exposure

Causes of altered heart rate associated with poisoning

- Bradycardia: beta-blockers; calcium channel blockers; opiates; digoxin
- Tachycardia: sympathomimetic agents (amphetamines, cocaine); alcohol; anticholinergic agents; salicylates; tricyclic antidepressants; theophylline

Causes of hypotension associated with poisoning

- Vasodilatation, with venous pooling in the lower limbs: ACE inhibitors; calcium channel blockers
- Myocardial depression: beta-blockers; calcium channel blockers; tricyclic antidepressants
- Reduced circulating blood volume: gastrointestinal losses (vomiting: diarrhea); increased insensible losses (salicylates)

Screening evaluation with overdoses

- History of overdose: what?, when?, how much?, what else?, why?
- Collateral information: family/friends; paramedics; notes; contents of pockets; empty bottles
- Recognition of medication: Toxbase; BNF; TICTAC (Tablet Identification Aids); NPIS; plant identification atlas

A. Banerjee, *Emergency Clinical Diagnosis*, DOI 10.1007/978-3-319-50718-7_10

Potential sources of caustics

- Acids: toilet bowl cleaners; anti-rust compounds; car battery fluid; stone cleaner; soldering fluxes
- Alkalis: drain cleaners; surface cleaners; disc batteries; laundry or dishwasher detergents; denture cleaners; industrial strength bleach

Causes of toxidromes (toxicological syndromes, consisting of a collection of physical signs that help identify the causative agent)

Sympathomimetic: beta adrenergic agonists (terbutaline); alpha adrenergic agonists (ergot alkaloids, phenylephrine), predominantly alpha-1 adrenergic agonists (ephedrine, pseudoephedrine); indirect acting (cocaine, amphetamines; methamphetamines); LSD; theophylline; caffeine; noradrenaline uptake inhibitors (MAOI);

Anticholinergic: antihistamines, antipsychotic agents, selective serotonin reuptake inhibitors, tricyclic antidepressants, atropine, scopolamine, benztropine

Cholinergic: organophosphate insecticides (nicotinic and muscarinic), neuromuscular blocking agents (nicotinic); chemical warfare nerve agents; carbamate insecticides (muscarinic); mushrooms (Boletus, Clitocybe and Inocybe species); nicotine containing products

Opiate (triad of miosis, hypoventilation and coma): codeine, heroin, methadone

Sedative-hypnotic: benzodiazepines; ethanol and other alcohols; barbiturates; quinazolines

Sedative withdrawal

Serotonin: serotonin breakdown inhibitors (monoamine oxidase inhibitors); serotonin reuptake inhibitors (SSRI; cocaine; opioids); serotonin precursors (LSD, L-tryptophan); serotonin release enhancers (amphetamine, atypical anti-psychotics: lithium, risperidone, olanzapine; atypical antidepressants: mirtazapine, venlafaxine); triptans

Alcohol withdrawal

Anti-muscarinic (anti-cholinergic) syndrome

- Tachycardia
- Dilated pupils(mydriasis)
- Dry, flushed, hot skin
- Dry mucous membranes/axilla
- Urinary retention
- Reduced bowel sounds: reduced peristalsis
- Hyperthermia
- Mild hypertension
- CNS: Confusion, hallucinations, seizures, sedation, agitated delirium, myoclonic jerking and choreoathetoid movement, lethargy, coma
- Cardiac arrhythmias
- Absent bowel sounds

"Hot as hades, dry as a bone, red as a beet, blind as a bat, and mad as a hatter"

Features of tricyclic antidepressant toxicity (the 3 Cs of cardiac complications, convulsions and coma)

Anticholinergic: dry mouth, dry and flushed skin, mydriasis, blurred vision, sinus tachycardia, hyperthermia, hallucinations, seizures, ileus, urinary retention

Sodium channel blockade: prolonged QT interval, AV blocks, widening of QRS complex with terminal R wave in aVR, ventricular arrhythmias (VT, VF)

Alpha-adrenergic blockade: hypotension; reflex tachycardia

Antihistamine: CNS sedation

Cholinergic (muscarinic) syndrome

- Excessive salivation
- Lacrimation
- Bronchorrhoea
- Bronchospasm; wheezing
- Abdominal cramps: hyper-peristalsis
- Urine and faecal incontinence
- Vomiting

- Sweating
- Miosis
- Bradycardia
- Muscle weakness and fasciculations
- Pulmonary oedema
- Confusion or lethargy; coma
- Seizures

Peripheral syndromes may be described as:

- SLUDGE: salivation; lacrimation; diarrhoea; gastro-intestinal motility, emesis
- BBB: bradycardia; bronchorrhoea; bronchospasm

Sympathomimetic (hyper-adrenergic) syndromes

- Tachycardia
- Tachypnoea
- Hypertension; with severe hypertension, reflex bradycardia may occur
- Hyperthermia
- Sweating (diaphoresis)
- Dry mucosae
- Piloerection
- Mydriasis
- Hyperreflexia
- Agitation
- Delirium
- Paranoid delusions
- Seizures
- Stroke
- Acute coronary syndrome
- Aortic dissection
- Cardiac arrhythmias
- Hyperactive bowel sounds
- Rhabdomyolysis

Potential presentations with cocaine toxicity

- CNS stimulation: tremors, euphoria, agitation, seizures, status epilepticus
- Cardiovascular: hypertension; chest pain (acute coronary syndrome: ST elevation myocardial infarction); rhythm disturbances: ventricular tachycardia; supraventricular tachycardia; aortic dissection; dilated cardiomyopathy
- Hallucinations; acute psychosis
- Acute cerebrovascular accidents: cerebral infarction; subarachnoid haemorrhage; cerebral vasculitis
- Pulmonary: bronchospasm; haemoptysis: alveolar haemorrhage; acute non-cardiogenic pulmonary oedema; hypersensitivity pneumonitis(crack lung); barotrauma: pneumothorax; pneumomediastinum (from coughing against a closed glottis while smoking or intranasally inhaling cocaine
- Rhabdomyolysis: acute kidney injury
- Gastrointestinal: bowel ischaemia; body packer syndrome; hepatitis
- Obstetric and perinatal: spontaneous miscarriage, abruptio placentae, premature labour, neonatal cerebral infarction, neonatal seizures, neonatal myocardial infarction

Opioid toxidrome

- Bradycardia
- CNS depression
- Reduced gastro-intestinal motility
- Hypotension
- Miosis
- Respiratory depression: bradypnoea, apnoea
- Hypothermia

Sedative-hypnotic toxidrome

- Bradycardia
- CNS depression-lethargy, obtundation
- Hypotension
- Hypothermia
- Respiratory depression
- Normal to large, sluggishly reactive, pupils
- Paradoxical excitement
- Slurred speech
- Ataxia

Benzodiazepines:

- CNS depression
- Normal vital signs
- No respiratory depression in oral overdose without concomitant CNS depressants

Features of sympatholytic syndrome

- Reduced blood pressure
- Reduced pulse rate
- Low body temperature
- Small or pinpoint pupils
- Reduced peristalsis

Serotonin syndrome (triad of altered mental state, autonomic nervous system dysfunction and neuro-muscular abnormalities)

- Agitation, restlessness, disorientation, confusion, coma
- Fever, sweating, shivering, tachypnoea, tachycardia, hypertension
- Ataxia, myoclonus, tremor, rigidity, akathisia, incoordination, hyperreflexia
- Diarrhoea

Causes of drug-induced hyperthermia

- Hyperthermic agitated delirium: anticholinergic agents; sympathomimetics
- Pharmacological hyperthermic syndromes

Serotonin syndrome: triad of altered mental state, autonomic instability, and muscle hyperactivity (tremor, shivering, hyperreflexia, clonus)

Neuroleptic malignant syndrome (dopamine receptor blockade): typical/atypical antipsychotic agents; tetrad of mental state changes (gradual onset catatonia); increased muscle tone (lead pipe rigidity and superimposed tremor causing cogwheeling; bradykinesia); hyperthermia; and autonomic dysfunction (tachycardia; alternating hypertension and hypotension)

Malignant hyperpyrexia: tachycardia, generalized skeletal muscle rigidity and masseter spasm, and hyperthermia, without muscle hyperactivity

- Status epilepticus inducing agents: theophylline

Risk factors for paracetamol toxicity

- Hepatic glutathione depletion: malnutrition; alcoholism; anorexia nervosa; bulimia; HIV; cystic fibrosis
- Cytochrome P450 system induction: alcoholism; anti-epileptic drug therapy; barbiturates

Features of paracetamol toxicity

- Onset of symptoms usually 24–72 h following ingestion, with right upper quadrant pain and rising serum transaminases
- Acute liver failure develops 72–96 h following ingestion, leading to jaundice, encephalopathy, acute kidney injury, coagulopathy, metabolic acidosis, multi-organ failure, sepsis, and cerebral oedema

Features of salicylate toxicity

- Salicylism: nausea and vomiting; tinnitus; hearing loss; tachypnoea; sweating; warm extremities
- Lethargy; seizures
- Non-cardiogenic pulmonary oedema
- Hypoglycaemia
- Upper gastrointestinal bleeding
- Respiratory alkalosis with high anion gap metabolic acidosis
- Coagulopathy
- Acute kidney injury

Features of digoxin toxicity

- Gastrointestinal symptoms: nausea; vomiting; diarrhoea; abdominal pain

- Visual symptoms: yellow-green chromatopsia; photophobia; blurred vision; haloes
- CNS symptoms: headache; lethargy; weakness; delirium; hallucinations; seizures
- Cardiac arrhythmias: ventricular premature beats; ventricular dysrhythmias (ventricular tachycardia; bidirectional ventricular tachycardia; torsades de pointes; ventricular fibrillation); bradyarrhythmias (sinus exit block or sinus arrest; sinus bradycardia; atrioventricular nodal block
- Hyperkalaemia, secondary to blockade of Na-K ATPase

Conditions contributing to digoxin toxicity

- Advanced age
- Chronic kidney disease
- Acute hypoxia
- Hypothyroidism
- Electrolyte disorder: hypokalemia; hypomagnesemia; hypercalcemia
- Respiratory alkalosis
- Drug interactions: slowed clearance (macrolides; quinine); cardioactive medications (beta blockers, calcium channel blockers)

Features of beta blocker toxicity

Cardiovascular
- Bradycardia, related to sino-atrial and atrio ventricular nodal blockade
- Hypotension; cardiogenic shock
- Asystole

Metabolic complications
- Hypoglycaemia
- Hyperkalaemia

Respiratory complications
- Respiratory depression
- Bronchospasm

Central nervous system toxicity
- Confusion
- Seizures
- Coma

Features of calcium channel blocker toxicity

- Bradycardia
- Hypotension; cardiogenic shock
- Hyperglycaemia

Features of acute cyanide toxicity

- CNS: excitement, dizziness, nausea and vomiting, headache, weakness, drowsiness, tetanic spasms, convulsions, hallucinations, loss of consciousness, coma
- Respiratory: shortness of breath, chest tightness
- Metabolic: high anion-gap metabolic acidosis

Club drugs associated with altered mental state

- Ketamine (vitamin K; Special K; Cat Valium)
- Flunitrazepam (Rohypnol; roofies;forget-me-pill; date-rape pill)
- Gamma-hydroxybutyrate (GHB; Grievous Bodily Harm; liquid ecstasy; liquid X, lollypops)
- Gamma-butyrolactone (GBL; Blue Nitro; Firewater; Gamma G; G3)
- Lysergic acid diethylamide (LSD; acid;boomers; yellow sunshines)
- Methamphetamine (meth; crystal; speed; ice; crank;fire; glass)
- Methylenedioxymethamphetamine (MDMA; ecstasy; X; XTC; Adam; Clarity; Lover's Speed)

Plant-induced toxidromes

- Gastrointestinal irritants: daffodil (bulbs); castor bean (seeds); pokeweed (roots and stem); Philodendron (leaves); Wisteria (seeds); laurel (leaves); Diffenbachia (leaves)

- Digitalis effects caused by cardiac glycosides: foxglove, lily-of-the-valley, white oleander, yew, red quill
- Nicotinic effects: poison hemlock (leaves, seeds), wild tobacco (leaves); golden chain tree (seeds)
- Atropinic (anticholinergic) effects: deadly nightshade, burdock, wild tomato, thorn apple (jimson weed)
- Cholinergic effects: physostigmine (Calabar bean)
- Epileptogenic effects: water hemlock
- Cyanogenic effects caused by cyanogenic glycosides: Prunus species (apricot, bitter almonds, wild black cherry, plum, peach); apple (seeds); pear (seeds); elderberry
- Sodium-channel blocking agents

Presentations of mushroom poisoning (usually related to wild mushroom collection by non-specialists)

- Protoplasmic poisons (cyclic octapeptides (amanitins); hydrazines (gyromitrin); orellanine): long latent period of 6–48 h followed by symptoms and irreversible liver, kidney and cardiac failure
- Neurotoxins: muscarine (sweating, salivation, lacrimation); ibotenic acid/muscimol; psilocybin (alcohol intoxication like syndrome)
- Disulfiram-like toxins (antabuse-like symptoms, only with alcohol consumption within 72 h of mushroom ingestion): coprine
- Gastrointestinal irritants: gastroenteritis

Categories of venomous snakes

- Elapidae (tropical and warm temperate zones): cobras, kraits, mambas, coral snakes
- Viperidae: Crotalidae (pit vipers) (North America): rattlesnake, cottonmouth, copperhead; Viperinae (true vipers) (Africa, Europe, Asia): vipers, adders
- Hydrophidae (sea snakes) (Indo-Pacific region): Hydrophinae

Presentations of venomous snake bites
The majority of venomous snake bites are dry, as systemic envenomation occurs in only 10–20% of cases

Local envenomation
- Local tissue damage: immediate pain; progressive swelling; ecchymoses; numbness; painful lymphadenopathy

Tissue-specific signs of systemic envenomation
- Paralytic neurotoxicity: ptosis, ophthalmoplegia, diplopia, dysphagia, dysarthria, drooling of saliva, limb weakness, respiratory muscle paralysis leading to respiratory failure and arrest
- Excitatory neurotoxicity: perioral paraesthesiae, sweating, salivation, piloerection, pulmonary oedema, autonomic storm
- Haemotoxicity: prolonged bleeding from wounds,bite or venipuncture sites; asymptomatic coagulopathy with prolonged INR; haematemesis; melaena; haematuria,
- Myotoxicity: muscle pain and tenderness, weakness, rhabdomyolysis, acute kidney injury

Causes of bites by terrestrial invertebrates
Phylum Arthropoda

Chelicerata
- Spiders
- Scorpions
- Ticks
- Mites

Mandibulata
- Insects
  - Hymenoptera
    - Bees
    - Wasps
    - Hornets
    - Yellow jackets
    - Ants: fire ants

Effects of spider bites

- Neurotoxic: widow spiders (Latrodectes); funnel web spiders (Atrax; Hadranyche); banana skin spiders (Phoneutria)
- Necrotising: violin or recluse spiders (Loxosceles)

Types of venomous marine invertebrates responsible for bites

Toxic marine sponges
Venomous coelenterates (Phylum Cnidaria)
- Hydrozoa: hydra; Portuguese man-of-war
- Scyphozoa: true jellyfish
- Anthozoa: soft corals; stone corals; sea anemones

Venomous echinoderms (Phylum Echinodermata)
- Sea stars or starfish (Asteroidea)
- Sea urchins (Echinoidea)
- Sea cucumbers (Holothuroidea)

Venomous molluscs (Phylum Mollusca)
- Cone shells
- Pteropods
- Cephalopods: octopus, squid, cuttlefish

Venomous sponges (Phylum Porifera)

Features of jellyfish envenomation

- Paraesthesiae; burning or stinging pain; pruritus
- Tentacle marks
- Vesicles; petechiae; urticaria
- Ulceration and necrosis in severe cases

Types of marine vertebrates responsible for bites and other injuries

- Stingrays
- Sharks
- Scorpaenidae family
  Zebrafish
  Scorpion fish
- Catfish

Types of diving emergencies
Barotrauma

- Mask barotrauma (mask squeeze)
- Pulmonary barotrauma: pneumothorax; pneumomediastinum; subcutaneous emphysema
- Otitic barotrauma
  External ear: pain; rupture of tympanic membrane
  Middle ear: middle ear haemorrhage; tympanic membrane rupture
  Inner ear: rupture of the round and oval windows
- Sinus barotrauma: pain; bleeding
- Dental barotrauma
- Gastrointestinal barotrauma

Decompression illness (gas bubble disease)

Features of alcohol intoxication

- Euphoria; behavioural disturbance; incoordination
- Ataxia; poor judgement; labile mood
- Marked ataxia; slurred speech; nausea and vomiting
- Stupor; coma

Risk factors for alcohol withdrawal include:

- Intake >15 units per day
- Previous severe withdrawal; seizures; delirium tremens
- Concomitant use of other psychotropic drugs

Features of alcohol withdrawal

- 6–12 h: autonomic hyperactivity (nausea, anorexia, agitation tremor, sweating, tachycardia, diarrhoea, insomnia)

- 12–24 h: auditory, visual and tactile hallucinations (alcoholic hallucinosis)
- 24–48 h: withdrawal seizures (single short generalized clonic-tonic seizures with short post-ictal period)
- 48–72 h: delirium tremens
- Wernicke's encephalopathy (thiamine deficiency): confusion; memory loss, ataxia and ophthalmoplegia (the triad is only seen in 10% cases)
- Korsakoff's psychosis: memory loss for current and recent events; confabulation

The CIWA (Clinical Institute Withdrawal Assessment Score) allows for scoring the potential for significant alcohol withdrawal based on ten withdrawal signs: nausea and vomiting; tremor; paroxysmal sweats; anxiety; agitation; tactile disturbances; auditory disturbances; visual disturbances; headache; and orientation and clouded sensorium

Features of delirium tremens

- Psychomotor agitation
- Clouded consciousness
- Disorientation
- Mood instability: anxiety, elation
- Autonomic hyperactivity and instability presenting as a hyperadrenergic state: tachycardia; tachypnoea; hyperthermia; excessive sweating; hypertension; tremor
- Illusions; delusions; transient visual (including Lilliputian-with diminutive people or animals), tactile and olfactory hallucinations
- Generalised tonic-clonic seizures
- Sudden cardiovascular collapse

Risk factors for delirium tremens include

- Previous history of delirium tremens
- Previous history of alcohol withdrawal seizures
- Older age
- Abnormal liver function
- Recent higher than normal levels of alcohol intake

Risk factors for Wernicke-Korsakoff psychosis

- Decompensated alcoholic liver disease
- Acute alcohol withdrawal
- Malnutrition; signs of weight loss
- Hospitalisation for concurrent acute illness

Seizures in alcoholic-dependent patient

- Withdrawal: alcohol; other drugs (benzodiazepines; opiates; barbiturates)
- Exacerbation of pre-existing epilepsy
- Acute overdose: alcohol; amphetamines; cocaine; anticholinergic; phenothiazines; tricyclic antidepressants
- Metabolic disorders: hypoglycaemia; hyponatraemia; hypomagnesaemia; hypocalcemia
- CNS disorders: acute head trauma; infections: meningitis, encephalitis; stroke
- Non-compliance with anticonvulsant medication

Causes of acute confusion in alcoholics

- Acute toxicity (alcohol intoxication)
- Acute alcohol withdrawal; delirium tremens; Wernicke's encephalopathy
- Head injury: diffuse; subdural haematoma
- Intracerebral haemorrhage
- Post-ictal folllowing seizure
- Hypoglycaemia
- Hepatic encephalopathy
- Sepsis

Alcohol dependence syndrome

The emergency department may allow for opportunistic screening for alcohol dependence (eg AUDIT-Alcohol Use Disorders Identification Test; CAGE questionnaire), the features of which include:

- A strong desire for, or the subjective awareness of the compulsion to take alcohol
- Repeated physical withdrawal symptoms, such as anxiety, tremor, excesive sweating, agitation, restlessness palpitations, headache, insomnia, nausea and vomiting)
- Increased tolerance to alcohol
- Preoccupation with drinking, associated with progressive neglect of alternative pleasures or interests, which may be social, occupational and recreational
- Stereotyping of pattern of alcohol consumption (narrowing of repertoire)
- Relief drinking to relieve or avoid withdrawal symptoms
- Rapid reinstatement of drinking pattern after a period of abstinence

11 Emergencies in the Elderly

Factors predisposing to falls
General:

- Advancing age
- Female gender
- Environmental hazards
- Previous falls
- Living alone

Physiological/functional

- Muscle weakness
- Impaired balance/gait
- Impaired mobility
- Use of assistive devices
- Sensory abnormality
- Impaired vision
- Impaired activities of daily living

Medical factors

- Number of diagnoses
- Acute illness
- Delirium
- Postural hypotension
- Carotid sinus hypersensitivity
- Cognitive impairment
- Neurological disease: Parkinson's disease/stroke
- Lower limb disease: peripheral neuropathy; peripheral vascular disease
- Depression
- Incontinence

Medication

- Polypharmacy
- Any psychotropic medication
- Sedatives-hypnotics, including benzodiazepines
- Antidepressants
- Digoxin
- Vasodilators
- Analgesics
- Diuretics
- Anti-hypertensives (postural hypotension)

Risk factors for falls in the elderly

- Accidental: environmental hazards (inadequate lighting, slippery floor, uneven carpet, steps, unsuitable footwear, electrical or extension cords, no grab bars, no handrails on stairways; falls from the bed)
- Motor problems
  Gait disturbance: Parkinsonism; cerebellar disorders
  Balance disorder
  Muscle weakness
- Sensory impairment
  - Lower limb proprioception: peripheral neuropathy
  - Vision impairment: glaucoma; cataract; refractive error; macular degeneration; diabetic retinopathy
  - Vestibular dysfunction

A. Banerjee, *Emergency Clinical Diagnosis*, DOI 10.1007/978-3-319-50718-7_11

- Medications/alcohol: sedatives; antidepressants; anti-psychotics; anti-hypertensive medication; polypharmacy (4 or more prescribed medications)
- Confusion and cognitive impairment: dementia; delirium; depression
- Cardiovascular
  - Cardiac arrhythmia
  - Carotid sinus hypersensitivity
  - Postural hypotension
- Pain related to arthritis

Causes of immobility in the elderly

- Musculoskeletal:
  Joints: arthritis (osteoarthritis; rheumatoid arthritis)
  Muscles: polymyalgia, hypothyroidism
  Bones: osteoporosis; osteomalacia; unsuspected fractures (hip, femur)
- Neurological: stroke; Parkinson's disease; peripheral neuropathy; cerebellar dysfunction
- Cardio-pulmonary causes: chronic ischaemic heart disease; COPD; severe heart failure; peripheral vascular disease
- Cognitive, psychological and sensory problems: advanced dementia; depression; fear of falling; pain; impaired vision
- Generalised weakness: malnutrition; neoplasm
- Endocrine-metabolic: electrolyte disorders; hypothyroidism
- Drug side effects
- Reduced effort tolerance: dyspnoea; anaemia
- Foot care disorders: podiatric problems

Causes of hypothermia

- Impaired thermoregulation: stroke; spinal cord injury; encephalopathy
- Reduced heat production: extremes of age; hypoglycaemia; malnutrition; immobilisation; inactivity; endocrine disorders: hypothyroidism, hypopituitarism, adrenal insufficiency
- Increased heat loss: environmental exposure; immersion; burns; exfoliative skin disease; vasodilatation: drug intoxication: alcohol, sedative-hypnotics, narcotics; shock; sepsis; iatrogenic: resuscitation with cold fluids; lack of active external rewarming in acute illness or injury

Risk factors for hypothermia in old age

- Cognitive impairment: dementia
- Chronic debilitating conditions, eg Parkinson's disease; stroke
- Malnutrition and self neglect
- Autonomic impairment
- Hypothalamic dysfunction
- Inadequate clothing
- Inadequate heating and home insulation
- Immobility
- Falls
- Alcohol: acute intoxication; chronic misuse
- Hypothyroidism; hypopituitarism; hypoadrenalism
- Drugs with vasodilator properties
- Socio-economic deprivation

Potential presentations of elder abuse

- Physical abuse: assault with infliction of pain or injury; inappropriate restraint; false imprisonment/confinement; misuse of medication; inadequate monitoring of prescriptions
- Psychological abuse: emotional abuse; threats of harm; threats of stopping care; ignoring
- Financial or material abuse: theft of money, property or other valuables; fraud; coercion regarding wills and any financial transaction
- Sexual abuse: all non-consensual sexual contact of any kind
- Violation of personal rights
- Neglect and acts of omission: depriving food, heating, clothing or essential medication

Historical and physical exam findings suggestive of elder abuse
Historical

- Functional dependence
- Depression
- Dementia (particularly a recent rapid decline in cognitive function)
- History of violence or aggression by either the victim or perpetrator
- Behavioural change
- Inadequate explanation or documentation of any injury

Physical examination

- Unexplained bruising
- Injuries to the trunk, head, and/or anogenital regions
- Evasive or defensive responses
- Malnutrition and dehydration
- Weight loss
- Pressure ulcers
- Genital infections
- Poor general hygiene

Features of senile squalor syndrome (Diogenes syndrome)

- Extreme self-neglect
- Domestic squalor; causes distress to neighbours, social and health professionals; syllogomania (hoarding of rubbish); offensive odour
- Social withdrawal
- Indifference to surroundings
- Inappropriate defaecation
- Normal or high intelligence; usually competent to decide to maintain their lifestyle, and decline offers of support; financial problems are rare

12 Gastrointestinal Emergencies

Causes of dysphagia
Oropharyngeal

- Neurological motility disorder: stroke; movement disorders (Parkinson's disease, progressive supranuclear palsy); amyotrophic lateral sclerosis; multiple sclerosis; bulbar palsy; brainstem tumour; pseudobulbar palsy
- Striated muscle disease: myasthenia gravis; myotonic dystrophy; polymyositis; dermatomyositis; inflammatory myopathy; muscular dystrophy
- Reduced salivary flow leading to dry mouth (xerostomia): Sjogren's syndrome; anticholinergics; antihistamines; ACE inhibitors; alpha-adrenergic blockers
- Structural lesions: inflammatory: pharyngitis, tonsillar abscess; head and neck tumours; pharyngeal diverticula; ulcerative stomatitis; painful glossitis; anterior marginal cervical osteophytes (especially with diffuse idiopathic skeletal hyperostosis)
- Metabolic: hypothyroidism; hyperthyroidism; steroid myopathy

Oesophageal

- Solids & liquids (neuromuscular motility disorders)
  Progressive: scleroderma; achalasia (progressive dysphagia for both solids and liquids; regurgitation of undigested food and saliva; chest pain; nocturnal cough and aspiration; minimal or no weight loss)
  Intermittent: diffuse oesophageal spasm; presby-esophagus (nutcracker oesophagus)
- Solids only (mechanical obstruction)
  Intermittent: lower oesophageal ring (Schatzki's ring); hypertensive lower oesophageal sphincter
  Progressive: peptic stricture (acid reflux due to gastro-oesophageal reflux disease); oesophageal cancer (progressive dysphagia, odynophagia, regurgitation, chest pain, weight loss, hoarseness of voice); foreign body impaction

Causes of mechanical obstruction

- Strictures
  Benign (peptic): reflux oesophagitis
  Malignant: carcinoma of oesophagus or gastric cardia
- Extrinsic compression: bronchial carcinoma; mediastinal lymph nodes; vascular compression; cervical osteoarthritis with vertebral osteophytes; mediastinal tumours
- Oesophageal web
- Foreign bodies (especially with pre-existing gastrointestinal abnormalities, such as diverticula, webs, rings): food bolus impaction; disc or button battery; coin (oesophageal coins are seen in a coronal alignment on an AP xray); toy parts, marbles

A. Banerjee, *Emergency Clinical Diagnosis*, DOI 10.1007/978-3-319-50718-7_12

- Extrinsic compression: goitre with retrosternal extension; mediastinal tumours; large left atrium

Odynophagia

- Oesophagitis: infective (candidal; herpetic; cytomegalovirus); pill-induced (associated with oesophageal dysmotility, stricture or extrinsic compression) (tetracycline, doxycycline; potassium chloride; NSAIDs, aspirin; alendronate); corrosive (caustic ingestion); radiation induced
- Oesophageal ulcer

Dysphagia checklist

- Evidence of weight loss
- Anaemia
- Hoarseness of voice
- Oral ulceration; signs of candidiasis
- Cervical lymphadenopathy
- Bulbar signs
- Chest signs

Features of caustic ingestion

- Oedema of the lips, tongue and palate
- Oropharyngeal burns
- Drooling of saliva
- Dysphagia
- Nausea and vomiting
- Haematemesis
- Shortness of breath
- Stridor
- Abdominal pain

Features of neurogenic dysphagia

- Drooling of saliva
- Difficulty in initiating swallowing
- Nasal regurgitation
- Choking or coughing while feeding
- Food sticking in the throat
- Nasal tone to speech
- Aspiration, with recurrent pneumonia

Features of oropharyngeal dysphagia

- Solids handled better than liquids
- Difficulty initiating swallowing
- Cough and choking during and after swallowing
- Nasal regurgitation of liquids
- Hesitancy and repeated attempts at the inititation of swallowing
- Food sticking in throat
- Nasal speech
- Changes in the character of the voice
- Constant drooling of saliva

Features of oesophageal dysphagia

- Sensation of food sticking in chest or throat after swallowing
- Recurrent pneumonia
- Gastro-oesophageal reflux disease: heartburn; belching; sour regurgitation; waterbrash

Red flags for dysphagia

- Progressive painless dysphagia
- Unintentional weight loss
- Persistent vomiting
- Haematemesis
- Hoarseness of voice
- Systemic symptoms: fever, night sweats
- Bulbar neurological signs
- Cervical lymphadenopathy

Risk factors for oesophageal cancer

- Age >70 years
- Smoking
- Alcohol consumption (SCC)
- Dietary factors
- Barrett oesophagus
- Gastro-oesophageal reflux disease (adenocarcinoma)
- Excessive ingestion of very hot liquids (SCC)
- Caustic ingestion (SCC)
- Achalasia (SCC)
- Plummer-Vinson syndrome (SCC)

Dysphagia evaluation checklist

- All: FBC, U&E, LFTs, bone profile, CXR (mediastinal widening, absence of gastric air bubble, extrinsic mass)
- Oropharyngeal: direct laryngoscopy; video fluoroscopy
- Oesophageal: endoscopy; barium swallow; oesophageal manometry

Possible presentations of gastro-oesophageal reflux disease

- Gastrointestinal: heartburn; regurgitation; waterbrash; globus sensation of lump in neck or throat; dysphagia (erosive oesophagitis; peptic stricture (intermittent solid food dysphagia in a patient with heartburn); adenocarcinoma of oesophagus); odynophagia; hiccups; epigastric pain, dyspepsia; vomiting; erosion of dental enamel
- Pulmonary: chronic nocturnal cough; asthma; sleep apnoea; aspiration; recurrent pneumonia; interstitial pulmonary fibrosis; acute life-threatening episodes
- ENT: sore throat; hoarseness; laryngitis; chronic sinusitis; vocal cord granulomas; sub-glottic stenosis
- Atypical chest pain
- Dystonic movements: Sandifer's syndrome (gastro-oesophageal reflux associated with torsional dystonia of the head, neck, eyes and trunk, and opithostonic posturing)

Risk factors for gastro-oesophageal reflux

- Smoking
- Alcohol ingestion
- Obesity
- Drugs: NSAIDs; calcium channel blockers; nitrates; benzodiazepines
- Systemic disease: diabetes mellitus with autonomic neuropathy; scleroderma
- Sleep apnoea

Causes of odynophagia

- Infectious oesophagitis
- Gastrooesophageal reflux/stricture
- Pill-induced ulceration
- Radiation oesophagitis
- Caustic stricture
- Foreign body
- Cancer

Causes of infective oesophagitis

- Fungal infections: candida albicans
  Risk factors
  Immunocompromised: HIV infection; transplant recipient; immunosuppressive therapy
  Immunocompetent: prolonged antibiotic therapy; acid suppressive therapy; oesophageal motility disorders; diabetes mellitus; head and neck radiation therapy
- Viral infections: herpes simplex; cytomegalovirus; Epstein-Barr virus
- Bacterial infections
- Protozoal infections

Abdominal pain mechanisms

Peritoneal irritation
Visceral obstruction
Visceral ischaemia
Visceral inflammation
Abdominal wall pain
Referred pain

Patterns of abdominal pain

Parietal: irritation of parietal peritoneum

- Pain in dermatome distribution
- Well localised
- Sharp
- Clear onset

Visceral: stretch, distension, contraction (spasm), compression or torsion of a hollow viscus

- Referred pain in embryonic distribution
- Poor localisation
- Dull and aching
- Insidious onset

Referred

Dermatomal perception of visceral pain

Organ	Site of pain	Dermatomes
Stomach	Epigastrium	T6-T10
Small bowel	Umbilical	T9-T10
Gallbladder	Epigastrium	T7-T9
Pancreas	Epigastrium	T6-T10
Colon up to splenic flexure	Umbilical	T11-L1
Colon from splenic flexure	Hypogastrium	L1-L2
Testis and ovary	Umbilical	T10-T11

Causes of abdominal pain (the site of origin of pain may be related to the source of the underlying causative pathology)

Diffuse pain

- Aortic aneurysm: leaking; ruptured
- Aortic dissection
- Early appendicitis
- Bowel obstruction
- Diabetic gastric paresis; diabetic ketoacidosis
- Gastroenteritis (vomiting precedes abdominal pain)
- Heavy metal poisoning
- Hereditary angioedema
- Mesenteric ischaemia
- Volvulus
- Metabolic disorder: Addisonian crisis, ketoacidosis (diabetic, alcoholic), acute intermittent porphyria (attacks of severe diffuse abdominal pain, associated with nausea and vomiting, constipation, muscle weakness, urine retention, and sometimes confusion, hallucinations and seizures; increased urine delta-aminolaevulinic acid and porphobilinogen; atatcks may be precipitated by hormonal changes, drugs, reduced calorie intake, alcohol, and emotional stress), uraemia
- Opioid withdrawal
- Pancreatitis
- Perforated bowel
- Peritonitis from any cause
- Sickle cell crisis
- Malaria
- Familial Mediterranean Fever

Abdominal wall pain (Carnett sign: pain is increased on tensing abdominal wall by lifting head and shoulders off the examination table while supine)

- Spiegelian, incisional hernia
- Rectus sheath haematoma (abdominal wall mass with bruising; risk factors include old age, anticoagulant therapy, trauma, injection procedures, physical exercise, and raised intra-abdominal pressure fro coughing, sneezing or vomiting)
- Muscle strain

Right upper quadrant pain

- Biliary disease: Biliary colic; acute cholecystitis (Murphy's sign of inspiratory arrest due to pain on inspiration during right subcostal palpation with hand or ultrasound probe; jaundice in 20–25% cases); choledocholithiasis, cholangitis
- Hepatic disease: acute hepatitis; liver abscess; hepatic congestion; liver tumour
- Perihepatitis (Fitzhugh-Curtis syndrome): may be associated with signs of salpingitis
- High retrocaecal appendicitis; appendicitis complicating pregnancy
- Perforated duodenal ulcer
- Perinephritis
- Pulmonary: right lower lobe pneumonia; pleuritis; pulmonary embolism; empyema
- Myocardial ischaemia
- Herpes zoster

Causes of tender palpable right subcostal mass

Empyema of gallbladder (suppurative cholecystistis).

Gall bladder perforation with abscess

Omental phlegmon

Carcinoma of the gall bladder

Risk factors for cholesterol gallstones
Increased bile cholesterol concentration

- Increasing age
- Female gender
- Obesity
- Pregnancy and multiparity
- Rapid weight loss (>1.5 kg/week), including during treatment for morbid obesity
- Hypertriglyceridaemia
- Low LDL cholesterol
- Diabetes mellitus
- Drugs: oestrogens, octreotide, ceftriaxone

Reduced bile acid pool

- Ileal disease (Crohn's disease; terminal ileal resection/ bypass)
- Primary biliary cirrhosis

Hepato-biliary causes of right upper quadrant pain in pregnancy
Not unique to pregnancy

- Viral hepatitis
- Budd-Chiari syndrome
- Hepatic malignancy
- Biliary colic
- Choledocholithiasis
- Cholangitis
- Cholecystitis

Unique to, or highly associated with, pregnancy

- Pre-eclampsia or eclampsia
- HELLP (haemolysis, elevated liver enzymes and low platelet count) syndrome (third trimester)
- Acute fatty liver of pregnancy
- Hepatic haemorrhage or rupture
- Symptomatic choledochal cysts

Left upper quadrant pain

- Splenic: splenic rupture/distension; splenic infarction; splenomegaly (spontaneous splenic rupture can present with referred left shoulder pain from diaphragmatic irritation-Kehr's sign, and a tender left upper quadrant mass-Ballance's sign, and is associated with infections (infectious mononucleosis and malaria) and haematological malignancy (lymphoma and leukaemia)
- Ruptured splenic artery aneurysm
- Gastritis
- Perforated gastric ulcer
- Jejunal diverticulitis; diverticulitis affecting the splenic flexure
- Pancreatitis
- Pulmonary: left lower lobe pneumonia; pleuritis; empyema
- Cardiac: pericarditis; myocardial ischaemia
- Herpes zoster

Right lower quadrant pain

- Colonic: acute appendicitis; acute enterocolitis; caecal diverticulitis; colonic obstruction; torsion of appendices epiploicae; epiploic appendagitis
- Small bowel: Crohn's disease (terminal ileitis); Meckel's diverticulitis; small bowel obstruction; intusussception (triad of vomiting, abdominal pain and currant jelly stools)
- Foreign body perforation
- Mesenteric adenitis
- Perforated peptic ulcer
- Gynaecological: ovarian cyst accident (including mittelschmerz)- rupture, torsion; endometriosis; pelvic inflammatory disease(salpingitis); ectopic pregnancy
- Cholecystitis
- Vascular: aortic aneurysm: leaking; ruptured; ruptured iliac artery aneurysm
- Renal: renal/ureteric colic; pyelonephritis
- Psoas abscess
- Inguinal hernia: incarcerated; strangulated
- Testicular torsion
- Seminal vesiculitis
- Rectus sheath haematoma
- Herpes zoster

Left lower quadrant pain

- Colonic: diverticulitis (sigmoid); acute appendicitis (with situs inversus); perforated colonic cancer; Crohn's colitis; ischaemic colitis; colonic obstruction

- Vascular: aortic aneurysm: leaking; ruptured; ruptured iliac artery aneurysm
- Gynaecological: ovarian cyst accident (including mittelschmerz),-torsion, rupture); endometriosis;pelvic inflammatory disease(salpingitis); ectopic pregnancy
- Renal: renal/ureteric colic; pyelonephritis
- Psoas abscess
- Testicular torsion
- Inguinal hernia: incarcerated; strangulated
- Seminal vesiculitis
- Rectus sheath haematoma
- Herpes zoster

Potential causes of non-specific abdominal pain (diagnosis of exclusion)

- Viral infection
- Parasitic infestation
- Gastroenteritis
- Mesenteric adenitis
- Ovulatory pain
- Lesions of appendices epiploicae of colon

Medical causes of acute abdominal pain

- Intra-thoracic: inferior ST elevation myocardial infarction; pericarditis; lower lobe pneumonia; pulmonary embolism; oesophageal disease
- Endocrine/ metabolic: diabetic ketoacidosis; acute adrenocortical insufficiency; acute intermittent porphyria; hyperlipidaemia; Familial Mediterranean Fever
- Drug induced: opioid withdrawal; lead poisoning
- Haematological: sickle cell crisis; acute leukaemia
- Central nervous system: pre-eruptive phase of herpes zoster; spinal nerve root compression

Causes of peritonitis

- Hollow viscus perforation: stomach (gastric ulcer; gastric cancer); duodenum (duodenal ulcer); small bowel (mesenteric ischaemia and infarction); colon (divericulitis; cancer; inflammatory bowel disease); appendix (appendicitis); gallbladder (cholecystitis)
- Abdominal trauma: blunt; penetrating
- Foreign body ingestion
- Anastomotic leakage
- Spontaneous bacterial peritonitis: ascites from portal hypertension; nephrotic syndrome
- Pelvic inflammatory disease

Abdominal pain evaluation
History
SOCRATES to characterize pain (allow the patient to describe the pain initially without any leading questions)

- Site and duration
- Onset: sudden versus gradual; sudden onset suggests a vascular emergency (mesenteric ischaemia; ruptured abdominal aortic aneurysm), volvulus, intestinal perforation or torsion of hollow viscus
- Character: sharp, dull, aching, colicky, burning
- Radiation: shoulder, back, groin or testicle
- Timing: intermittent, constant
- Exacerbating (aggravating factors): movement (worsens pain in peritonitis), position, food, medications, and alleviating factors: rest.
- Severity

Associated symptoms: fever; nausea and vomiting; diarrhoea/constipation; haematemesis/ melaena; fresh rectal bleeding; dysuria/ haematuria
Physical examination checklist

- Vital signs; tachypnoea may be related to metabolic acidosis, hypoxaemia, or catecholamine-induced pain response; signs of hypovolaemia: tachycardia, postural hypotension
- Localisation of maximal tenderness and guarding
- Signs of peritonitis: tenderness, guarding (abdominal wall rigidity), percussion tenderness, rebound tenderness (gentle depression of the abdominal wall for 15 to 30 minutes, followed by sudden release of pressure), generalised ileus, fever

- Specific signs: Carnett's sign: increased pain on tensing abdominal wall when a supine patient lifts the head and shoulders off the bed; Murphy's sign: inspiratory arrest on deep palpation of right upper quadrant; psoas sign (passive hip extension is painful, with the patient in the lateral decubitus position); Rovsing's sign (pressure in the left lower quadrant produces rebound pain in the right lower quadrant on release of the pressure); obturator sign (flexion with external and internal rotation of the hip is painful)
- Abdominal mass
- Aortic tenderness or enlargement (bedside ultrasound may be useful)
- Hernial orifices
- External genitalia
- Bowel sounds: absent; normal; hyperactive; tinkling
- Rectal examination
- Bimanual pelvic examination

Special considerations with assessment of acute abdominal pain in the elderly

- Difficulty in obtaining a history caused by impaired cognitive function (eg dementia)
- Atypical presentations
- Lack of typical clinical findings (eg peritonitis without peritonism)
- Multiple co-morbidities
- Medications that block physiological responses leading to difficulty in assessment (eg beta-blockers)
- Decreased immune function, leading to increased severity of disease

Causes of acute abdominal pain and shock (indicative of hypovolaemia and/or sepsis)

- Perforated hollow viscus: perforated peptic ulcer
- Massive haemorrhage: spontaneous splenic rupture; leaking abdominal aortic aneurysm; ruptured ectopic pregnancy
- Acute arterial occlusion: mesenteric accident (superior mesenteric artery embolism/thrombosis, mesenteric venous thrombosis, non-occlusive mesenteric ischaemia); strangulation obstruction
- Third space losses of fluid: acute pancreatitis
- Cardiac: acute inferior STEMI

Causes of haemoperitoneum

- Trauma: penetrating; blunt (liver, spleen)
- Vascular accident: ruptured aneurysm of abdominal aorta, splenic artery, or iliac artery
- Gynaecological: ruptured ectopic pregnancy; ruptured ovarian cyst (follicular cyst; endometriotic cyst)
- Ruptured intra-abdominal neoplasm: hepatocellular carcinoma; hepatic adenoma; pelvic tumours (malignant ovarian masses; uterine sarcomas)
- Spontaneous rupture of spleen
- Anticoagulant therapy

Causes of referred abdominal pain

- Cardiac: inferior STEMI; congestive heart failure with hepatic congestion
- Pulmonary: lower lobe pneumonia; pulmonary embolism

Presentations of ruptured abdominal aortic aneurysm (infra-renal aortic diameter 3 cm or more)

- Triad of abdominal, flank or back pain, acute hypotension and pulsatile abdominal mass; a tender aneurysmal mass is indicative of an aortic emergency
- Ureteric colic
- Rupture into inferior vena cava (aorto-caval fistula): high-output congestive heart failure
- Rupture into duodenum (aorto-duodenal fistula): upper gastrointestinal bleeding
- Acute testicular pain and bruising
- Inguinoscrotal mass mimicking hernia
- Rupture into left renal vein: massive haematuria
- Iliofemoral venous thrombosis from ilio-caval compression

- Acute lower limb ischaemia
- Chronic contained rupture, with lumbar neuropathy

Other potential presentation of abdominal aortic aneurysm:

- Duodenal compression
- Hydronephrosis
- Ureteric obstruction and renal pain
- Thrombo-embolic phenomena: femoral; popliteal; microemboli(trash foot: tip necrosis of toes; small punctate pretibial ischaemic lesions
- Acute thrombosis, resembling saddle embolus

Bedside ultrasound diagnosis of abdominal aortic aneurysm
Abdominal aortic aneurysm is dilatation of the aorta greater than 3 cm or 1.5 times the normal diameter for that person

Maximum aortic diameters at different levels

- Level of diaphragm 2.5 cm
- Level of renal arteries 2 cm
- Bifurcation 1.5–2 cm
- Iliac arteries just distal to the bifurcation 1 cm

Atypical presentations of acute appendicitis

- Acute right upper quadrant or loin pain: retro-caecal or retro-colic appendicitis
- Gastroenteritis: diarrhea and vomiting: pre-and post-ileal appendicitis
- Acute right lower quadrant pain with psoas irritation
- Acute small bowel obstruction
- Dysuria and pyuria; microscopic haematuria: sub-caecal and pelvic appendicitis

Alvarado Score (MANTRELS) for diagnosis of acute appendicitis
SYMPTOMS

Migration of pain to the right lower quadrant = 1
Anorexia = 1
Nausea or vomiting = 1

SIGNS

Tenderness in the right lower quadrant = 2
Rebound tenderness = 1
Elevated temperature: fever of 37.3 C or more = 1

LABORATORY TESTS

Leukocytosis >10,000 white blood cells per microlitre in the serum = 2
Left shift of leukocytes = 1

Total = 10

Score
5 or 6: Compatible with the diagnosis of acute appendicitis
7 or 8: Probable appendicitis
9 or 10: Very probable acute appendicitis

Investigations for abdominal pain

- Venous blood: full blood count, urea and electrolytes, CRP, liver function tests (right upper quadrant pain), amylase/lipase, glucose; blood gas analysis
- 12 lead ECG
- Ultrasound/CT
- Urine dipstick
- Urine beta-HCG (all women of child bearing age)

Red flags for abdominal pain

Severe pain
Signs of shock
Abdominal distension
Signs of peritonitis
Failed initial treatment
Haemodynamic disturbance

Causes of loin pain

- Renal: pyelonephritis; calculus; neoplasm; infected obstructed kidney; abscess; infarction; pelvi-ureteric obstruction
- Aortic: leaking aneurysm; dissection
- Radiculopathy

- Muscle strain
- Herpes zoster
- Retroperitoneal fibrosis

Causes of hyperamylasemia (rises 2–12 h after initiating insult, and remains elevated 3–5 days).
Pancreatic causes

- Acute pancreatitis; acute exacerbation of chronic pancreatitis
- Pancreatic cancer

Non-pancreatic intra-abdominal emergencies

- Ruptured ectopic pregnancy
- Peritonitis
- Perforated hollow viscus (peptic ulcer disease with perforation
- Intestinal obstruction
- Mesenteric ischaemia/infarction
- Biliary tract disease; acute cholecystitis; choledocholiathiasis
- Aortic dissection
- Acute appendicitis
- Acute salpingitis

Miscellaneous

- Salivary gland disease
- Pregnancy
- Tumour
- Burns
- Renal disease: chronic kidney disease
- Diabetes ketoacidosis
- Macroamylasaemia

Features of acute pancreatitis

- Sudden onset of upper abdominal pain, radiating to the mid-thoracic area of the back; continuous, severe, reduced on sitting up or leaning forwards
- Nausea and vomiting
- Upper abdominal distension
- Low grade fever (high fever indicates infected pancreatic necrosis or coexistent cholangitis)
- Epigastric tenderness
- Paralytic ileus, with absent bowel sounds
- Intravascular volume depletion due to retroperitoneal fluid loss: hypovolaemic shock
- Ecchymoses around the umbilicus and in the flanks, associated with severe haemorrhagic pancreatitis
- Signs of peritoneal irritation
- Painless pancreatitis can be seen in patients undergoing peritoneal dialysis or following renal transplantation
- Serum amylase or lipase is at least three times greater than the upper limit of normal. Lower diagnostic levels are associated with delayed presentation and with relapsing acute pancreatitis, where there is loss of pancreatic exocrine cell mass; lipase is a preferable investigation. The absolute level does not correlate with severity of the underlying disease.

Causes of acute pancreatitis
Toxic/metabolic
- Chronic alcohol abuse
- Toxic alcohols
- Metabolic: hypertriglyceridaemia; hypercalcaemia
- Toxins: scorpion venom; snake venom

Obstructive causes (biliary tract disease)
- Gallstones; ampullary obstruction (carcinoma, adenoma, peri-ampullary diverticulum)
- Structural abnormalities: choledochocele; pancreas divisum; annular pancreas

Abdominal trauma: penetrating/blunt (bicycle handlebar injury to upper abdomen)
Penetrating peptic ulcer
Drugs: thiazide diuretics; glucocorticoids; immunosuppressants (azathioprine, 6-mercaptopurine); oestrogens; gliptins; anti-epileptic drugs (valproate)
Necrotising vasculitis: systemic lupus erythematosus, thrombotic thrombocytopenic purpura
Infections: viral (mumps; cytomegalovirus; Epstein-Barr virus; varicella-zoster virus); bacterial (mycobacteria); parasitic (Ascaris lumbricoides; liver flukes-Clonorchis sinensis; Fasciola hepatica)

Eating disorders: anorexia; bulimia
Iatrogenic: post-ERCP; post-sphincterotomy
Hereditary
Idiopathic

Adverse prognostic features on admission with acute pancreatitis (modified Glasgow criteria)

- Age >55 years
- Pa02 on room air <8 kPa
- White cell count >15,000/cu mm
- Glucose >10.0 mmol/L
- Serum calcium <2.0 mmol/L
- Serum albumin <32 g/dl
- Enzymes: aspartate transaminase >250 IU/L; lactate dehydrogenase >600 IU/L
- Serum urea nitrogen >16.1 mmol/L

Causes of mesenteric ischaemia
Occlusive

- Arterial: embolism (cardiac or aortic emboli-usually from mural thrombus in left atrium or left ventricle); thrombosis (atherosclerosis; aortic aneurysm; aortic dissection)
- Venous: thrombosis-hypercoagulable states (neoplasm, oral contraceptive pill, thrombophilia, thrombocytosis, polycythaemia vera); intra-abdominal sepsis with portal pyaemia; pancreatitis; malignancy; portal hypertension
- Strangulation: adhesive band; volvulus; internal hernia; intusussception

Non-occlusive: low-flow states with hypotension (congestive heart failure, cardiogenic shock, septic shock); vasopressor therapy; drug-induced mesenteric vasoconstriction (cocaine, alpha-agonists, beta blockers, ergotamines).

Features of mesenteric ischaemia

- Age usually over 60 years
- Sudden onset of severe diffuse abdominal pain out of proportion to findings on physical examination and unresponsive to opiate analgesia
- Nausea, vomiting, diarrhoea ("gut emptying")
- Later development of peritoneal signs secondary to generalized peritonitis associated with bowel infarction
- Gastrointestinal bleeding
- A preceding history of post-prandial abdominal discomfort (abdominal angina), food avoidance and weight loss may indicate pre-existing chronic mesenteric ischaemia, with superimposed thrombosis. Typically, abdominal discomfort occurs 10–15 min after eating, and lasts from one to 4 h.
- Leukocytosis
- Metabolic acidosis with high anion gap and elevated venous lactate

Risk factors for mesenteric arterial embolism

- Cardiac arrhythmias: atrial fibrillation; atrial flutter
- Post-myocardial infarction: mural thrombus; ventricular aneurysm
- Valvular heart disease: mitral stenosis; infective endocarditis
- Structural heart defects: right-to-left intracardiac shunts
- Dilated cardiomyopathy
- Iatrogenic: post-angiography or endovascular procedures

Acute gastroenteritis syndromes (triad of diarrhea, vomiting and fever).
Bloody diarrhoea

- Invasive bacterial pathogens: Salmonella enterica serotypes; Campylobacter jejuni; Shigella; Entero-invasive Escherichia coli; Entero-haemorrhagic E. coli; Yersinia enterocolitica; Clostridium difficile
- Protozoal: Entamoeba histolytica; Balantidium coli
- Miscellaneous: Schistosoma mansoni; Trichuris trichiura

Acute watery diarrhoea

- Viruses: rotavirus; enteric adenoviruses; calciciviruses; astroviruses; coronaviruses; Norwalk agent

- Preformed bacterial toxin (symptoms within 6 hours of ingestion): Salmonella enterica serotypes; Campylobacter jejuni; Entero-pathogenic Escherichia coli; Entero-toxigenic E.coli; Entero-aggregative E.coli; Vibrio cholerae; Vibrio parahaemolyticus; Clostridium difficile; Staphylococcus aureus(toxin b); Bacillus cereus; Yersinia enterocolitica
- Protozoa: Giardia lamblia; Cryptosporidium parvum; Isospora belli; Cyclospora cayetanensis; Dientamoeba fragilis; Entamoeba histolytica
- Non-infective: food allergy/intolerance (cow's milk protein intolerance; lactose intolerance); chemotherapy/ radiation therapy

Persistent diarrhoea

- Viruses: recurrent infections with rotavirus
- Bacteria: Mycobacterium tuberculosis; recurrent and relapsing infections with other bacterial pathogens
- Protozoa: Giardia lamblia; Entamoeba histolytica; Cryptosporidium parvum; Isospora belli; Cyclospora cayetanensis
- Miscellaneous: post-infectious irritable bowel syndrome; disaccharidase deficiency

Mechanisms of infective diarrhoea

- Non-inflammatory, or secretory, diarrhoea
- Viral infections: Rotavirus, Norwalk agent, astrovirus
  - Vibrio cholerae
  - Preformed toxins: Staphylococcus aureus, Bacillus cereus
  - Parasites: Giardia lamblia, Cryptosporidium parvum, Isospora belli
  - Inflammatory diarrhea (dysenteric syndromes) (small volume bloody diarrhea, lower abdominal cramps, faecal urgency, tenesmus, fever)
- Bacterial dysentery: Shigella, Salmonella, Escherichia coli 0157, Campylobacter
- Amoebic dysentery
- Invasive gastrointestinal infections (enteric fever syndromes)

Potential sources of food poisoning

- Campylobacter: raw or undercooked meat (especially poultry); unpasteurised milk; untreated water
- Salmonella: raw or undercooked meat; raw eggs, milk, and other dairy products
- Listeria: chilled "ready-to-eat" foods, including cooked sliced meats and pate, soft cheeses (Brie, Camembert, feta); and pre-packed sandwiches
- Escherichia coli: undercooked beef (especially mince, burgers, meatballs); unpasteurised milk; contaminated raw leaf green vegetables
- Bacillus cereus: fried rice dishes sitting at room temperature (eg in a buffet)
- Vibrio cholerae and vibrio parahaemolyticus: contaminated water; undercooked seafood (fish and shellfish)
- Norovirus: person-to-person spread, through contaminated food or water; raw shellfish (especially oysters)

Risk factors for complications following acute gastroenteritis

- Age 60 years or older
- Pregnancy
- Co-morbidities: immunosuppression; chronic kidney disease; inflammatory bowel disease; diabetes mellitus; connective tissue diseases; gastric achlorhydria (proton pump inhibitor or histamine 2 receptor antagonist treatment)

Causes of blood in the stool associated with diarrhoea

Infectious colitis

- Campylobacter
- Escherichia coli 0157
- Shigella
- Salmonella

Inflammatory bowel disease

- Ulcerative colitis (severity can be graded by Truelove and Witts' severity index into mild, moderate and severe)
- Crohn's disease

Risk factors for infectious colitis

- Antimicrobial therapy: broad spectrum antibiotics
- Immunodeficiency: HIV; cancer chemotherapy
- Enteropathogen exposure: travel to the developing world; food and water contamination; water sports
- Extremes of age: infancy; elderly
- Gastric achlorhydria; proton pump inhibitor therapy

Acute presentations of inflammatory bowel disease

- Bloody diarrhoea
- Acute right lower quadrant abdominal pain
- Lower gastrointestinal bleeding
- Acute small bowel or large bowel obstruction
- Bowel perforation; intra-abdominal abscess
- Toxic megacolon: a life-threatening complication with systemic toxicity; abdominal distension; bloody diarrhoea; signs of peritonitis; septic shock; acute dilatation of the colon (usually transverse colon) to a diameter of 6 cm or greater, with loss of haustral markings, thumbprinting from haustral thickening at regular intervals (caused by mucosal oedema) and pseudopolyps
- Perianal disease: abscess; fistula; fissure (wide, deep, with undermined edges, multiple, often lateral to the midline)
- Extra-intestinal manifestations: erythema nodosum; acute red eye (iritis, episcleritis); acute arthritis; pyoderma gangrenosum

Criteria for severe ulcerative colitis

- More than 6 bowel movements per day
- Temperature >37.8 degrees Centigrade
- Heart rate >90 beats per minute
- Haemoglobin <10.5 g/dl
- ESR >30 mm/hour

Causes of toxic megacolon

- Inflammatory bowel disease: ulcerative colitis; Crohn's disease
- Infectious colitis: bacterial (Clostridium difficile; Salmonella; Shigella; Campylobacter; Yersinia; Pseudomonas); viral (cytomegalovirus); parasitic (amoebic colitis; Cryptosporidium)
- Ischaemic colitis
- Obstructing colon cancer

Risk factors for clostridium difficile colitis

- Age >65 years
- Antibiotic therapy: clindamycin; cephalosporins, fluoroquinolones
- Immunosuppression
- Gastric acid suppression: proton pump inhibitors; H2-receptor blockers
- Gastrointestinal tract surgery
- Colonic disease: colorectal cancer; inflammatory bowel disease
- Previous Clostridium difficile infection
- Chemotherapy for haematological and solid organ malignancy

Causes of Traveller's diarrhoea

- Gram negative bacilli: Enterotoxigenic Escherichia coli; Salmonella species; Shigella species
- Curved motile Gram negative bacilli: Vibrio species; Campylobacter species; Plesiomonas shigelloides; Aeromonas hydrophila
- Protozoa: Entamoeba histolytica; Giardia lamblia; Cryptosporidium
- Viruses: Norwalk agent

Mechanisms of diarrhoea

Osmotic (high osmotic load of intraluminal content)

- Lactase deficiency
- Disaccharidase deficiencies
- Magnesium induced
- Short bowel
- Extensive mucosal disease: celiac disease; Crohn's disease
- Bile salt malabsorption
- Pancreatic insufficiency
- Drugs, eg lactulose

Secretory (active chloride secretion)

- Toxins: cholera; clostridium
- Excess gut hormones
- Stimulant laxatives
- Bacterial overgrowth
- Inflammatory bowel disease
- Diabetic neuropathy
- Villous adenoma of the rectum
- Carcinoma of the rectum
- Neural crest tumours, eg carcinoid, VIPoma

Dysmotility

- Functional bowel disease
- Endocrine disorders
- Autonomic neuropathies

Inflammatory

- Infections
- Inflammatory bowel disease
- Ischaemic bowel disease

Diarrhoea and vomiting checklist

- The presence of blood in the stool indicates an invasive infection
- Volume of stool: large volume watery diarrhea, diffuse abdominal cramps, bloating and borborygmi (bowel sounds audible at a distance) indicate small bowel disease, while small volume bloody diarrhea with lower abdominal cramping and tenesmus (sensation of incomplete bowel evacuation) indicates large bowel disease
- Travel history
- Exposure history: exposure to a known source of enteric infection (contaminated food or water)-eating meals out, farm visit; contacts who are ill
- Ingestion of specific dietary items during food-borne outbreaks: dairy products; eggs; chicken; seafood
- Recent hospitalization or antimicrobial use: consider Clostridium difficile
- Risk factors for HIV infection and other co-morbid illnesses resulting in immunosuppression, including cancer chemotherapy, will lead to a wider differential diagnosis

Causes of flushing and diarrhoea

- Anxiety attacks
- Diabetic autonomic neuropathy
- Thyrotoxicosis
- Carcinoid syndrome
- Phaeochromocytoma
- Systemic mastocytosis

Causes of faecal incontinence (involuntary loss of solid or liquid faeces of flatus)

- Constipation; faecal impaction with overflow incontinence
- Diarrhoea: gastroenteritis; inflammatory bowel disease; irritable bowel syndrome
- Obstetric injury to the pelvic floor: instrumental vaginal delivery; third degree perineal tear with sphincter involvement; prolonged second stage of labour; large baby; occipito-posterior presentation
- Post-gastrointestinal surgery: colectomy with ileoanal anastomosis; internal anal sphincterotomy for chronic anal fissure; haemorrhoidectomy; anal dilatation
- Neurological causes: spinal cord injury; multiple sclerosis; spina bifida; stroke
- Post radiation for pelvic cancer
- Congenital anorectal anomalies

Causes of constipation
Features:

- Hard pellet-like stools
- Infrequent defaecation
- Excessive straining at stool with difficulty in evacuation (dyschezia)

Dietary factors: insufficient dietary fibre (low residue diet); insufficient fluid intake (dehydration).
Motility disorders: irritable bowel syndrome; idiopathic slow transit
Drugs:

- Aluminium- and calcium- containing antacids
- Tricyclic antidepressants
- Anti-cholinergic agents: amitriptyline
- Iron supplements
- Opioid analgesics: codeine, dihydrocodeine, morphine
- Lead poisoning
- Long-term laxative abuse
- Anti-Parkinsonian agents
- Phenothiazines
- Diuretics
- Calcium channel blockers: verapamil
- Beta blockers
- Calcium supplements

Metabolic/endocrine diseases:

- Hypercalcemia; hypomagnesemia
- Diabetic autonomic neuropathy
- Hypothyroidism
- Hypokalemia
- Uraemia

Anorectal disease:

- Painful anal conditions: anal fissure; anorectal abscess; thrombosed haemorrhoids; proctitis
- Pelvic outlet syndrome

Colonic obstruction

- Colorectal carcinoma
- Benign colonic stricture (diverticular; ischaemic)
- Myenteric plexus aganglionosis-Hirschsprung's disease(congenital); Chagas disease(acquired)
- Chronic intestinal pseudo-obstruction
- Faecal impaction

Neurological conditions

- Spinal cord injury
- Cerebrovascular disease
- Multiple sclerosis
- Parkinson's disease

Immobility and lack of exercise
Depression

Red flag symptoms in constipation

- New onset of severe constipation or recent change of bowel habit in elderly patient
- Rectal bleeding
- Unexplained anaemia
- Family history of colorectal cancer or inflammatory bowel disease
- Tenesmus
- Weight loss
- Vomiting

Rome II criteria for constipation
Adults
Two or more of the following for at least 12 weeks in the preceding 12 months:

- Straining during >25% of bowel movements
- Lumpy or hard stools for >25% of bowel movements
- Sensation of incomplete evacuation for >25% of bowel movements
- Sensation of anorectal blockage for >25% of bowel movements
- Manual manoeuvres to facilitate >25% of bowel movements
- <3 bowel movements per week
- Loose stools not present, and insufficient criteria for irritable bowel syndrome met

Evaluation of constipation

- Digital rectal examination
- Full blood count
- Serum calcium
- Thyroid function tests

Features associated with faecal impaction

- Diarrhoea
- Faecal incontinence
- Urinary frequency/incontinence
- Rectal pain
- Abdominal pain
- Large bowel obstruction

Risk factors

- Immobility
- Inadequate diet
- Medication: opiates; anticholinergic agents
- Chronic kidney disease

Causes of small bowel obstruction (colicky abdominal pain, nausea, vomiting-often bilious, diarrhoea, and later constipation).

Adynamic ileus: generalised peritonitis (perforated viscus); acute pancreatitis; postoperative ileus; electrolyte disease; intra-abdominal infection; acute diverticulitis; acute appendicitis; pelvic inflammatory disease

Mechanical obstruction

Luminal: gallstone ileus (Rigler's triad of mechanical small bowel obstruction, pneumobilia and ectopic gallstone within the intestinal lumen); neoplasm; bezoar; foreign body; parasites

Intramural (in the bowel wall): Meckel's diverticulum; Crohn's disease; neoplasm (leiomyoma carcinoid, adenocarcinoma); intussusception (triad of pain, currant jelly stool and palpable sausage-shaped abdominal mass –in 20 to 25% of children); volvulus; radiation enteritis; haematoma; ischaemic stricture

Extrinsic: post-operative adhesions; incarcerated groin (inguinal or femoral) hernia; obturator hernia (acute small bowel obstruction, associated with medial thigh pain due to obturator nerve compression in the obturator canal, often in frail elderly women-Howship-Romberg sign); abscess; metastatic disease; congenital bands

Risk factors for intraperitoneal adhesions

- Open abdominal or pelvic surgery
- Peritonitis
- Foreign body: talc, starch, cellulose
- Inflammatory bowel disease
- Radiation enteritis
- Sclerosing peritonitis (drug-induced: beta blocker)

Radiological features of small bowel obstruction

- Multiple central dilated loops of bowel (>3 cm in diameter, measured outer wall to outer wall)
- Valvulae conniventes (stacked coin appearance) in jejunal loops
- Tubular featureless appearance of ileal loops
- Absence of gas in the colon
- Air-fluid levels
- String of beads sign caused by trapping of gas in valvulae conniventes along the walls of dilated fluid-filled loops

Causes of pneumobilia

- Gallstone ileus
- Biliary-enteric anastomosis
- Recent ERCP
- Emphysematous cholecystitis
- Incompetence of sphincter of Oddi: sphincterotomy

Causes of large bowel obstruction (triad of colicky abdominal pain, constipation or obstipation (absolute constipation for stool and flatus) and abdominal distension). Continuous pain may indicate bowel ischaemia. An abrupt onset suggests an acute obstructive event, while a subacute history associated with altered bowel habit may indicate malignancy. Caecal tenderness implies impending perforation.

- Luminal; faecal impaction; foreign body
- Intramural: colorectal malignancy; diverticulitis with stricture; Crohn's disease; sigmoid volvulus (dilated ahaustral closed large bowel loop extending into the right upper quadrant; coffee bean sign produced by central thicker wall caused by double thickness of opposed bowel loops, separating the loop into two compartments lined by thinner outer walls); caecal volvulus (dilated large bowel loop extending into left upper quadrant, with preserved haustral pattern, and associated small bowel dilatation); endometriosis
- Extrinsic: hernias; adhesions
- Intestinal pseudo-obstruction (Ogilvie's syndrome) (acute massive colonic dilatation in the absence of mechanical obstruction; caecum diameter >10 cm is associated with a risk of perforation)

Radiological features of large bowel obstruction

- Dilated peripheral colonic loops (>6 cm, except in caecum, where >9 cm is abnormal dilatation)
- Collapsed distal colon
- Small bowel dilatation depends on the competence of the ileocaecal valve
- Incomplete haustral markings

Features suggesting strangulation obstruction with bowel ischaemia

- Constant pain
- Tender irreducible external hernia
- Signs of peritonism
- Reduced bowel sounds
- Fever; tachycardia
- Raised WCC and CRP
- Acidosis; raised lactate

Risk factors for sigmoid volvulus

- Elderly
- Chronic constipation; laxative abuse
- Chronic neurological and psychiatric disease: Parkinson's disease; multiple sclerosis; chronic schizophrenia; Alzheimer's dementia
- Megacolon; Chagas' disease

Percutaneous endoscopic gastrostomy complications in emergency practice

- Peri-stomal wound infection: cellulitis (pain, redness, induration), discharge, fluctuant mass at the site; may progress to necrotising fasciitis, peritonitis, deep wound abscess
- Buried bumper syndrome (internal bumper buried within gastric mucosa): peri-stomal leakage/infection; immobile catheter; abdominal pain and flow resistance on attempted flushing
- Inadvertent removal: if the PEG tube has been in situ for more than 1 month, a mature tract may be assumed to be present
- Gastric outlet obstruction: intermittent vomiting, cramping abdominal pain; aspiration pneumonia

Dyspepsia

A group of symptoms indicative of the presence of upper gastro-intestinal tract disease

There are four categories:

- Ulcer-like: abdominal pain
- Reflux-like (gastro-oesophageal reflux): heartburn; regurgitation; retrosternal discomfort
- Dysmotility-like (delayed gastric emptying): early satiety; post-prandial fullness and bloating
- Non-specific or unspecified

Alarm symptoms in dyspepsia (indicating the need for early endoscopy)

- Age >50 years with recent onset dyspepsia
- Anorexia
- Progressive unintentional weight loss
- Unexplained iron deficiency anaemia (except in pre-menopausal women)

- Gastrointestinal bleeding: overt or occult (positive stool occult blood)
- Progressive dysphagia or odynophagia
- Persistent or recurrent vomiting
- Previous gastric ulcer
- Previous gastric surgery
- Ulcerogenic medication: NSAID/aspirin/ steroid therapy
- Epigastric mass
- Epigastric pain severe enough to hospitalise patient
- Strong history of familial gastrointestinal cancer
- Concomitant disease with possible gastrointestinal involvement

Risk factors for gastric cancer

- Alcohol abuse
- Smoking
- Helicobacter pylori infection
- Autoimmune gastritis (pernicious anaemia)
- Menetrier's disease
- Previous partial gastrectomy (>20 years ago)
- Positive family history of gastric cancer
- Familial adenomatous polyposis

Causes of unintentional weight loss

- Chronic infection: tuberculosis; fungal; AIDS; infective endocarditis
- Malignancy: carcinoma; lymphoma; leukaemia
- Inadequate dietary intake: immobility; dementia; impaired consciousness; anorexia; anorexia nervosa
- Endocrine: thyrotoxicosis, diabetes mellitus, adrenocortical insufficiency
- Behavioural: depression, eating disorders, psychosis
- Social: isolation; financial difficulties
- Gastrointestinal:
  Gastrointestinal obstruction: neoplasm; stricture; adhesions
  Motility disorders: achalasia, gastroparesis
  Pancreaticoduodenal: pancreatic cancer, chronic pancreatitis
  Small intestinal malabsorption
  Bacterial overgrowth

Lower gastrointestinal bleeding

Usually originates distal to the duodenojejunal flexure

Bright red blood, with or without clots, usually indicates bleeding low in the colon or rectum

Dark red or maroon blood usually indicates bleeding higher in the colon or the small bowel

Melaena usually indicates bleeding in the stomach

Causes of lower gastrointestinal bleeding

Small bowel:

- Diverticular disease: Meckel's diverticulum; pseudo-diverticula; jejunal diverticula
- Intususception
- Mesenteric infarction
- Aorto-enteric fistula: primary/ secondary
- Vascular lesions: angiodysplasia; telangiectasia; arteriovenous malformation
- Tumours: lymphoma; gastrointestinal stromal tumours; carcinoid; adenocarcinoma
- Ulceration: Crohn's disease; Zollinger-Ellison syndrome; NSAIDs, potassium supplements; vasculitis

Large bowel:

- Colonic diverticular disease (diverticulosis)
- Angiodysplasia (vascular ectasias); arteriovenous malformations
- Colitis
  - Ulcerative proctocolitis
  - Chronic radiation proctocolitis
  - Ischaemic colitis
  - Crohn's colitis (granulomatous)
- Carcinoma
- Hamartomatous and neoplastic polyps
- Endometriosis
- Aorto-colonic fistula

Ano-rectal
Haemorrhoids; rectal/colonic varices
Anal fissure
Radiation proctitis
Solitary rectal ulcer syndrome

Associated symptoms with acute lower gastrointestinal bleeding
Abdominal pain:

- Ischaemic bowel: ischaemic colitis
- Inflammatory bowel disease: Crohn's disease; ulcerative colitis
- Ruptured abdominal aortic aneurysm

Painless bleeding:

- Diverticuli (diverticular disease)
- Angiodysplasia
- Polyps
- Haemorrhoids

Bloody diarrhoea:

- Inflammatory bowel disease
- Infection: infectious colitis (E coli O157: H7; Shigella; Salmonella; Campylobacter jejuni)

Rectal pain:

- Anal fissure
- Haemorrhoids

Constipation:

- Colorectal malignancy
- Haemorrhoids

Causes of upper gastrointestinal bleeding (bleeding proximal to the ligament of Treitz at the duodeno-jejunal flexure).

Upper gastrointestinal bleeding can present with the vomiting of frank blood (haeamatemesis) or of coffee ground vomitus (dark coloured vomit containing altered blood), with or without melaena (passage of dark and tarry stools).

- Peptic ulcer disease: gastric; duodenal
- Drug-associated upper gastrointestinal tract erosive disease: aspirin, NSAIDs, steroids, bisphosphonates
- Oesophagitis
- Mallory-Weiss tear (haematemesis following repeated episodes of retching and vomiting, caused by longitudinal mucosal tear in distal oesophagus or gastric cardia; usually self limiting with spontaneous healing)
- Gastric/oesophageal varices (may have jaundice, ascites, hepatic encephalopathy, and stigmata of chronic liver disease-spider naevi, palmar erythema, splenomegaly)
- Stress ulceration
- Gastritis/ gastric erosions; haemorrhagic gastritis
- Tumours: gastric; oesophageal
- Cameron ulcers within hiatus hernia
- Swallowed blood from nasal bleeding
- Rare:

Aneurysms: aortic; splenic artery
Aorto-duodenal fistula: prior aortic surgery; abdominal aortic aneurysm
Aorto-oesophageal fistula (Chiari's triad of mid-thoracic pain, sentinel upper gastrointestinal bleeding, and exsanguination after a symptom-free interval; associated with thoracic aortic aneurysm, foreign body ingestion, oesophageal malignancy, and prosthetic graft erosion)
Arterial malformations of stomach (Dieulafoy lesion-a large tortous superficial mucosal arteriole)
Pancreatic tumours; chronic pancreatitis; pancreatic pseudocysts; pancreatic pseudoaneurysms
Haemobilia: bleeding from gallbladder or biliary tree; abdominal trauma, biliary tract instrumentation, pancreatic pseudocyst
Hereditary haemorrhagic telangiectasia
Pseudoxanthoma elasticum
Angiodysplasia
Ehlers-Danlos syndrome
Haemostatic disorders

Pitfalls in the diagnosis of gastro-intestinal bleeding

Exogenous blood
- Epistaxis
- Uncooked meat

Black stools
- Iron preparations
- Grape juice; purple grapes
- Spinach
- Chocolate

Pseudo-blood
- Medications in red syrup
- Beets; tomato skin/juice
- Red diaper syndrome
- Peach skin; red cherries
- Cranberry juice

Clinical evaluation of upper gastrointestinal bleeding

- Haemodynamic status: vital signs and postural changes
- Signs of generalized vascular malformations/ disorders: petechiae; telangiectasia
- Signs of chronic liver disease (digital clubbing, leukonychia, palmar erythema, spider naevi, scratch marks, hepatosplenomegaly, ascites, peripheral oedema)
- Signs of portal hypertension: ascites
- Signs of hepatic encephalopathy
- Source of bleeding in pharynx or anterior nares
- History of dyspepsia, dysphagia or odynophagia

Risk stratification in acute upper gastrointestinal bleeding

- Age
- Presence of shock
- Co-morbidities
- Major stigmata of recent haemorrhage
- Cause of bleeding

Potential sources of obscure gastro-intestinal bleeding

- Vascular ectasias
- Small intestinal neoplastic lesions
- Hemosuccus pancreaticus: bleeding from peri-pancreatic blood vessels into a pancreatic duct
- Haemobilia: haemorrhage into a biliary duct (triad of right upper abdominal pain, jaundice and acute upper gastrointestinal bleeding)
- Aorto-enteric fistula
- Dieulafoy's lesion (erosion of, and bleeding from, a gastric submucosal arteriole)
- Meckel's diverticulum
- Extra-oesophageal varices: gastric; small intestinal; colonic
- Diverticula, especially small intestinal
- Cameron lesions (linear erosions or ulcers of gastric mucosal folds) within hiatus hernia, caused by diaphragmatic compression

Clinical presentations of colorectal cancer

Right sided lesions

- Occult blood loss, with insidious onset of unexplained iron deficiency anaemia
- Distal ileal obstruction
- Palpable right iliac fossa mass
- Fever of unknown origin
- Acute appendicitis
- Left-sided lesions
- Visible blood in stool
- Altered bowel habit
- Large bowel bbstruction

Clinical risk factors for colorectal cancer

- Genetic
- Polyposis syndromes: familial polyposis coli; Gardner's syndrome; Turcot syndrome; Oldfield's syndrome; Peutz-Jeghers syndrome
  - Hereditary non-polyposis syndromes: Lynch syndrome I; Lynch
  - syndrome II

- Pre-existing disease
- Inflammatory bowel disease: ulcerative colitis; Crohn's disease
- Prior colorectal cancer
- Adenomatous polyps
- Pelvic irradiation
- Breast or genital tract cancer
- Schistosomiasis
- General
- Age of onset of symptoms >40 years
- Positive family history of colorectal cancer: 1st degree relative with colorectal cancer or adenomatous polyps diagnosed before the age of 60

Presentations of rectal cancer

Persistent or recurrent rectal bleeding, especially with onset aged over 40 years
Altered bowel habit
Tenesmus
Atypical presentations: "piles"; anal pain from anoderm involvement; secondary deposits: chest; liver
Local complications
Perforation: local abscess; generalised peritonitis
Intestinal obstruction
Abscess: sacral/perineal pain
Fistula: bladder (male); vagina (female)

Causes of pruritus ani

Anorectal disease: inflammatory bowel disease (Crohn's disease); haemorrhoids (external, internal); fistulae
Infections: bacterial infections; Candida; pinworms (Enterobius vermicularis); viral infections (anal warts)
Hygiene: inadequate or overzealous (soap, scent, lotion)
Skin conditions: psoriasis, seborrhoeic dermatitis, contact dermatitis, lichen planus, lichen simplex, lichen sclerosus, Bowen's disease

Causes of anal and rectal pain

- Thrombosed external haemorrhoid: acute severe pain; bluish purple tender swelling, covered with perianal skin and with minimal induration, at the anal verge
- Anal fissure: linear ulcer in epithelial lining of anal canal distal to the dentate line, usually in the posterior midline; pain and bright red bleeding during and after defaecation; with chronicity, sentinel tag at distal pole, hypertrophied anal papilla in the anal canal proximal to the fissure, and circular fibres of the internal anal sphinter visible in the base
- Ano-rectal abscess: perianal pain, worse on sitting and with defaecation and indurated swelling at the anal verge; fever and chills; associated with diabetes mellitus, Crohn's disease and chronic corticosteroid therapy. Fluctuation is a late feature and is not required in order to make the diagnosis. Ischiorectal abscess presents with gluteal pain and induration. With supralevator or intersphincteric abscesses, no visible external manifestations may be present, and severe rectal pain may be accompanied by urinary symptoms (eg dysuria; inability to void, and urinary retention)
- Prolapsed strangulated or thrombosed internal haemorrhoid: rectal bleeding, pruritus
- Acute proctitis
- Rectal foreign body
- Anal cancer
- Proctalgia fugax

Causes of ascites
Normal peritoneum

Portal hypertension

- Parenchymal liver disease: cirrhosis; alcoholic hepatitis; fulminant hepatic failure; massive liver metastases
- Hepatic congestion: congestive heart failure; constrictive pericarditis; veno-occlusive disease; Budd-Chiari syndrome; tricuspid regurgitation

Hypoalbuminaemic states: nephrotic syndrome; severe malnutrition, protein-losing enteropathy

Miscellaneous: chylous ascites (lymphatic leak), pancreatic ascites, biliary ascites, nephrogenic ascites, urine ascites, ovarian tumours; myxoedema

Diseased peritoneum

Infections: bacterial peritonitis, tuberculous peritonitis, fungal peritonitis, HIV-associated peritonitis

Malignancy: peritoneal carcinomatosis; hepatocelllular carcinoma; metastatic disease; primary mesothelioma

Other: granulomatous peritonitis, vasculitis, Familial Mediterranean Fever, eosinophilic peritonitis (Mnemonic for causes of abdominal swelling: fat, fluid, flatus, faeces, foetus)

Causes of abnormal gas patterns on plain abdominal x-ray

Air inside the bowel (intra-luminal air):

- Ileus
- Obstruction
- Gas outlining mucosal lesion

Extra-luminal:

- Free peritoneal
- Retroperitoneal
- Loculated peritoneal, ie abscess

Air following known anatomical structures:

- Intramural air
- Biliary air
- Portal venous air

Causes of intestinal intramural gas

Linear pattern associated with ischaemia or infarction

- Mesenteric vascular disease
- Obstruction
- Toxic colon, eg colitis; necrotising enterocolitis

Linear gas without infarction

- Connective tissue disorders, eg scleroderma
- Caustic ingestion
- Iatrogenic, eg post-surgery catheterisation, stenting, endoscopic biopsy
- Immunosuppression

Cystic gas pattern

- Pneumatosis cystoids intestinalis
- Associated with chronic obstructive lung disease

Causes of pneumoperitoneum

Perforated abdominal hollow viscus: duodenal ulcer; ischaemic bowel; bowel obstruction; inflammatory bowel disease; diverticulitis

Mechanical perforation: trauma; colonoscopy; foreign body; iatrogenic

Post-operative free intra-peritoneal gas: laparotomy; laparoscopy

Peritoneal dialysis

Vaginal aspiration: vaginal douching, vaginal insufflation with air during sexual activity (coitus; oral sex); waterskiing

Mechanical ventilation

Pneumatosis cystoides intestinalis

Features of pneumoperitoneum on supine x-rays

- Gas in the right upper quadrant, which may be peri-hepatic, sub-hepatic, or in the hepato-renal space
- Visualisation of the falciform and medial umbilical ligaments
- Double wall (Rigler's) sign

Causes of pseudo-peritoneum

Sub-diaphragmatic extraperitoneal fat

Multicontoured diaphragm

Interposition of transverse colon or small bowel between liver and diaphragm (Chilaiditi syndrome)

Basilar horizontal plate atelectasis

Interposition of omental fat between liver and diaphragm

Diaphragmatic hernia

Large diverticulum arising in subdiaphragmatic oesophagus, stomach, or duodenum

Sub-pleural air

Causes of nausea and vomiting

Upper gastrointestinal disorder

- Reflux oesophagitis
- Gastric outlet obstruction
- Small bowel obstruction
- Acute gastritis (alcoholic)/gastroenteritis (viral, bacterial, parasitic)
- Acute cholecystitis
- Acute pancreatitis
- Acute hepatitis
- Diabetic gastroparesis

Therapeutic drug use:
- Opiates
- Cardiac glycosides: digoxin
- Cancer chemotherapy
- Antibiotics

Drug toxicity: paracetamol; digoxin; theophylline

Drug abuse: narcotics; alcohol; narcotic withdrawal

CNS:

- Migraine
- Labyrinthine disease: acute labyrinthitis; motion sickness
- Raised intracranial pressure
- Head injury

Psychological (self-induced)-eating disorders:

- Anorexia nervosa
- Bulimia
- Psychogenic vomiting

Metabolic/endocrine

- Hyperparathyroidism
- Chronic kidney disease
- Acute adrenocortical insufficiency
- Diabetic ketoacidosis
- Acute liver failure

Pregnancy:
- Physiological
- Hyperemesis gravidarum

Genitourinary: pyelonephritis

Miscellaneous; electrolyte disorder; glaucoma

Causes of small intestinal fluid levels on plain abdominal xray:

- Large intestinal obstruction
- Small intestinal obstruction
- Paralytic ileus
- Cleansing enemas
- Gastroenteritis
- Hypokalaemia
- Uraemia
- Jejunal diverticulosis
- Mesenteric thrombosis
- Normal (always <2.5 cm long)
- Peritoneal metastases

Causes of hiccups

Gastrointestinal: gastric distension; gastro-esophageal reflux; hepatitis; cholecystitis; cholelithiasis; bowel obstruction; pancreatitis

Diaphragmatic irritation: hiatal hernia; abdominal mass; peritonitis

CNS: stroke; infection; ventriculo-peritoneal shunt

Chest: pneumonia

Metabolic: uraemia; hyponatraemia; hypocalcaemia

Toxic/ drug induced: alcohol; chemotherapeutic agents

Psychogenic: stress; grief

Idiopathic

Causes of jaundice

Pre-hepatic (increased production of bilirubin) (unconjugated hyperbilirubinaemia)
- Genetic diseases: sickle cell disease; thalassemia (ineffective erythropoeisis); glucose 6 phosphate dehydrogenase deficiency
- Increased breakdown of red blood cells (increased reticulocyte count): haemolytic anaemias (eg, hereditary spherocytosis) (unconjugated hyperbilirubinaemia, anaemia with reticulocytosis)

Intra-hepatic

Hepatocellular (reduced hepatic uptake of, or conjugation of, bilurubin)

- Viral hepatitis (hepatitis A, B, C, D, E)

- Autoimmune hepatitis
- Alcoholic liver disease: acute alcoholic hepatitis; cirrhosis
- Leptospirosis
- Disorders of bilirubin metabolism (impaired hepatocellular conjugation of bilirubin): Gilbert's syndrome; Crigler-Najjar syndrome; Dubin-Johnson syndrome; Rotor syndrome

Cholestasis

- Familial and congenital: benign recurrent intrahepatic cholestasis, Caroli's disease
- Viral hepatitis
- Infiltration: granuloma; cancer
- Hepatotoxic drugs: anabolic steroids; oral contraceptive
- Primary biliary cirrhosis
- Cholangiocarcinoma
- Primary sclerosing cholangitis; autoimmune cholangiopathy
- Vanishing bile duct syndrome (complication of drug-induced liver injury leading to progressive destruction of the intra-hepatic bile ducts and chronic cholestasis)
- Sepsis

Post-hepatic cholestasis (extrahepatic biliary obstruction).
Inside bile duct (intra-ductal)

- Gallstones in common bile duct
- Parasites

Inside wall:

- Biliary tract tumours: gallbladder cancer; cholangiocarcinoma
- Common bile duct stricture
- AIDS cholangiopathy

Outside duct wall:

- Cancer in head of pancreas
- Pancreatitis (acute; chronic)
- Tumour/lymph nodes in porta hepatis: lymphoma, cholangiocarcinoma, metastatic carcinoma
- Pancreatic pseudocyst

Causes of biliary obstruction
Intrahepatic

- Hepatitis
- Cirrhosis: post-hepatitic; primary biliary cirrhosis
- Drugs: anabolic steroids; chlorpromazine

Extrahepatic

- Intra-ductal: neoplasm; stone; parasite (Ascaris lumbricoides); biliary stricture; primary sclerosing cholangitis; AIDS-related cholangiopathy; biliary tuberculosis
- Extra-ductal: neoplasm (cholangiocarcinoma; metastases; cance of head of pancreas); pancreatitis; parasites (Ascaris lumbricoides; liver flukes)

Risk factors for jaundice

- Liver disease
- Previous episodes of jaundice
- Blood transfusion
- Intravenous drug use
- Alcohol history
- Sexual history
- Travel history
- Drug history, including over-the-counter, recreational and herbal
- Contacts: environmental and food exposure

Causes of jaundice with fever
Pre-hepatic jaundice

- Haemolysis: severe malaria; Mycoplasma pneumoniae; sickle cell crisis

Hepatic jaundice

- Viral hepatitis
- Enteric fever: Salmonella hepatitis
- Viral haemorrhagic fever
- Liver abscess (amoebic; pyogenic)
- Rickettsial infections
- Infectious mononucleosis
- Leptospirosis (biphasic illness of initial flu-like illness with fever, anorexia, nausea and vomiting, headache and myalgia, followed by haemorrhages, jaundice,

hepatorenal syndrome (acute kidney injury)) (occupational risk factors include sewage workers, veterinarians, abattoir workers, rodent control workers, and famers; recreational risk factors include activities in freshwater such as swimming, sailing, water skiing and wind surfing)
- Drug induced hepatitis: amoxicillin with clavulanic acid, NSAIDs, carbamazepine

Post-hepatic jaundice
- Biliary tract infection: acute cholecystitis; choledocholithiasis with ascending cholangitis (Charcot's triad of intermittent fever with chills, right upper quadrant abdominal pain and jaundice); biliary ascariasis

Bedside ultrasound evaluation of the biliary tract
Gallstones

- Echogenic objects within the echo-free gallbladder lumen
- Distal acoustic shadowing
- Mobile, and move with changes in position of the patient: demonstrate gravitational dependency, seeking the most dependent portion of the gallbladder
- The lumen of the gallbladder may contain lithogenic bile, known as **sludge,** which has low-level echogenicity (it appears less white than stones), tends to layer out in the dependent portion of the gallbladder with a flat fluid: fluid interface, and fails to shadow.

Acute cholecystitis

- Symmetrical thickening of the entire gall bladder wall >3 mm
- Dilated gall bladder: >10 cm in length; >4 cm in width
- Echo-poor halo around the gallbladder-due to intramural oedema-alternating echogenic and hypo-echoic layers within the wall
- Gallstones
- Impacted stone in neck of gallbladder
- Gas in gallbladder wall
- The sonographic Murphy sign represents local tenderness and inspiratory arrest over the sonographically visualised gallbladder
- Increased flow with colour Doppler
- Peri-cholecystic fluid: focal anechoic collection adjacent to the gallbladder, especially in the region of the fundus; collection >1 cm indicates gallbladder perforation

Acute Liver Failure
Features
- Jaundice
- Ascites
- Peripheral oedema
- Encephalopathy (confusion, flapping tremor, constructional apraxia); cerebral oedema
- Coagulopathy
- Upper gastrointestinal bleeding
- Acute kidney injury
- Sepsis
- Previously normal liver function

Causes
- Hepatotoxicity: dose dependent: paracetamol overdose, methyldioxymethamphetamine; idiosyncratic drug reactions (isoniazid; NSAIDs, antiepileptic drugs, antibi otics-rifampicin)
- Acute viral hepatitis: hepatitis A, B, C, D, E; cytomegalovirus, adenovirus, haemorrhagic fever viruses, herpes simplex virus, Epstein-Barr virus, paramyxovirus
- Autoimmune hepatitis
- Acute steatosis syndromes (extensive hepatocyte infiltration with fat microdroplets and minimal hepatocellular necrosis): acute fatty liver of pregnancy; Reye's syndrome; acute alcoholic hepatitis
- Toxins: Amanita phalloides (mushroom ingestion), Bacillus cereus, yellow phosphorus, organic solvents (hydrocarbons, eg carbon tetrachloride)
- Vascular: ischaemic hepatitis (shock liver); hepatic vein thrombosis (Budd-Chiari

syndrome); hepatic veno-occlusive disease; portal vein thrombosis; hepatic artery thrombosis; congestive heart failure; right heart failure

Metabolic: α1-antitrypsin deficiency; hereditary fructose intolerance; galactosaemia; LCAT (lecithin-cholesterol acyltransferase) deficiency; Reye's syndrome; hepatolenticular degeneration; tyrosinaemia

Malignancy: primary liver tumours (hepatocellular carcinoma, cholangiocarcinoma); secondary tumours (extensive hepatic metastases from adenocarcinoma, melanoma, lymphoma); leukaemia

Miscellaneous: adult-onset Still's disease; heatstroke

Laboratory findings

- Hepatic injury: elevated transaminases (ALT, AST, GGT)
- Hepatic dysfunction: coagulopathy not correctable with vitamin K; hypoglycaemia; hypoalbuminaemia; increasing bilirubin; hyperammonaemia; high lactate

Causes of coagulopathy in liver disease

- Cholestasis causing vitamin K malabsorption, with impaired synthesis of vitamin K-dependent coagulation factors II, VII, IX and X)
- Hepatocellular disease leading to failure of γ carboxylation of coagulation factors and reduced synthesis of all coagulation factors except Factor VIII and von Willebrand factor

Factors precipitating hepatic encephalopathy

- Gastrointestinal bleeding
- Sepsis; spontaneous bacterial peritonitis
- Azotemia and hypovolaemia (diuretic-induced)
- Hypokalaemia; alkalosis
- CNS depressant drugs: sedatives (benzodiazepines); opiates; tricyclic antidepressant drugs
- Hepatocellular injury
- Constipation
- High protein diet
- Hypoglycaemia
- Post-portosystemic shunt placement

Causes of hepatomegaly

- Infection: viral: hepatitis (acute; chronic), infectious mononucleosis; parasitic: malaria; abscess: pyogenic, amoebic
- Vascular congestion: supra-hepatic: congestive heart failure, right ventricular failure, constrictive pericarditis, Budd-Chiari syndrome; intra-hepatic: veno-occlusive disease
- Infiltration: neoplasm (primary: hepatocellular carcinoma; metastases); haematological malignancy: lymphoma, leukaemia; granuloma: sarcoidosis, tuberculosis; extramedullary haematopoeisis: haemolytic anaemias, haemoglobinopathies – thalassaemia, sickle cell disease)
- Storage disorders: fat: non-alcoholic hepatic steatosis, diabetes mellitus, obesity, mucopolysaacharidoses; lipid-lipidoses (Niemann-Pick; Gaucher); metals: copper (hepatolenticular degeneration), iron (haemochromatosis); abnormal protein: alpha1-antitrypsin; glycogen: glycogen storage disease
- Biliary tract obstruction: extra-hepatic biliary obstruction (cholelithiasis; tumour)

Causes of splenomegaly

- Infection: viral: infectious mononucleosis, cytomegalovirus, HIV; bacterial: tuberculosis, infective endocarditis, brucellosis, syphilis, typhoid; fungal: histoplasmosis; parasitic: malaria, visceral leishmaniasis, hydatid disease, schistosomiasis; rickettsial: typhus
- Congestive splenomegaly due to portal hypertension: cirrhosis (alcoholic liver disease; primary biliary cirrhosis; hepatitis B/C); portal vein thrombosis; splenic vein thrombosis
- Haematological causes: haemolytic anaemias ; haemoglobinopathies (early sickle cell disease, thalassaemia); haemoglobin-

opathies; myeloproliferative disorders: chronic leukaemia, acute leukaemia, polycythaemia vera, lymphoma, essential thrombocytosis; extramedullary haematopoiesis: myelofibrosis (agnogenic myeloid metaplasia)
- Space occupying lesions: cyst; haemangioma
- Trauma: subcapsular haematoma

The 3 Ms of massive splenomegaly are chronic myeloid leukaemia, myelofibrosis, and malaria

Significant findings with blunt abdominal trauma

- Hypovolaemic shock
- Evidence of intraperitoneal penetration: signs of peritonism (guarding, rebound tenderness); free intraperitoneal air; omental evisceration; implement in situ
- Gastrointestinal bleeding
- Seat belt marks
- Steering wheel contusion
- Bicycle handlebar marks on the upper abdomen
- Macroscopic haematuria
- Flank (Grey Turner) or peri-umbilical (Cullen) ecchymosis
- Abdominal bruit

Confounding factors in the evaluation of abdominal trauma

- Head injury with altered level of consciousness
- Alcohol/drug intoxication
- Spinal cord injury
- Distracting injury

Potential involvement with blunt abdominal trauma

- Solid viscus: liver, spleen, kidneys, pancreas
- Hollow viscus: small intestine; large intestine; stomach; oesophagus; urinary bladder
- Vascular injuries: aorta; inferior vena cava
- Bones: pelvis; lumbar spine
- Diaphragm

Features of seat belt syndrome

- Abdominal wall contusion
- Iliac or pubic fractures
- Lumbar spine fractures: wedge compression fracture; Chance fracture
- Intra-abdominal injuries: small bowel perforation; mesenteric tears; bladder rupture

13 Renal and Urological Emergencies

Causes of red urine

- Macroscopic haematuria
- Haemoglobinuria (haemolysis)
- Myoglobinuria
- Drugs: rifampicin; metronidazole; warfarin; nitrofurantoin
- Menstruation
- Food: beetroot (anthrocyanin); red cabbage; blackberries; food colourants (paprika; rhodamine B)
- Urate crystals: 'brick dust' in a baby's nappy

Types of haematuria

The timing of haematuria during micturition is an aid in the localization of the source of bleeding.

- Initial: anterior urethra
- Terminal: posterior urethra; bladder, including neck and trigone; prostate; seminal vesicles
- Total: bladder; upper urinary tract (kidney or ureter)

Checklist for haematuria assessment

- Timing: initial, total, terminal
- Lower urinary tract symptoms: dysuria, increased urinary frequency, urgency, urethral discharge
- Obstructive urinary symptoms: hesitancy, straining to void, sensation of incomplete emptying
- Flank pain: renal stone disease; pyelonephritis
- Suprabic pain: bladder outlet obstruction; haemorrhagic cystitis
- Signs associated with glomerular origin: peripheral and periorbital oedema; oliguria; hypertension; weight gain
- Features of vasculitis: skin rash; arthralgia; fever
- Recent urological intervention, such as bladder catheterization, prostate biopsy, ureteral stent placement, nephrostomy, or trans-urethral surgery
- Drug history: anticoagulants; nephrotoxic medications (eg NSAIDs)
- Family history of renal disease
- Occupational history: exposure to chemicals and smoking
- Travel history
- Urine dip stick analysis for blood, protein, leucocytes, nitrites. Dipstick tests do not distinguish between intact red blood cells, free haemoglobin or free myoglobin.
- Urine microscopy for red blood cells; red cell casts; dysmorphic red blood cells. Three or more red blood cells per high power field on at least two out of three correctly collected urine specimens indicates microscopic haematuria.
- Renal function: plasma creatinine/eGFR
- Upper urinary tract imaging: CT scan

A. Banerjee, *Emergency Clinical Diagnosis*, DOI 10.1007/978-3-319-50718-7_13

Red flags with haematuria

- Painless macroscopic haematuria (which has a high diagnostic yield for urological malignancy)
- Symptomatic microscopic haematuria in absence of urinary tract infection
- Unexplained microscopic haematuria in patient aged >50 years

Causes of haematuria
Glomerular disease

- IgA nephropathy (Berger's disease)
- Acute post-infectious glomerulonephritis (nephritogenic strains of Group A streptococcus) (hypertension; skin rash)
- Alport's syndrome (hereditary nephritis)
- Membrano-proliferative glomerulonephritis
- Systemic vasculitis/ lupus
- Thin glomerular basement membrane disease (benign familial haematuria)
- Rapidly progressive glomerulonephritis

Non-glomerular
Upper urinary tract (kidney and ureter)

Tumours: renal cell carcinoma; transitional cell carcinoma.

Medullary/ interstitial disease: papillary necrosis; medullary sponge kidney; tuberculosis

Urolithiasis

Trauma to kidneys/ureters

Miscellaneous

- Arterio-venous malformation
- Loin pain-haematuria syndrome (recurent loin pain and intermittent macroscopic or microscopic haemturia); nutcracker syndrome (compression of left renal vein between abdominal aorta and superior mesenteric artery)
- Renal artery thrombosis
- Hereditary haemorrhagic telangiectasia

Lower urinary tract (bladder and urethra)

Bladder: haemorrhagic cystitis; transitional cell carcinoma; stone; schistosomiasis; radiation cystitis

Prostate: benign prostatic hyperplasia; cancer; prostatitis

Urethra: urethritis

Coagulopathies: anticoagulants; haemophilia; sickle cell disease

Features suggesting glomerular origin of haematuria

A fresh, midstream, clean-catch or cather specimen of urine should be analysed

- Smoky brown coloured urine; no clots
- Red blood cell casts
- Dysmorphic red blood cells
- Significant proteinuria (>500 mg/24 h)

Risk factors for urothelial cancer presenting with haematuria

- Age > 40 years
- Male gender
- History of cigarette smoking, past or current
- History of occupational chemical or dye exposure (aromatic amines, benzenes)
- Cyclophosphamide therapy
- History of pelvic radiation
- Chronic irritative voiding lower urinary tract symptoms (urgency, frequency, dysuria, nocturia, hesitancy, sensation of incomplete emptying)
- Prior urological disease or treatment
- Chronic indwelling foreign body

Retention of urine

Urinary retention can be acute or chronic. Acute urinary retention refers to the sudden inability to pass urine and empty the bladder during voluntary voiding.

Causes of acute urinary retention

Anatomical causes resulting in mechanical obstruction to the flow of urine

- Penis: phimosis; paraphimosis; foreign body constriction
- Urethra: foreign body, calculus; urethritis; stricture; tumour; thrombosed urethral car-

uncle; meatal stenosis; pelvic trauma with disruption of posterior urethra or bladder neck; peri-urethral abscess

- Extrinsic compression: pelvic mass (gynaecological malignancy, ovarian cyst, uterine fibroid); pelvic organ prolapse (cystocele, rectocele, uterine prolapse); haematoma; retroverted impacted gravid uterus; faecal impaction (causing pressure on the bladder trigone)
- Prostate: benign prostatic hyperplasia; cancer; prostatitis; bladder neck contracture; prostatic infarction; prostatic abscess

Neuropathic Causes

- Motor/paralytic: spinal shock; spinal cord syndromes; cauda equina syndrome
- Sensory/ paralytic: diabetes mellitus; multiple sclerosis; spinal cord syndromes

Drugs causing dynamic obstruction to urine flow: anticholinergic, anti-spasmodic, tricyclic antidepressants, alpha-adrenergic agonists, antihistamines, opiates, anti-psychotics.

Infective/inflammatory: urinary tract infection; acute vulvovaginitis; genital herpes.

Causes of acute urinary retention in women
Neurological:

- Diabetes mellitus
- Multiple sclerosis
- Spinal cord lesions: trauma, tumours
- Transverse myelitis
- Cerebrovascular accident
- Fowler's syndrome: impaired relaxation of external sphincter in post-menopausal women

Non-neurological:

Urethral Obstruction:

- Cystocoele; rectocoele; uterine prolapse
- Stricture; diverticulum
- Previous incontinence surgery
- Herpetic vulvo-vaginitis
- Previous total abdominal hysterectomy

Lower urinary tract symptoms in men which can be predictive for the development of acute urinary retention

- Storage symptoms: frequency; urgency; nocturia; incontinence
- Voiding symptoms: slow stream; spraying; intermittent flow; terminal dribbling
- Post-micturition symptoms: incomplete emptying; dribbling

Urinary retention checklist

- Time of last voiding
- Previous episodes of acute urinary retention
- Preceding lower urinary tract symptoms
- Haematuria, leading to clot retention
- Neurological symptoms and signs
- Drug history
- Constipation
- Recent abdominal or pelvic surgery
- Bladder distension, recognized by a palpable tender suprapubic mass and confirmed on bedside ultrasound scan
- Urine dip stick analysis
- Renal function
- Bladder ultrasound for residual urine post-voiding
- Digital rectal examination after catherisation to evaluate anal tone, size and texture of the prostate, presence of faecal impaction

Complications of long-term indwelling urethral catheters presenting in emergency practice Blocked catheter: encrustation (crystal precipitation), often associated with urease-producing bacteria (Proteus mirabilis); kinks; stones

- Infection (asymptomatic bacteriuria; urethritis; cystitis; pyelonephritis; seminal vesiculitis; epididymo-orchitis; bacteraemia; urosepsis). Catheter-related infection can present with
  - Fever < 38.4 degrees centigrade
  - Unusually cloudy urine
  - Mental state changes
  - More frequent catheter blockage

  - Increased detrusor spasms
  - Hypotension
  - >5–10 WBCs per high-power field on microscopy
- Gross haematuria
- Leakage of urine (bypassing) around catheter: detrusor overactivity causing spasms (overactive bladder, cystitis, bladder outlet obstruction) (may respond to anticholinergic medication); catheter blockage
- Failure of balloon deflation: secondary lumen obstruction; valve malfunction (cut off side-arm and remove valve)
- Paraphimosis

Causes of renal pain
Urinary obstruction
- Calculus
- Necrotic papilla
- Blood clot
- Tumour
- Pelvi-ureteric junction dyssynergia

Rapid renal swelling
- Acute pyelonephritis
- Bleeding into renal cyst
- Infection in renal cyst
- Renal tumour (primary/secondary)

Renal infarction
- Arterial embolism
- Acute arterial thrombosis
- Acute venous thrombosis
- Arteritis

Causes of acute renal vein thrombosis (nausea and vomiting; loin and groin pain; macroscopic or microscopic haematuria)

- Hypercoagulable states: hypovolaemia; pregnancy; oral contraceptive pill; thrombophilia; nephrotic syndrome
- Renal vein compression: tumour; lymphadenopathy; retroperitoneal fibrosis; aortic aneurysm
- Renal cell carcinoma
- Sickle cell disease

Indications for hospital admission with renal colic

- Intractable pain and vomiting
- Infected obstructed urinary tract
- Bilateral obstruction
- Anuria
- Chronic kidney disease
- Known single kidney
- Renal transplant

Risk factors for renal stones

- Biochemical: hypercalciuria; hyperoxaluria; hyperuricosuria; cystinuria
- Anatomical lesions: pelvi-ureteric junction obstruction; hydronephrosis; calyceal diverticulum; horseshoe kidney; vesico-ureteric reflux; medullary sponge kidney

Factors predisposing to renal injury following trauma

- Paediatric kidney: more mobile; less perinephric fat
- Congenital renal abnormalities: pelvi-ureteric junction obstruction; malrotation; duplex collecting systems; horseshoe kidney

Causes of unilateral ureteric obstruction
Mechanical:

Lumen:
- Stone
- Blood clot
- Sloughed papilla

In wall:
- Transitional cell carcinoma
- Stricture (eg, tuberculosis)

Outside wall:
- Metastatic carcinoma
- Lymphoma
- Cervical cancer
- Retroperitoneal fibrosis

Functional:
- Pregnancy
- Pelvi-ureteric junction obstruction
- Vesico-ureteric junction obstruction (primary obstructive megaureter)

Causes of dysuria

Dysuria refers to discomfort, burning or pain on urination. The most common cause is urinary tract infection. External dysuria is related to the irritation of inflamed external genitalia by urine (as in vulvovaginitis), while internal dysuria is felt within the urethra.

- Infection: cystitis, urethritis (clear, mucopurulent or purulent urethral discharge, dysuria, urethral pruritus), prostatitis (penile, perineal or pelvic pain, dysuria, pain with ejaculation, premature ejaculation), vulvo-vaginitis, cervicitis, epididymo-orchitis
- Inflammation: interstitial cystitis; atrophic vaginitis
- Contact irritants or allergens: soap, tampon, spermicide, lubricant, bubble baths
- Drugs: NSAIDs, anticholinergics
- Foreign bodies in bladder; calculi
- Tumours: bladder, prostate
- Spondyloarthropathy: reactive arthritis; Behcet syndrome

Red flags for dysuria

- Fever
- Flank pain
- Recent genitourinary tract instrumentation
- Immunocompromised
- Known urological abnormalities
- Male sex

Dysuria checklist

- Other lower urinary tract symptoms: frequency, urgency, hesitation, urethral discharge
- Sexual history: new sexual partner; multiple sexual partners; frequent sex; partner with urethritis
- Vaginal discharge
- Drug history: prescribed medication; topical hygiene products (vaginal sprays'douches; bubble baths)
- Recent urinary tract instrumentation
- Urine dip stick analysis
- Urine microscopy

Causes of dysuria-frequency of micturition

- Urinary tract infection
- Genital infection: Trichomonas, gonococcus, Candidiasis
- Non-specific urethritis(Chlamydia)
- Bladder base irritation (calculus, idiopathic interstitial cystitis)
- Urethral syndrome

Categorisation of urinary tract infections

- Asymptomatic bacteriuria
- Uncomplicated lower urinary tract infection (irritative symptoms: frequency, urgency, dysuria, suprapubic discomfort, new or increased incontinence)
- Uncomplicated upper urinary tract infection
- Complicated urinary tract infection: associated structural or functional urinary tract abnormalities
- Recurrent uncomplicated urinary tract infection

Clinical presentations of urinary tract infections

Lower urinary tract
- Cystitis; urethritis: dysuria, frequency, urgency, suprapubic or urethral pain, turbid and foul-smelling urine, haematuria
- Prostatitis: perineal, sacral or suprapubic pain, frequency, urgency, fever, acute urinary retention, tender enlarged indurated prostate on rectal examination

Upper urinary tract
- Pyelonephritis: fever, with or without chills, loin pain, nausea and vomiting, frequency, urgency, dysuria

- Renal abscess
- Perinephric abscess

Risk factors for acute uncomplicated cystitis in women

- Sexual intercourse
- Delayed post-coital micturition
- Diaphragm and spermicide use
- Recent urinary tract infection

Risk factors for serious underlying pathology in the presence of confirmed childhood urinary tract infection (NICE guidelines)

- Poor urine flow
- History suggesting previous or confirmed previous urinary tract infection
- Recurrent fever of uncertain origin
- Antenatally-diagnosed renal abnormality
- Family history of vesico-ureteric reflux or renal disease
- Constipation
- Dysfunctional voiding
- Enlarged bladder
- Abdominal mass
- Evidence of spinal lesion
- Poor growth
- Hypertension

Causes of recurrent urinary tract infection (3 or more episodes in a 6 month period) (recurrence is associated with different organisms, whilst relapse is caused by the same initial organism)

- Premenopausal women: sexual intercourse; spermicide exposure; diaphragm use; new sexual partner
- Postmenopausal women: atrophic vaginitis; incontinence; pelvic floor prolapse; diabetes mellitus
- Men: lower urinary tract obstruction-bladder outlet obstruction (benign prostatic hyperplasia); urethral stricture; bladder neck obstruction; bladder stone; tumour; diverticula; foreign bodies; prostate cancer; detrusor-sphincter dyssynergia

Defining features of complicated urinary tract infection

- Associated anatomical abnormalities: entero-vesical fistula (associated with pneumaturia), diverticula, cystocele; stricture
- Iatrogenic: long-term indwelling urethral catheter, surgery, ureteric stent, nephrostomy tube
- Voiding dysfunction: vesico-ureteric reflux; neurogenic bladder; pelvic floor dysfunction; incontinence
- Urinary tract obstruction: bladder outlet obstruction; urethral stricture; pelvi-ureteric junction obstruction

  Other: pregnancy; urolithiasis; diabetes mellitus; renal failure; renal transplantation; multi-drug resistant uropathogens.

Considerations for treating catheter-associated bacteriuria

- Fever, with or without chills
- Loin pain
- Altered mental state: confusion
- Acute haematuria

Causes of sterile pyuria

- Stone disease
- Uroepithelial tumour
- Interstitial nephritis
- Tuberculosis
- Leukocytes from other sources
- Chlamydia trachomatis

Causes of acute scrotal pain and swelling
It is important to consider the diagnosis of testicular torsion in all patients presenting with acute scrotal pain and swelling. This is guided primarily by the history and physical examination findings. A history of trauma does not exclude testicular torsion. Scrotal imaging should not delay definitive treatment for testicular torsion.

Ischaemia

- Testicular torsion (torsion of spermatic cord) (high, tender swollen testis; swollen, shortened and tender spermatic cord; abnormal lie, usually transverse, of contralateral testis; late reactive hydrocoele, scrotal oedema; absent cremasteric reflex)
- Torsion of testicular (hydatid of Morgagni) or epididymal appendage (blue dot sign, with bluish discolouration at the superior pole of the testis, related to infarction)

Infection

- Acute epididymitis
- Acute orchitis
- Acute epididymo-orchitis (unilateral scrotal pain and swelling; tenderness of epididymis and testis; symptoms of urethritis-urethral discharge; symptoms of urinary tract infection-dysuria, frequency; scrotal erythema and/or oedema; secondary hydrocoele; relief of pain on scrotal elevation; cremasteric reflex present)
- Abscess: intra-testicular, intra-vaginal; scrotal skin
- Gangrenous infections: Fournier's gangrene (acute necrotizing infection of the scrotum, penis, or perineum)

Acute on Chronic Events

- Testicular tumour with rupture, haemorrhage, infarction or infection
- Hydrocele: rupture, haemorrhage, infection
- Spermatocele: rupture, haemorrhage

Inflammatory Conditions

- Fat necrosis of scrotal wall
- Henoch-Schonlein vasculitis of scrotal wall
- Idiopathic scrotal oedema (age 5–9 years; insidious onset of swelling and redness starting in the perineum or inguinal region and spreading to the hemi-scrotum; the testis is not tender)

Hernia

Incarcerated strangulated inguinal hernia.

Trauma

- Testicular rupture
- Haematocoele

Checklist for acute scrotum

- Lower urinary tract symptoms: dysuria; frequency, urgency
- Sexual history
- History of trauma
- Medical history: urinary tract abnormality; urinary tract infection
- Recent urinary tract catheterization or instrumentation
- Position, size and symmetry of testes
- Signs of cellulitis
- Site of maximal tenderness: testis; epididymis, superior pole of testis
- Presence or absence of cremasteric reflex
- Failure of relief of pain with scrotal elevation makes testicular torsion more likely
- Hernial orifices
- Urine dipstick analysis

Causes of acute epididymo-orchitis

- Sexually transmitted infections (high risk sexual activity: multiple sexual partners, unprotected sexual intercourse, insertive anal intercourse): Chlamydia trachomatis; Neisseria gonorrhoeae; Gram negative enteric organisms
- Non-sexually transmitted infections: mumps; Gram negative enteric organisms (obstructive urinary tract disease; urinary tract instrumentation); tuberculosis

Penile emergencies

Features of paraphimosis

- Caused by failure to reduce foreskin retraction after urethral catheterization, penile examination, sexual activity

- Penile pain
- Enlarged congested glans penis with a tight ring of preputial skin proximal to the glans
- The rest of the penile shaft is normal
- May cause acute urinary retention in children

Causes of priapism

Priapism is penile erection that lasts more than 4 h and is unrelated to sexual interest or stimulation. Ischaemic or low-flow priapism accounts for more than 95% of all presentations and is considered a compartment syndrome, requiring urgent decompression of the corpora cavernosa, ideally preceded by colour Doppler ultrasound scanning. The presentation is with a painful fully rigid penile shaft and a soft glans penis. High-flow priapism presents with an erection that is not fully rigid and is not painful.

- Low-flow (ischaemic; veno-occlusive)

  Haematological disorders: sickle cell disease; leukaemia; thalassemia; multiple myeloma.

  Prescription medications: oral vasoactive medications used to manage erectile dysfunction, eg sildenafil; alpha-adrenergic receptor antagonists, eg tamsulosin; antidepressants, eg fluoxetine; anti-psychotic agents, eg risperidone; oral anticoagulants, eg warfarin.

  Spinal cord trauma.

  Neoplasm: prostate cancer; bladder cancer.

  Poisonous venom: black widow spider or scorpion bites.

  Recreational drug abuse: marijuana, cocaine
- High-flow (non-ischaemic; arterial)

  Perineal straddle injury.

  Intracavernous injections for erectile dysfunction (papaverine, alprostadil).

Checklist for priapism

- Duration of erection
- Previous episodes of priapism and treatment given
- Drug history: prescribed medication including erectogenic therapy; recreational drugs
- History of haemoglobinopathy, such as sickle cell disease, thalassemia
- Trauma to penis, perineum (straddle injury) or pelvis
- Cavernosal blood gases

Acute kidney injury

Diagnosis

- Serum creatinine rise $\geq$ 26 micromol/l from baseline within a 48 h period, or an increase of more than or equal to 1.5 to 2 fold from baseline
- Serum creatinine rise by 50% or more in 7 days
- Urine output <0.5 ml/kg/h for six consecutive hours in adults

Causes

Pre-renal

- Intravascular fluid volume depletion: **extracellular fluid loss**: haemorrhage; gastrointestinal losses (diarrhoea and vomiting); skin losses: burns, Stevens-Johnson syndrome; renal salt- and water-wasting states; excessive diuresis; loss of intravascular fluid into extravascular space (**extracellular fluid sequestration**): peritonitis, ascites, pancreatitis, crush injury
- Low cardiac output: heart failure; cardiomyopathy; ischaemic heart disease; positive pressure ventilation; abdominal compartment syndrome (tense ascites leading to intra-abdominal pressure > 20 mm Hg); pulmonary embolism
- Low systemic vascular resistance with peripheral vasodilatation: septic shock; liver failure; anti-hypertensive medication; anaphylaxis
- Increased renal vascular resistance (afferent arteriolar vasoconstriction): drugs-NSAIDs, radiocontrast agents, tacrolimus; renal artery obstruction; renal vein thrombosis; hepatorenal syndrome
- Reduced efferent arteriolar tone: ACE inhibitors; angiotensin II receptor blockers

Renal

- Glomeruli: acute glomerulonephritis, rapidly progressive glomerulonephritis
- Tubules: acute tubular necrosis (hypoxic-ischaemic injury, from prolonged hypotension); nephrotoxic (intravenous iodinated radiocontrast media; aminoglycosides; lithium; pentamidine; platinum-based chemotherapeutic agents) (endogenous toxins-heme pigment-myoglobin-rhabdomyolysis, haemoglobin-intravascular haemolysis) (urate crystals-tumour lysis syndrome); multiple myeloma cast nephropathy
- Interstitium: acute interstitial nephritis (pyuria and white cell casts); drugs: β-lactam antibiotics-penicillins and cephalosporins, NSAIDs, proton pump inhibitors, allourinol, ACE inhibitors, sulphonamides; infection: pyelonephritis
- Vascular: renal artery obstruction-thrombosis, emboli, vasculitis, dissection; renal vein obstruction-thrombosis, thromboembolic disease including haemolytic uraemic syndrome and thrombotic thrombocytopenic purpura

Post-renal (obstruction in the renal pelvis, ureters, bladder or urethra)

- Ureteric obstruction: lumen: stone, papillary necrosis, blood clot; intramural: tumour, post-radiation fibrosis, stricture; extrinsic: retroperitoneal tumour/fibrosis, pelvic malignancy
- Bladder neck obstruction: benign prostatic hyperplasia; prostate cancer; neurogenic bladder; bladder tumour; stone disease; haemorrhage/clot
- Urethral obstruction: stricture, tumour; phimosis

Risk factors for acute kidney injury

- Age >75 years
- Pre-existing chronic kidney disease (eGFR < 60 ml/min/1.73 m squared)
- Previous history of acute kidney injury
- Symptoms/history of obstructive uropathy
- Chronic conditions: heart failure; liver disease; diabetes mellitus
- Atherosclerotic peripheral vascular disease
- Nephrotoxic medication use within last week: NSAIDs; ACE inhibitors; angiotensin II receptor antagonists; diuretics
- Hypovolaemia
- Sepsis
- Oliguria (urine output <0.5 ml/kg/h)
- Cardiac surgery
- Exposure to iodinated contrast agents within last week

Evaluation of acute kidney injury

- General: current symptoms; skin rash; eyes: uveitis; joint swelling
- Volume status: heart rate, blood pressure, peripheral perfusion; jugular venous pressure, core temperature, skin turgor, moistness of mucous membranes
- Lower urinary tract symptoms
- Drug history, including over-the-counter, recreational drugs and herbal remedies
- Signs of renovascular disease: bruits
- Abdominal examination: palpable bladder; pelvic or rectal masses

Causes of uraemia

- Acute kidney injury
- End-stage renal disease
- Increased dietary protein load
- Catabolic state with fever: sepsis; rhabdomyolysis
- Gastrointestinal haemorrhage
- Hypovolaemia; dehydration; low cardiac output

Potential acute presentations with end-stage renal disease

- Anaemia (erythropoietin deficiency)
- Bleeding disorder
- Gastrointestinal symptoms: anorexia, nausea, vomiting; gastrointestinal bleeding
- Volume overload: pulmonary oedema

- Neuromuscular presentations: muscle cramps; peripheral neuropathy; asterixis; seizures; encephalopathy
- Cardiovascular: pericarditis; cardiac tamponade; congestive heart failure

Reversible causes of acute deterioration in renal function in the presence of chronic kidney disease

- Infection: urinary tract infection; sepsis
- Reduced renal perfusion: hypovolaemia; heart failure
- Nephrotoxins: endogenous (myoglobin, haemoglobin, calcium, uric acid); exogenous (drugs, contrast media)
- Malignant hypertension

Complications of arteriovenous fistula for intermittent haemodialysis that can present acutely

- **Thrombosis**: severe pain; palpable thrombus
- Stenosis: difficulty in cannulation; arm oedema
- Aneurysm: pseudoaneurysm; venous aneurysm
- Steal syndrome: hand ischaemia during exercise and/or haemodialysis
- Congestive heart failure
- Infection at vascular access site

Features of urethral trauma

- Blood at the external urethal meatus or vaginal introitus
- Macroscopic haematuria
- Perineal (butterfly pattern), penile or scrotal haematoma
- Inability to pass urine
- Distended bladder
- Urine extravasation in the scrotum

14 Haematological and Oncological Emergencies

Causes of neutropenia (total neutrophil count <1 × 10/L regardless of total white cell count)

- Infections: bacterial; viral; rickettsial; parasitic
- Drugs: antibiotics; chemotherapy agents; anti-metabolites; antipsychotics; anti-thyroid drugs; anti-epileptic drugs; heavy metals
- Ionizing radiation
- Haematopoeitic disease: leukaemia; aplastic anaemia
- Autoimmune: SLE
- Hypersplenism
- Nutritional: alcoholism; B12/folate deficiency

Neutropenic sepsis should be considered with presentations within 6 weeks of last administration of chemotherapy or radiotherapy for cancer.

Evaluation of neutropenic sepsis (febrile neutropenia is defined as a single oral temperature greater than 38.3 degrees Centigrade, or a temperature greater than 38.0 degrees Centigrade sustained over 1 h, in association with a neutrophil count <0.5 × 10^9/L)

- Inspect intravenous access sites
- Skin sepsis
- Oropharyngeal sepsis: gums; pharynx
- Palpate maxillary and frontal sinuses
- Chest auscultation; chest xray
- Inspect perianal area for cellulitis and abscess; avoid rectal examination as may cause bacteraemia
- Urine dipstick analysis
- Cultures from each intravenous port and from peripheral blood

Causes of neutrophilia

- Infections: bacterial; parasitic; viral; fungal
- Inflammation
- Drugs: glucocorticoids; lithium
- Haemorrhage
- Burns
- Gangrene
- Myelo-proliferative disorders: leukaemia; polycythaemia rubra vera
- Physiological: exercise, stress; menstruation
- Metabolic: diabetic ketoacidosis; acute kidney injury

Causes of leukaemoid reactions (WBC count >50,000/cu mm)

- Haemorrhage
- Drugs: glucocorticoids; all-trans retinoic acid
- Infections: tuberculosis; pertussis; infectious mononucleosis
- Asplenia
- Acute haemolysis

A. Banerjee, *Emergency Clinical Diagnosis*, DOI 10.1007/978-3-319-50718-7_14

- Diabetic ketoacidosis
- Organ necrosis: ischaemic colitis

Causes of eosinophilia (eosinophil count >500/μl)

- Allergic/atopic disease: asthma; allergic rhinitis; urticaria
- Parasitic infestations: helminths (ascariasis); filariasis; toxocara; trichinella; strongyloides; visceral larva migrans; ankylostomiasis
- Fungal disease
- Drug reaction with eosinophilia and systemic symptoms (DRESS)
- Skin disease: dermatitis herpetiformis
- Pulmonary infiltration with eosinophilia (eosinophilic pulmonary infiltration with peripheral blood eosinophilia): Loeffler's syndrome; tropical eosinophilia; Churg-Strauss syndrome (eosinophilic granuloma with polyangiitis); nitrofurantoin lung
- Myeloproliferative disease: chronic myeloid leukaemia; polycythaemia vera
- Lymphoproliferative disease: acute lymphoblastic leukaemia; lymphoma (Hodgkin; non-Hodgkin; T-cell); mycosis fungoides

Hypereosinophilic syndrome is characterized by:

- Eosinophil count >1500/μl for longer than 6 months
- Signs of end-organ involvement attributable to eosinophilic infiltration
- No identifiable cause

Causes of lymphocytosis (lymphocyte count >5,000/μl)

- Transient, reactive: acute viral infections (infectious mononucleosis; CMV; hepatitis); acute bacterial infections (pertussis; typhoid)
- Chronic intracellular bacterial infection (tuberculosis; brucellosis); secondary syphilis
- Protozoal infection: toxoplasmosis; American trypanosomiasis (Chagas disease)
- Haematological malignancy: chronic lymphocytic leukaemia; lymphoma (non-Hodgkin); acute lymphoblastic leukaemia

Causes of lymphocytopenia (lymphocyte count <1500/μl)

- Reduced production: aplastic anaemia; thymic dysplasia; ataxia telangiectasia; Wiskott-Aldrich syndrome
- Increased destruction: radiation therapy; cancer chemotherapy (alkylating agents); glucocorticoids
- Increased loss: intestinal lymphangiectasia (protein-losing enteropathy); impaired intestinal lymphatic drainage (Whipple disease); thoracic duct leak

Causes of thrombocytopenia

Artifactual: platelet clumping

Reduced production of platelets

- Diminished or absent megakaryoctes in bone marrow: aplastic anaemia; leukaemia or other infiltrative bone marrow disease; dose-dependent bone marrow suppression (chemotherapeutic agents); paroxysmal nocturnal haemoglobinuria
- Diminished platelet production despite the presence of megakaryocytes in bone marrow: alcohol-induced thrombocytopenia; HIV-associated thrombocytopenia; B12 or folate deficiency

Altered distribution: platelet sequestration in enlarged spleen (hypersplenism)

Cirrhosis with portal hypertension and congestive splenomegaly

Myelofibrosis with myeloid metaplasia

Increased destruction of platelets

(a) **Immunological**

- Idiopathic thrombocytopenic purpura
- Systemic lupus erythematosus
- Anti-phospholipid syndrome
- Post-transfusion purpura (allo-immune)

- Drug-mediated: immune-mediated platelet destruction (heparin-heparin dependent IgG antibodies bind to heparin/platelet factor 4 complexes; falling platelet count during or following heparin treatment, with or without thrombosis-venous or arterial), trimethoprim
- Lymphoproliferative disorders

(b) **Non-immunological**
Systemic infections (hepatitis; Epstein-Barr virus, cytomegalovirus)
Disseminated intravascular coagulation
Sepsis
Pregnancy (gestational thrombocytopenia)
Thrombotic microangiopathies associated with consumptive thrombocytopenia, microangiopathic haemolytic anaemia, and thrombosis: thrombotic thrombocytopenic purpura; haemolytic uraemic syndrome; disseminated intravascular coagulation

Dilution
Massive red blood cell replacement or exchange transfusion

Causes of multiple bruising

- Purpura simplex
- Alcohol abuse
- Non-accidental injury; elder abuse
- Senile purpura: transient red to purple patches on the forearms and dorsal aspects of hands
- Vitamin C deficiency
- Cushing's syndrome
- Connective tissue disease: Ehlers-Danlos syndrome
- Medication: aspirin, clopidogrel, oral anticoagulants, NSAIDs

Features of non-accidental bruising in children

- Children not independently mobile
- Babies
- Away from bony prominences
- Bruises on the face, back, abdomen, arms, buttocks, ears, hands
- Multiple bruises in clusters
- Multiple bruises of uniform shape
- Bruises carrying the imprint of the implement used (linear marks from sticks or belts) or ligature marks
- Symmetrical bruising
- Human bite marks

Features of acute idiopathic thrombocytopenic purpura

- Abrupt onset; occasional preceding upper respiratory tract infection
- Skin bruising with ecchymoses
- Mucosal bleeding: epistaxis; bleeding gums; vaginal bleeding
- Subconjunctival haemorrhage
- No splenomegaly

Causes of thrombocytosis (platelet count >450,000/μl)

- Spurious: cryoglobulinaemia; red cell fragmentation syndromes
- Primary: clonal myeloproliferative disorders (associated with increased risk of thrombotic (arterial and venous) and haemorrhagic events): essential thrombocythaemia (isolated thrombocytosis); polycythaemia vera; chronic myeloid leukaemia; chronic myelomonocytic leukaemia; myelodysplastic syndrome; refractory anaemia with ringed sideroblasts associated with thrombocytosis; primary myelofibrosis
- Secondary, or reactive (associated with raised inflammatory markers or acute/chronic blood loss)
- Transient causes: acute blood loss; recovery (rebound) from myelosuppression (cancer chemotherapy); acute infection/inflammation; extreme physical exertion
- Sustained causes: asplenia: post-splenectomy; functional; chronic inflammation: rheumatoid arthritis, vasculitis, connective

tissue disease, tuberculosis, inflammatory bowel disease; Iron deficiency anaemia; haemolytic anaemia; drugs: glucocorticoids, vinca alkaloids, adrenaline; lymphoma

Presentations of coagulation disorders

- Small vessel bleeding in the skin (petchiae), mucosae, including gastrointestinal and genital tracts is associated with thrombocytopenia, qualitative platelet defects and von Willebrand's disease
- Large vessel bleeding into muscles, joints and solid organs is associated with coagulation factor deficiencies, such as haemophilia
- A bleeding history checklist should include note of spontaneous bruising, epistaxis, bleeding with dental extraction or after surgery, bleeding after accidental trauma, and in women abnormal menstrual bleeding (menorrhagia) and pregnancy-related building. A family history of bleeding disorder should also be obtained.

Possible acute presentations of haemophilia include:

- Acute haemarthrosis (knee, ankle, elbow) (an aura of tingling and tightness within the joint often precedes rapid joint swelling)
- Intramuscular bleeding (quadriceps, hamstrings, iliopsoas, biceps, triceps, forearm flexors), producing acute compartment syndrome, or spontaneous ilio-psoas haematoma (triad of groin pain, hip flexion, and femoral neuropathy)
- Intracranial haemorrhage
- Gastrointestinal bleeding
- Post-traumatic bleeding

Causes of microcytic hypochromic anaemia

- Iron deficiency
- Sideroblastic anaemia
- Thalassaemia
- Anaemia of chronic disease

Iron deficiency (low serum ferritin; low serum iron with increased iron-binding capacity and raised transferrin)

Chronic blood loss
- Gastrointestinal tract: carcinoma-colon/gastric; gastric or duodenal ulceration; NSAIDs; hookworm infestation; angiodysplasia; inflammatory bowel disease
- Uterine: menorrhagia

Dietary iron deficiency: vegans, elderly
Failure of iron absorption
- Antacids; proton pump inhibitors

Increased losses:
- Chronic intravascular haemolysis with haemosiderin loss in the urine

Excessive iron requirements
- Pregnancy
- Exfoliative skin disease

Features suggesting haemolytic anaemia

- Anaemia with reticulocytosis (evidence of increased erythropoeitic activity)
- Evidence of increased red blood cell destruction: raised serum unconjugated bilirubin, lactate dehydrogenase; decreased serum haptoglobin and detection of urine haemosiderin indicate intravascular haemolysis
- Abnormal red blood cell morphology: microspherocytes
- Evidence of intravascular haemolysis: red blood cell fragments (schistocytes) on peripheal smear

Causes of haemolytic anaemia
Normal red blood cells; autologous and transfused cells are both destroyed

- Immunological: autoimmune haemolytic anaemia (autoantibodies to red cell surface antigens: warm antibody-IgG; cold agglutinin-IgM); alloimmune haemolytic

anaemia: induced by red cell antigens: haemolytic transfusion reaction, post-stem cell grafts, or drug-induced. Cold agglutinin haemolytic anaemias can be caused by infections (Mycoplasma pneumoniae; infectious mononucleosis), lymphoproliferative disorders-lymphoma and chronic lymphocytic leukaemia, and paroxysmal cold haemoglobinuria.
- Reticuloendothelial hyperactivity: hypersplenism
- Microangiopathic (mechanical destruction of red cells in the circulation): thrombotic thrombocytopenic purpura; haemolytic uraemic syndrome (triad of microangiopathy haemolytic anaemia, thrombocytopenia and acute kidney injury); DIC; defective prosthetic heart valves-with peri-valvular leaks; malignant hypertension; pre-eclampsia/HELLP
- Infections: toxin-mediated (alpha- and beta-haemolytic streptococci; meningococcus; Clostridium perfringens); red cell invasion and destruction (Plasmodium falciparum; Bartonella; Babesiosis)
- Snake bite

Abnormal red blood cells

- Cell membrane disorders: hereditary spherocytosis; hereditary elliptocytosis
- Enzyme disorders: G6PD deficiency; pyruvate kinase deficiency
- Haemoglobinopathies: sickle cell disease; thalassaemia; unstable haemoglobins

Causes of macrocytic anaemia (MCV >1OO femtolitres)

Normal erythropoeisis
- Liver disease
- Reticulocytosis: haemorrhage; haemolysis
- Severe hypothyroidism/hypopituitarism
- Alcohol abuse

Megaloblastic erythropoeisis or dyserthyr opoeisis
- Nutritional deficiency: B12/folate deficiency
- Haemolytic anaemia
- Haematological malignancy
- Myelodysplastic syndrome

Causes of folate deficiency

- Dietary deficiency, especially in alcoholics
- Increased requirements: pregnancy; haemolysis
- Malabsorption: gluten-induced enteropathy; jejunal resection
- Increased loss
- Drugs: folic acid antagonists; purine analogues; pyrimidine analogues; ribonucleotide reductase inhibitors; anti-epileptic drugs (phenytoin)

Causes of vitamin B12 deficiency

- Gastric: intrinsic factor deficiency with atrophic gastritis (pernicious anaemia); gastrectomy
- Terminal ileal disease: Crohn's disease; resection; parasitic infestation: Diphyllobothrium latum
- Dietary deficiency, in vegans

Causes of polycythaemia

True polycythaemia (increased red cell mass)
- Primary: polycythaemia vera (splenomegaly; thromboembolism; headache; pruritus; gout)
- Secondary
  - Central hypoxia: high altitude; chronic lung disease (COPD); congenital cyanotic heart disease (right to left shunts); heavy smoking; chronic carbon monoxide exposure; hypoventilation syndromes (obstructive sleep apnoea)
  - Renal hypoxia: renal artery stenosis; polycystic kidney disease; end stage renal disease
  - Exogenous EPO: drugs used in doping: recombinant EPO; androgens (anabolic steroids)
  - Pathological EPO production: neoplasm (hepatocellular carcinoma; renal cell cancer; cerebellar haemangioblastoma; uterine leiomyoma)
  - Congenital: high oxygen-affinity haemoglobins (may be familial)

Apparent (relative) polycythaemia

- Dehydration or plasma loss: diarrhea and vomiting; burns
- Chronic apparent polycythaemia (stress polycythaemia): associated with obesity, hypertension, diuretic therapy, heavy smoking, and high alcohol intake

Causes of acquired methaemoglobinaemia (>1% of haemoglobin in red blood cells is replaced by methaemoglobin)-due to exposure to oxidizing agents

- Drugs: antimicrobial agents (dapsone; sulphonamides); local anaesthetics (benzocaine-contained in over-the-counter gels and liquids, lidocaine, prilocaine, EMLA cream)
- Toxins: aniline dyes; nitrates; nitrites (used as preservatives and dyes in food industry); amyl nitrate (recreational drug in poppers)
- Nitric oxide donors: glyceryl trinitrate; nitric oxide; nitrous oxide; nitroprusside
- Industrial chemicals: nitrobenzene; nitroethane
- Pesticides

Presenting features of methaemoglobinaemia

- Central cyanosis unresponsive to oxygen administration
- Cardiovascular: dyspnoea; dizziness, syncope; cardiac arrhythmias
- Neurological: lethargy; headache; seizures; coma

Causes of raised carboxyhaemoglobin levels

- Smoking
- Carbon monoxide inhalation: carbon monoxide is produced by the incomplete combustion of hydrocarbon-containing material, such as fossil fuels (coal, natural gas, petroleum, diesel) and biomass fuels (wood). Gas stoves, fires and boilers, charcoal grills, gas powered water heaters, paraffin heaters, solid fuel powered stoves, boilers and room heaters are all potential sources. The risk increases in enclosed or poorly ventilated spaces. Carbon monoxide detectors allow for early recognition of potential toxic exposure. There is a poor correlation between COHb levels and symptom severity
- Methylene chloride (dichloromethane) toxicity (solvent in paint and varnish strippers and in degreasing agents; propellant for insecticides, air fresheners and paints; exposure usually occupational, but may also be environmental or household)

Clues to the diagnosis of domestic carbon monoxide poisoning

The diagnosis can be difficult to suspect, as the early symptoms (headache, confusion, nausea, vomiting, dizziness, weakness, and shortness of breath) are non-specific, but can be suggested in the following circumstances:

- More than one person in the house affected with non-specific illness, including pets
- Symptoms better when away from the house, eg on holiday, but recur on returning home
- Symptoms related to cooking, with a stove in use; wood burning stove
- Seasonal symptoms, worse in winter, with heating in use-fossil fuel use; minimised ventilation

Causes of supra-therapeutic INR (international normalized ratio) while on warfarin therapy

- Warfarin dosage and compliance, including inadvertent over-medication
- Drug history, including prescribed drugs, over-the-counter drugs and herbal supplements (check INR 3–5 days after commencing any drug interacting with warfarin that will be administered for longer than 7 days)
- Alcohol intake
- Changes to diet: reduction in vitamin K rich foods, such as leafy green vegetables; consumption of fruit juices, especially cranberry or grapefruit
- Liver disease
- Cancer

Presentations of sickle cell crisis

- Bone crisis (vaso-occlusive crisis)
- Acute chest syndrome: low grade fever, non-productive cough, shortness of breath, haemoptysis, acute chest pain, signs of consolidation, new infiltrate on chest xray
- Acute splenic sequestration: pallor; lethargy; hypotension; rapid splenic enlargement
- CNS complications: stroke, presenting with hemiparesis, monoparesis, aphasia/dysphasia, cranial nerve palsies or coma
- Acute anaemia, presenting with pallor, tachycardia, tachypnoea, jaundice, enlarged spleen/liver, S3 gallop, congestive heart failure: bone marrow suppression (viral or other infections); sequestration of blood in the liver or spleen; increased intravascular haemolysis (hyper-haemolytic crisis)

Precipitants for sickle cell crises include

- Infection
- Dehydration
- Hypoxia
- Acidosis
- Sedatives
- Alcohol
- Excessive physical exercise

Categories of oncological emergencies

- Metabolic: malignant hypercalcaemia (osteolytic metastases; humoral hypercalcaemia); acute tumour lysis syndrome (abrupt and massive release of cellular metabolites into the circulation after rapid lysis of malignant cells, producing the metabolic triad of hyperkalaemia, hyperphosphatemia, hyperuricaemia; secondary hypocalcaemia; acute kidney injury); SIADH
- Neurological: metastatic spinal cord compression; brain metastases (raised intracranial pressure; seizures)
- Cardiovascular: malignant pericardial effusion (cardiac tamponade); superior vena cava obstruction
- Haematological: hyperviscosity syndrome (triad of bleeding, including mucosal bleeding-epistaxis, bleeding gums gastrointestinal bleeding, and purpura; visual disturbance, including central retinal vein occlusion, retinal haemorrhages and papilloedema; and focal neurological signs); hyper-leukocytosis (leukostasis; WCC >100,000/cu. mm.; CNS manifestations, such as headache, blurred vision, visual field defects and papilloedema; and lung manifestations, including effort dyspnoea, hypoxaemia and respiratory distress); DIC
- Infections: febrile neutropenia; septic shock
- Chemotherapy agent side effects
  - Extravasation injuries: vesicants (anthracyclines; vinca alkaloids, mitomycin C); irritants (taxanes; platinums; epipodphyllotoxins; topoisomerase I inhibitors)
  - Gastrointestinal: mucositis; enteritis with diarrhea and dehydration; obstipation

Causes of hyperviscosity syndrome

- Myeloma (especially IgA)
- Waldenstrom's macroglobulinaemia
- Polycythaemia vera
- Hyper-leukocytosis

Features of hyperviscosity syndrome

- Neurological: confusion; ataxia; nystagmus; vertigo; coma
- Visual disturbance: blurred vision; amaurosis fugax; central retinal vein occlusion
- Genitourinary and gastrointestinal bleeding

Risk factors for tumour lysis syndrome

The metabolic triad of tumour lysis syndrome comprises hyperuricaemia, hyperkalaemia and hyperphosphataemia

- Tumour related: rapid progression; large tumour burden

(LDH >1500 IU/ml, WCC >50 × 10^3/L); extensive bone marrow involvement; high tumour sensitivity to cancer chemotherapy agents
- Host factors: intravascular volume depletion (dehydration); pre-existing hyperuricaemia; obstructive uropathy; chronic kidney disease; concurrent potentially nephrotoxic medication

Features of malignant spinal cord compression (extradural tumour growth; peri-tumoral oedema and thecal compression; pathological fracture with angulation of the spinal cord; tumour induced spinal arterial occlusion)

- Back pain is the most common initial symptom, preceding neurological symptoms in 95% of cases. In cervical region compression, subscapular pain is noted, in the thoracic region thoracic pain, and in the lumbosacral region lumbosacral or hip pain. The back pain can be multi-segmental or band-like, and is increasing in severity, with poor response to analgesic medication. The pain is increased on lying on the back.
- Radicular pain
- Motor: progressive weakness (heaviness of legs), gait abnormalities; paraparesis (thoracic level compression)
- Conus medullaris syndrome (upper lumbar spine compression): distal lower limb weakness, saddle anaesthesia, overflow incontinence of bladder and bowel)
- Loss of bladder and bowel function is generally a late sign
- The spine should be considered to be unstable unless proven otherwise

Checklist for causes of nausea and vomiting in patients with cancer

- Medication: cancer chemotherapy; opioids
- Mucosal irritation: NSAIDs; gastro-oesophageal reflux
- Mechanical obstruction of bowel
- Metastatic disease: cerebral; liver
- Metabolic complications: hypercalcaemia; hyponatraemia
- Meningeal irritation: raised intracranial pressure
- Sepsis: gastrointestinal; systemic
- Cardiac: myocardial ischaemia; congestive heart failure
- Anxiety

Emergency presentations and manifestations of acute leukaemia include

- Bone marrow failure (secondary to infiltration), presenting with features of the triad of anaemia (fatigue, effort intolerance, pallor, congestive heart failure), thrombocytopenia (spontaneous mucosal and skin (petchiae, purpura) bleeding) and neutropenia (recurrent infections; neutropenic sepsis)
- Visceral infiltration:
  Hepatomegaly, splenomegaly, lymphadenopathy (ALL)
  Mediastinal mass with superior vena cava syndrme (T-ALL)
  Gingival hyperplasia (monocytic subtype of AML)
  Bone and joint pain, occasionally with limp (ALL)
  Testicular swelling
- CNS involvement: chloroma (myelosarcoma)- orbit, spinal extradural compression with cauda equina syndrome; intracranial haemorrhage; leukaemic meningitis (meningeal syndrome)
- Leukostasis (CNS: stroke; pulmonary: infiltrates, hypoxaemia)
- Constitutional symptoms: fever; weight loss
- Spontaneous tumour lysis syndrome (mature B-ALL)

Infectious Disease Emergencies 15

Sepsis definitions
SYSTEMIC INFLAMMATORY RESPONSE SYNDROME

CRITERIA: Requires two or more of the following:

- Temperature >38 C or <36 degrees Centigrade
- Heart rate >90 beats/minute in the absence of beta-blocker
- Respiratory rate >20 breaths/minute or paCO2<4.2 kPa (32 mmHg)
- White blood cell count >12,000/cu.mm, <4000/cu mm or >10% immature forms (left shift)

SEPSIS

- SIRS in a patient with a confirmed source of infection

SEVERE SEPSIS

- Sepsis in the presence of organ dysfunction and hypotension (<90 mmHg or 40 mmHg reduction from normal blood pressure in the absence of other causes of hypotension)

SEPTIC SHOCK

Sepsis (SIRS + infection) with a systolic blood pressure <90 mmHg or a drop of >30 mmHg, despite adequate resuscitation and signs of perfusion deficits (i.e. lactic acidosis, oliguria, depressed mental status)

May not be hypotensive if vasopressors or inotropes are being used.

Causes of fever of unknown origin

- Infection
  Bacterial: tuberculosis; infective endocarditis; liver abscess; perinephric abscess; subphrenic abscess; bone and joint infections
  Viral: Epstein Barr virus; AIDS
  Chlamydial
  Rickettsial
  Fungal
  Protozoal: amoebic liver abscess
- Connective tissue disease: polyarteritis nodosa; systemic lupus erythematosus; Still's disease; polymyalgia rheumatica; temporal arteritis
- Malignancy: lymphoma; leukaemia; solid tumours: renal cell carcinoma; hepatocellular carcinoma
- Inflammatory bowel disease
- Drug fever
- Factitious fever (failure of temperature to follow normal diurnal cycle; health care professional; normal pulse and respiratory rate with fever, rapid defervescence without sweating; very high temperature 106 F or greater)

Fever check list

- Localising symptoms
- Pattern and duration of fever

A. Banerjee, *Emergency Clinical Diagnosis*, DOI 10.1007/978-3-319-50718-7_15

- Temperature-pulse relationship (relative bradycardia)
- Drug history, including intravenous drug use
- Travel history
- Sexual history
- Sick contacts
- Animal contacts
- Occupational history
- Immunisation history
- Implanted medical devices and prostheses
- Past history of serious, protracted, unusual recurrent infections

Sources of infection in sepsis

- Lungs: pneumonia, lung abscess
- Cardiovascular system: infective endocarditis
- Genitourinary system: urinary tract infection, pyelonephritis
- Gastrointestinal system: cholecystitis, diverticulitis, appendicitis, colitis, pelvic abscess
- Gynaecological: retained tampon; pelvic inflammatory disease
- Skin and soft tissue: cellulitis, necrotizing fasciitis, abscess
- Oral cavity: teeth, gums, pharynx, retropharyngeal space
- Ears, paranasal sinuses, nose
- Musculoskeletal: osteomyelitis; septic arthritis
- Indwelling intravascular devices: peripherally inserted central venous catheters
- CNS: meningitis

Fever in the returned traveller
Travel related illnesses include fever, diarrhoea, dysentery, skin and soft tissue infections, respiratory infections and meningoencephalitis, sometimes leading to coma

Checklist for history taking
- Countries of travel, including stopovers in transit
- Destinations within countries travelled to: rural/urban
- Prophylaxis; pre-travel immunisation
- Treatments or procedures: injections, blood transfusions, surgery
- Drugs: prescribed; over the counter; recreational
- Diet: seafood; raw or undercooked food; dairy products
- Sexual activity: protection; multiple partners; commercial sex
- Bites: insect; animal; snake; spider; human
- Freshwater skin contact

Clinical findings of relevance
- Maculopapular skin rash: dengue; acute HIV infection; syphilis; rickettsial infections
- Petechial skin rash: meningoccal infection; viral haemorrhagic fevers; leptospirosis; rickettsial infections
- Eschar: typhus; anthrax; spider bite; cutaneous diphtheria
- Ulcer: leishmaniasis; mycobacterial infection
- Jaundice: viral hepatitis; malaria; cholangitis; liver abscess (amoebic/ pyogenic)
- Lymphadenopathy: leishmaniasis; typhoid; acute HIV infection
- Hepatomegaly: viral hepatitis; malaria; schistosomiasis; amoebic liver abscess
- Splenomegaly: malaria; visceral leishmaniasis; brucellosis

Malaria should be suspected in the presence of:

- A flu-like illness (fever, chills, sweating, anorexia, headache, myalgia, arthralgia, nausea, abdominal pain, vomiting, diarrhea) in anyone who has visited a malaria endemic zone within the preceding 3 months. Malaria is endemic in sub-Saharan, central and west Africa, South and Central Asia, the Middle East, Korea, Central (including Mexico) and South America, Haiti and the Dominican Republic (Hispaniola), Oceania and Papua New Guinea
- Leukopenia, anaemia and thrombocytopenia are common

Severe malaria is recognized by the presence of one or more of the following

- Cerebral malaria (unrousable coma with peripheral Plasmodium falciparum parasitaemia after exclusion of other causes of encephalopathy)
- Severe normocytic anaemia (haemoglobin<5 g/dl)
- Acute kidney injury (serum creatinine >265 mmol/L)
- Acute pulmonary oedema/adult respiratory distress syndrome
- Hypotension/shock (systolic blood pressure <80 mmHg)
- Spontaneous bleeding and /or laboratory evidence of disseminated intravascular coagulation
- Generalised convulsions: more than two episodes in 24 h
- Jaundice
- Hyperpyrexia
- Hypoglycaemia (blood glucose <2.5 mmol/L)
- Metabolic acidosis (plasma bicarbonate <15 mmol/L)
- Hyperlactataemia (lactate >5 mmol/L)
- Macroscopic haemoglobinuria

Causes of fever and coma after foreign travel

- Cerebral malaria
- Viral encephalitis (herpes simplex, HIV, enteroviral, arboviral)
- Bacterial meningoencephalitis (pyogenic, tuberculous)
- Fungal and protozoal meningoencephalitis (African trypanosomiasis)
- Brain abscess

Causes of haemorrhagic fever in travellers

- Viral haemorrhagic fever; Dengue haemorrhagic fever
- Yellow fever
- Severe Gram negative or Gram positive sepsis; meningococcaemia
- Fulminant viral hepatitis
- Severe malaria
- Rickettsial infection
- Leptospirosis

Viral haemorrhagic fever should be suspected in the presence of:

- Travel to an area of endemic infection within 21 days
- Acute severe febrile flu-like illness, with malaise, fatigue, anorexia, headache, arthralgia, myalgia, nausea and vomiting
- Evidence of vascular involvement caused by virus-induced endothelial damage leading to increased vascular permeability: conjunctival injection and haemorrhage; petechiae, ecchymoses; bleeding from orifices (mouth-gingival, nose, ears, haematemesis and melaena); non-dependent oedema; shock; DIC
- An erythematous non-pruritic maculopapular rash (followed by desquamation of the affected skin 3–4 days after onset) and severe posterior pharyngeal oedema can be seen with Ebola and Marburg haemorrhagic fevers
- Arenavirus infection can be associated with pharyngitis, retrosternal chest pain and proteinuria

Causes of hyperthermic syndromes (core temperature > 41 C)

- Intracranial haemorrhage: pontine haemorrhage
- Heat stroke: exertional; non-exertional
- Drug-induced hyperthermia: amphetamines; monoamine oxidase inhibitors; cocaine; phencyclidine; tricyclic antidepressants; LSD
- Neuroleptic malignant syndrome: phenothiazines; butyrophenones; metoclopramide; domperidone
- Serotonin syndrome
- Malignant hyperthermia: inhalational anaesthetics; succinylcholine
- Endocrine: thyrotoxicosis (thyroid storm); phaeochromocytoma
- Delirium tremens

Features of heat stroke

- Exposure to heat stress: exogenous or endogenous
- Signs of severe CNS dysfunction: seizures; delirium; coma
- Core temperature >40.5 C (105 F)
- Dry, hot skin is common; sweating may persist
- Marked rise in liver transaminases

HIV-associated diseases leading to acute presentation

Central and peripheral nervous systems

- Cerebral toxoplasmosis
- Cryptococcal meningitis
- HIV myelopathy
- HIV encephalopathy
- Progressive multifocal leukoencephalopathy
- Primary brain lymphoma
- Viral encephalitis (CMV, HSV, VZV)
- Viral myelitis (CMV, HSV, VZV)

Respiratory tract

- Pneumocysis jiroveci pneumonia
- Pulmonary tuberculosis
- Bacterial pneumonia
- Kaposi sarcoma

Gastrointestinal tract

- Candidal stomatitis and oesophagitis
- Oral hairy leukoplakia
- Cryptosporidiosis; isosporiasis
- Anorectal herpes simplex

16 Paediatric Emergencies

Assessment of child with fever

Measurement of temperature:

- Age <4 weeks: electronic thermometer in axilla
- 4 weeks to 5 years: electronic thermometer or chemical dot thermometer in axilla, or infrared tympanic thermometer

Life-threatening features

- Compromise of airway, breathing or circulation
- Decreased level of consciousness

Low risk for serious illness (nice guidelines)

- Normal colour of skin, lips and tongue
- Normal response to social cues
- Content/smiles
- Stays awake or awakens quickly
- Strong normal cry or absence of crying
- Moist mucous membranes

Signs of toxicity

- A: reduced alertness, arousal or activity (no response to social cues)
- B: breathing difficulties: tachypnoea, increased work of breathing
- C: colour (pale, blue, ashen or mottled), circulation (cool peripheries), cry (weak, high pitched or continuous)
- D: decreased fluid intake or decreased urine output (fewer than four nappies a day)

Other concerning features

- Persistent fever despite anti-pyretic treatment
- Fever more than 5 days
- Presence of vomiting, including bile-stained vomit

Localising signs in sepsis

- Respiratory: localized crepitations, signs of consolidation
- Gastrointestinal: focal/ rebound tenderness and guarding
- CNS: signs of meningeal irritation, encephalopathy
- Bone and soft tissue: focal redness, tenderness and oedema
- Head and neck: cervical lymphadenopathy, paranasal sinus tenderness, stridor, tonsillo-pharyngeal exudate
- Skin: pustular lesions
- Cardiovascular: changing murmurs

Causes of fever without focus

- Viral infection
- Urinary tract infection
- Malaria

A. Banerjee, *Emergency Clinical Diagnosis*, DOI 10.1007/978-3-319-50718-7_16

- Connective tissue disease
- Occult abscess
- Occult bacteraemia
- Drug fever

Diagnostic criteria for Kawasaki Disease

Fever of at least 38.5 degrees Centigrade, lasting at least 5 days and typically unresponsive to antipyretics and antibiotics

At least four out of the following five

- Bilateral non-purulent conjunctivitis; primarily bulbar
- Mucosal changes of the oropharynx: dry red lips with fissures, strawberry tongue, oropharyngeal erythema; no discrete oral lesions or exudates
- Changes in extremities: oedema and/or erythema of the palms of the hands and the soles of the feet; desquamation, beginning peri-ungually around the nail bed
- Rash: usually truncal, polymorphous, erythematous or maculo-papular; no petechial, vesicular or bullous lesions
- Cervical lymphadenopathy, often unilateral and large (>1.5 cm in diameter)

Exclusion of other diagnoses, including measles, rubella, adenovirus infection, streptococcal scarlet fever, toxic shock syndrome, Stevens-Johnson syndrome, leptospirosis, parvovirus infection

Recognition of the sick child

- Airway: partial obstruction (bubbly noises, snoring, stridor)
- Breathing: apnoeic episodes, bradypnoea, tachypnoea, chest recession (supraclavicular, intercostal, subcostal or substernal), tracheal tug, use of accessory muscles of respiration, head bobbing (neck extension during inspiration and neck flexion during expiration) in infants, nasal flaring(exaggerated opening of nostrils during breathing), end-expiratory grunting, cyanosis, gasping, wheezing, silent chest
- Circulation: tachycardia, pallor, reduced level of consciousness, confusion, agitation, reduced urine output, prolonged capillary refill time, mottled skin, cold extremities
- Disability: reduced alertness, high pitched or other abnormal quality of cry, seizure, floppiness, posturing

Normal values for children

Blood pressure in mmHg

Age	Systolic	Diastolic	Mean
Neonate (<1 kg)	40–60	15–35	25–45
(3 kg)	50–70	25–45	35–55
Infant (6 months)	85–105	55–65	65–80
Child (2 years)	95–105	55–65	65–80
(7 years)	100–110	55–70	70–85
Adolescent	110–130	65–80	80–95

Normal systolic blood pressure = 70 mmHg + age in years × 2

Normal diastolic blood pressure = 2/3rds systolic blood pressure

Age (years)	Respiratory rate	Heart rate	Blood volume (ml/kg)
<1	30–40	110–160	85–90
1–2	23–35	100–150	80–85
2–5	25–30	95–140	75–80
5–12	20–25	80–120	65–70
>12	15–20	60–100	65–70

The key elements of initial assessment of a child involve:

Appearance: The **TICLS** ("tickles") mnemonic summarises the main components of assessment of the general appearance of a child:

- Tone
- Interactiveness
- Consolability
- Look/gaze
- Speech/cry

Work of breathing: abnormal positioning; abnormal airway sounds; retractions; nasal flaring.

Circulation to skin: pallor; mottling; cyanosis.

Recognition of increased work of breathing in children

- Abnormal airway sounds: altered voice; wheeze; stridor; grunting
- Abnormal positioning: head bobbing; tripoding
- Chest wall retractions: supraclavicular, intercostal, subcostal and sternal
- Nasal flaring

Causes of reduced level of consciousness in childhood

- Shock (hypovolaemic, distributive, cardio genic)
- Sepsis
- Metabolic diseases
- Intracranial infections
- Raised intracranial pressure
- Convulsions; post-ictal state
- Intoxication/poisoning
- Trauma
- Hypertension
- Stroke
- Acute hydrocephalus

Causes of incessant crying in infants and young children

- Infantile colic: characterized by paroxysmal episodes of incessant crying (usually daily), high-pitched cry, generalized hypertonicity and inconsolability. The onset is at 1–4 weeks of age, and there is spontaneous improvement by the age of 3–4 months
- Infections: otitis media; meningitis; encephalitis; systemic sepsis; urinary tract infection, osteomyelitis, septic arthritis, pneumonia, gastroenteritis
- Trauma: limb fracture; shaken baby
- Gastrointestinal: intusussuception; gastro-oesophageal reflux; constipation; anal fissure; incarcerated inguinal hernia; testicular torsion; appendicitis
- Metabolic: hyponatraemia; hypernatraemia; hypoglycaemia; hyperglycaemia
- Skin: nappy rash; atopic eczema

Red flags with incessant crying

- Fever: temperature greater than 38 degrees Centigrade in infant less than 12 weeks' age
- Paradoxical irritability: unwillingness to be held
- Poor feeding
- Cyanotic or apneic spells
- Bilious or projectile vomiting
- Bloody stools
- Antibiotic pre-treatment
- Meningism
- Abnormal limb movement
- Abdominal tenderness or mass

Risk Factors for Non-accidental Injury

Parental

- Young parental age: teenage parents
- Single parent family; separation/divorce
- Deprivation
- Lack of social support
- Low self esteem
- Drug or alcohol abuse
- Domestic violence
- Mental health problem
- Financial stress
- Parent abused or neglected in childhood
- Non-biological parents in the home

Child

- Learning difficulties
- Behavioural difficulties
- Physical disability
- Chronic illness
- Prematurity; low birth weight

Historical features indicating non-accidental injury

- History not consistent with pattern of injury
- Inconsistent history between different family members
- Injuries that are not consistent with developmental age of child
- Unwitnessed injury
- Delayed presentation to health care
- Different history from carers at different times
- Repeated attendance to hospital

Signs of non-accidental injury

- Any bruising to young babies
- Long bone fractures in children aged <18 months
- Spiral fractures in long bones, especially humerus
- Rib fractures (especially) posterior in very young children
- Bruising on unusual places away from bony prominences, including the ears, cheeks, chin, buttocks, trunk and posterior thigh
- Bruising patterns: multiple clusters; patterned (in shape of causative objects); linear marks (from belt or cane); fingerprint bruises
- Small deep, circular burns (cigarette burns) or other contact burns
- Immersion scalds to either feet or buttocks
- Red lines to wrists or ankles (from ligatures)
- Human bite marks (U shaped)
- Isolated tear of upper lip fraenulum
- General neglect
- Failure to thrive without organic causes
- Multiple injuries of different ages
- Injuries to genitalia
- Subdural haematoma in children aged under 1 year
- Regression to younger behaviour patterns

Features suggestive of sexual abuse

- Vaginal discharge/bleeding in a pre-pubertal child
- Recurrent vulvovaginitis
- Genital or anal injury
- Rectal bleeding
- Pregnancy and terminations
- Sexually transmitted infections
- Soiling or wetting in a previously toilet-trained child

X-ray features of non-accidental injury

- Epiphyseal-metaphyseal junction fractures (bucket-handle or corner fractures)
- Metaphyseal chip fractures
- Diaphyseal fractures: spiral/oblique; multiple fractures in various stages of healing
- Fracture patterns incompatible with the history of causation
- Rib fractures, especially multiple posterior fractures
- Lower limb fractures in non-ambulatory children
- Complex skull fractures (bilateral, crossing suture lines, stellate)

Indicators of Emotional Abuse

- Behavioural problems: aggression; eating disorders; toileting problems; regression
- Mental health problems: withdrawal; depression; deliberate self harm; alcohol and substance misuse
- Problems with social interaction: school refusal; bullying; running away from home; frozen watchfulness
- Problems with parental interaction: verbal abuse; over-disciplining; over-protection; fabricated and induced illness

Indicators of fabricated illness

- Carer reports symptoms that are not explicable medically
- Poor response to medication or other standard therapy

- Symptoms exclusively observed by or in presence of carer
- Multiple hospitalizations, with extensive investigation
- Caring and concerned mother who is comfortable in a medical setting, and often involved with other families or with hospital staff
- Carers seeking multiple medical opinions
- Dead sibling or sibling with complicated medical history
- Poor school attendance

Potential presentations of fabricated or induced illness

- Suffocation, which may present as an acute life threatening event
- Administration of noxious substances or poisons
- Excessive or unnecessary administration of ordinary substances (e.g. excess salt)
- Excess or unnecessary use of medication (prescribed for the child or others)
- The use of medically provided portals of entry (e.g. gastrostomy, central lines) for administration of infected or toxic material

Apparent life threatening events in children

Defined as episodes involving some combination of apnoea, colour change (cyanosis, pallor, plethora), change in muscle tone (floppy or stiff) and chaking or gagging. The parent or carer is very alarmed and may think that the child is dying, and usually initiates some form of life support

Most infants will be 2–4 months of age.

ALTE is commoner in babies born prematurely.

Causes of apparent life threatening events

- Infection: viral: upper respiratory tract infection- respiratory syncytial virus; bacterial infections: pertussis, meningitis, septicaemia
- Gastro-intestinal: gastro-oesophageal reflux disease
- Non-accidental injury (shaken baby; drug overdose; intentional suffocation; Munchausen by proxy syndrome; head injury)
- Airway obstruction: congenital abnormalities (Pierre Robin syndrome); infection
- Abdominal causes: intusussception; strangulated hernia; testicular torsion
- Metabolic causes: hypoglycaemia; hypocalcaemia; hypokalaemia; inborn errors of metabolism
- Cardiac disease: congenital heart disease; cardiac arrhythmias; long QT syndrome; vascular ring
- Toxin/drugs: accidental or non-accidental
- Neurological causes: head injury, seizures; infections (meningitis, encephalitis); cerebral malformations
- Breath-holding spells

Evaluation of ALTE

- Circumstances of the event
- Activity at time of event: feeding, coughing, gagging, choking, vomiting
- Breathing effort
- Colour
- Movement and tone
- Observed cough or vomiting
- Duration of event

Checklist for physical examination

- Skin: rash
- CVS: cardiac murmur
- Respiratory system: respiratory rate and pattern; adventitious sounds
- Neurological: responsiveness; muscle tone; reflexes; focal signs
- Abdomen: distension; tenderness

Causes of apnoeic episodes in children

- Central: prematurity; CNS: head injury, toxic overdose (opiates, benzodiazepines, barbiturates); sepsis
- Obstructive: obstructive sleep apnoea

- Mixed: gastro-oesophageal reflux, with or without aspiration
- Seizures; intracranial haemorrhage
- Metabolic disease
- Undiagnosed neuromuscular weakness
- Cardiac arrhythmia

Acute presentations of inborn errors of metabolism in children (organic acidurias; fatty acid oxidation disorders; urea cycle defects; amino acid metabolism defects; carbohydrate metabolism defects)

- Unexplained, overwhelming or progressive neonatal disease
- Symptoms emerge or worsen with a normally self-limited illness
- Altered level of consciousness: coma; lethargy
- Acute heart failure
- Acute liver failure or Reye-like syndrome (acute non-inflammatory encephalopathy, fatty degeneration of the liver accompanied by marked elevation of serum transaminases, in the absence of clinical signs of liver involvement)
- Acute cerebral oedema
- Acute encephalopathy
- Seizures

Triggering factors

- Fever
- Acute gastroenteritis
- Low caloric intake
- Excessive protein intake
- Excessive exercise

Historical clues

- Parental consanguinity
- Unexplained death among sibling (s) in early life
- Unexplained disorders in other family members (progressive neurological disease); family history of metabolic disease
- Unusual smell of the body or urine: burn sugar (maple syrup urine disease), sweaty feet (isovaleric acidaemia)
- Neonatal illness without an adequate explanation
- Poor feeding; persistent or recurrent vomiting
- Symptoms worse after feeds or improved on glucose/saline
- Short stature
- Malformations: characteristic facies; abnormal hair or alopecia; dysmorphic features

Biochemical clues

- Hypoglycaemia; ketotic hypoglycaemia; hypoketotic hypoglycaemia (fatty acid oxidation disorders)
- High anion gap metabolic acidosis (ketones: beta-hydroxybutyrate and acetoacetate, lactate, methylmalonic acid); ketoacidosis is seen with organic acidurias
- Hyponatraemia
- Primary respiratory alkalosis
- Raised serum creatine kinase
- Hyperammonaemia
- Elevated liver enzymes

Causes of hyperammonaemia

- Urea cycle defects
- Organic acidurias: branched chain organic acid defects
- Liver disease: cirrhosis; porta-systemic shunts
- Drugs: Reye's syndrome; valproate encephalopathy

Neonatal emergencies

Normal neonatal characteristics

- Heart rate: 110–160 beats per minute, as measured by auscultation over the cardiac apex using a stethoscope. A heart rate below 100 beats per minute is abnormal.

With a heart rate below 60 beats per minute external chest compressions should be commenced.

- Respiratory rate: 40–60 breaths per minute

Recognition of the sick neonate

- Airway: obstruction
- Breathing: apnoea (cessation of breathing >15 s); bradypnoea; tachypnoea (respiratory rate>60/minute); use of accessory muscles of ventilation; chest wall recessions; nasal flaring; grunting and/or gasping; central cyanosis
- Circulation: pale, mottled or grey skin; tachycardia; bradycardia; peripheral or cyanosis; capillary refill time >3 s; hypotension
- Disability: unresponsiveness; hypotonia or hypertonia; excessive crying, weak cry, high pitched cry; poor suck and swallow; poor response to the environment; tremors; jitteriness; seizures
- Temperature >38 or <35.5 degrees Centigrade

Risk factors for neonatal illness

- Maternal: Infection: primary chorioamnio nitis, Group B streptococcus, Listeria monocytogenes, HIV, herpes simplex, syphilis, toxoplasmosis, rubella, hepatitis B; Alcohol/drug abuse; Rhesus isoimmunization; Chronic disease: diabetes mellitus, hypertension; Toxaemia of pregnancy
- Labour/delivery (intrapartum): prolonged rupture of membranes (>18 h prior to delivery); meconium stained amniotic liquor; abnormal presentation; cord prolapse; prolonged labour or precipitate delivery; analgesia before or during delivery (narcotic use within 4 h of delivery)
- Foetal/newborn: preterm (<37 weeks): post-term (>41 weeks); low birth weight (<2500 g); large for gestational age (>4200 g); birth trauma; need for resuscitation

Neonatal history checklist

- Maternal medical and social history: age; chronic disease; medications in pregnancy; alcohol intake; smoking; occupational exposures
- Family history of genetic disease
- Maternal past obstetric history: gravidity; parity; blood type; pregnancy outcomes
- Pregnancy-related maternal complications: urinary tract infection; pregnancy-related hypertension; gestational diabetes mellitus; pre-term labour
- Current antepartum and intrapartum obstetric history: procedures (ultrasound scanning; aminocentesis); screening tests (rubella antibody, HBsAg, HIV)
- Antepartum tests of foetal wellbeing: Doppler assessment of foetal blood flow patterns
- Peripartum events: maternal fever; premature or prolonged rupture of membranes; foetal distress; meconium-stained amniotic fluid; type of delivery; anaesthesia and analgesia during labour; infant status at birth; resuscitative measures; Apgar score

Features of neonatal sepsis

- Apnoea; tachypnoea
- Respiratory distress
- Lethargy
- Irritability
- Seizures
- Poor feeding
- Abdominal distension; vomiting
- Fever; hypothermia; temperature instability
- Jaundice
- Hepatosplenomegaly
- Congestive heart failure
- Hypoglycaemia; hyperglycaemia

Causes of neonatal respiratory distress

- Upper respiratory tract obstruction: nasal (posterior choanal atresia): pharyngeal

(Pierre-Robin syndrome); laryngeal (vocal cord paralysis, laryngeal web or cyst); tracheal (tracheomalacia; vascular ring); cystic hygroma
- Lower respiratory tract obstruction: meconium aspiration; aspiration of gastric contents
- Alveolar disease: respiratory distress syndrome; pneumonia; pulmonary oedema; congenital heart disease
- Pulmonary compression: pneumothorax; repaired omphalocele; congenital diaphragmatic hernia; congenital lobar emphysema

Causes of neonatal cyanosis

- Cardiac lesions:
- Reduced pulmonary blood flow and intracardiac right-to-left shunt: critical pulmonary stenosis; tetralogy of Fallot.
- Normal or increased pulmonary blood flow, intracardiac mixing: hypoplastic left heart syndrome; transposition of the great arteries; truncus arteriosus
- Pulmonary lesions
- Primary parenchymal lung disease: aspiration syndromes; respiratory distress syndrome; pneumonia.
- Airway obstruction: choanal atresia; tracheal stenosis.
- Extrinsic compression of lungs: pneumothorax; congenital diaphragmatic hernia; pleural effusion.
- Hypoventilation: central nervous system lesions; sedation; sepsis; neuromuscular disease
- Cyanosis with normal paO2: methaemoglobinaemia; polycythaemia

Features of congestive heart failure in neonates

- Tachypnoea
- Tachycardia
- Poor or slow feeding
- Sweating or colour change with feeding
- Hepatomegaly
- Poor weight gain

Presentations of neonatal seizures

- Subtle seizures (without tonic or clonic movements of the limbs): ocular phenomena (tonic eye deviation upwards or to one side; nystagmoid eye movements; sustained eye opening); oro-bucco-lingual movements (chewing, lip smacking, sucking); alternating limb movements (boxing, pedalling, rowing, swimming); autonomic phenomena (sudden changes in skin colour); apnoea with tonic stiffening of the body
- Clonic seizures: focal or multi-focal clonic limb movements
- Tonic seizures: tonic stiffening of the body
- Myoclonic jerks

Causes of neonatal seizures

- Transient metabolic disturbances: hypoglycaemia; hypocalcaemia; hyponatraemia
- Inborn errors of metabolism (inherited and persistent metabolic disturbances)
- Hypoxic ischaemic encephalopathy (perinatal asphyxia)
- Focal cerebral ischaemic injury: neonatal arterial stroke; dural venous sinus thrombosis
- Intracranial haemorrhage: subarachnoid haemorrhage; subdural haematoma; intraventricular haemorrhage
- Central nervous system infections: congenital encephalitis (intrauterine infection with CMV, toxoplasmosis); bacterial meningitis (Group B streptococcal; Escherichia coli)

Features of neonatal hypoglycaemia

- Lethargy; apathy
- Weak or high-pitched cry
- Hypotonia
- Tremors; irritability
- Apnoea
- Cyanosis
- Poor feeding; vomiting
- Seizures
- Coma

Causes of neonatal hypoglycaemia

- Increased utilization of glucose (hyperinsulinism): diabetic mother; large for gestational age infant; discordant twin; islet cell hyperplasia; insulin-producing tumours; erythroblastosis foetalis; maternal beta-sympathomimetic therapy
- Reduced production/ stores of glucose: prematurity; intrauterine growth retardation
- Increased utilization and/or decreased production: perinatal stress (sepsis; shock; hypothermia; respiratory distress); defects in carbohydrate metabolism (glycogen storage disease; galactosaemia; hereditary fructose intolerance); endocrine disorders (adrenocortical insufficiency; hypothalamic deficiency; glucagon deficiency); disorders of amino acid metabolism; maternal therapy with beta blockers

Causes of neonatal jaundice

- Increased production of bilirubin: haemolytic disease of the newborn (Rhesus or ABO isoimmunisation); haemolytic anaemias (red cell defects; G6PD deficiency); acquired drug-induced haemolysis; extravascular blood (cephalhaematoma); polycythaemia
- Reduced conjugation of bilirubin: galactosaemia: familial non-haemolytic jaundice; Gilbert's disease; α-1 antitrypsin deficiency
- Obstruction to biliary flow: biliary atresia; choledochal cysts; cystic fibrosis; tumour; band; increased enterohepatic circulation of bile: duodenal atresia, annular pancreas, meconium plug
- Mixed: sepsis; intrauterine infections: respiratory distress syndrome

Causes of eye discharge in the neonate

- Conjunctivitis: gonococcal (purulent discharge, tense oedema of eyelids, chemosis); chlamydial (watery discharge)
- Dacryocystitis: redness, swelling in region of lacrimal sac; green discharge
- Dacryostenosis: unilateral watery discharge, with crusting

Printed by Printforce, the Netherlands